Genitourinary Imaging

Mukesh G. Harisinghani • Arumugam Rajesh

Genitourinary Imaging

A Case Based Approach

Springer

Mukesh G. Harisinghani
Department of Radiology
Harvard Medical School Massachusetts
General Hospital
Boston, Massachusetts
USA

Arumugam Rajesh
Department of Radiology
University Hospitals of Leicester NHS Tr
Leicester General Hospital
Leicester
UK

ISBN 978-1-4471-7228-4 ISBN 978-1-4471-4772-5 (eBook)
DOI 10.1007/978-1-4471-4772-5
Springer London Heidelberg New York Dordrecht

Printed on acid-free paper

Springer is part of Springer Science+Business Media (www.springer.com)

Preface

The concept of this case based GU Imaging text stems from the daily "interesting case" rounds we have in the Division of Abdominal Imaging at the Massachusetts General Hospital. This interesting case conference provides a platform for showcasing the optimal use of multiple modalities to answer clinical questions posed in the GU realm. This daily routine benefits all cadres of audience including residents, fellows and faculty in the division and has resulted in a multitude of clinical research projects, journal discussions and teaching points. The current text is a cross section of interesting GU cases from this daily conference. The goal of this text is to not only show interesting GU cases but also provide a brief synopsis of the salient teaching points associated with each case that one should consider when one comes across them. We have tried to encompass the common GU clinical entities in these case discussions. We hope the reader will find the text easy to read providing a quick overview of all common areas in the GU system.

In addition to the contributors listed in the acknowledgement section, we would like to especially thank Dr. Jennifer Uyeda for helping us in compiling the cases.

Boston, MA, USA — Mukesh G. Harisinghani
Leicester, UK — Arumugam Rajesh

Contents

Contributors

Himani Agarwal, MBBS, DNB Kovai Medical Centre and Hospital, Coimbatore, TN, India

Ala Alsherbini, MD Radiology Department, Hamad Medical Corporation, Doha, Qatar

Seetharaman Cannane, DMRD, DNB Kovai Medical Centre and Hospital, Coimbatore, TN, India

Prapruttam Duangkamon, MD Department of Abdominal Imaging and Intervention, Massachusetts General Hospital, Boston, MA, USA

Amit Nandan Dhar Dwivedi, MD Department of Radiodiagnosis and Imaging, Institute of Medical Sciences, Banaras Hindu University, Varanasi, UP, India

Prashant Gupta, DNB Kovai Medical Centre and Hospital, Coimbatore, TN, India

Sandeep Hedgire, MD Department of Abdominal Imaging and Intervention, Massachusetts General Hospital, Boston, MA, USA

Tejas Kalyanpur, DMRD, DNB Kovai Medical Centre and Hospital, Coimbatore, TN, India

Ruhi Karwal, DMRD, DNB OrthoOne Orthopedic Specialty Centre, Singanallur, Coimbatore, TN, India

Susanna Lee, MD Department of Abdominal Imaging and Intervention, Massachusetts General Hospital, Boston, MA, USA

Yun Mao, MD Department of Abdominal Imaging and Intervention, Massachusetts General Hospital, Boston, MA, USA

Mahan Mathur, MD Department of Body Imaging, Department of Diagnostic Radiology, Yale School of Medicine, New Haven, CT, USA

Pritesh Patel, MD Department of Abdominal Imaging and Intervention, Massachusetts General Hospital, Boston, MA, USA

Santhosh Poyyamoli, MD Kovai Medical Centre and Hospital, Coimbatore, TN, India

Anuradha Shenoy-Bhangle, MD Department of Abdominal Imaging and Intervention, Massachusetts General Hospital, Boston, MA, USA

Ahmed Monier Sherif, MD Radiology Department, Hamad Medical Corporation, Doha, Qatar

Jennifer Uyeda, MD Department of Radiology, Brigham and Women's Hospital, Boston, MA, USA

Mathias D. Van Borsel, MD Department of Radiology and Medical Imaging, Ghent University Hospital, Ghent, Belgium

Chapter 1
Adrenal Gland

Case 1.1

Brief Case Summary: 35 year old male with abdominal pain

Imaging Findings An axial non-contrast CT scan demonstrates a hypodense nodule in the right adrenal gland with attenuation value of 3 Hounsfield units (Fig. 1.1).

Axial non-contrast, contrast enhanced images at 1 and 15 min CT images from another patient demonstrate a right adrenal nodule with absolute washout of 67 % (Fig. 1.2a–c).

Differential Diagnosis Adrenal adenoma, pheochromocytoma, adrenocortical carcinoma, adrenal cyst, adrenal metastasis

Diagnosis and Discussion: Adrenal adenoma

Adrenal adenomas are the most common primary benign adrenal neoplasm, typically found as an incidental finding. The prevalence increases with age, ranging from 0.14 % in patients 20–29 years up to 7 % in patients older than 70 years. Functioning adenomas which secrete cortisol (Cushing syndrome) or aldosterone (Conn syndrome) can occasionally be encountered. Although the majority of functioning adenomas will be unilateral, bilateral lesions can be seen in up to 20 % of patients.

Imaging findings typically demonstrate a well-defined, homogenous mass less than or equal to 3 cm. Histologically, the majority (ranging from 70 to 90 %) of adrenal adenomas will contain intracellular lipid. As a result, the majority of adrenal adenomas will demonstrate an attenuation value of less than 10 Hounsfield units on a non-contrast CT examination, and can be confidently diagnosed as a lipid rich adenoma. The remaining lesions (also known as lipid poor adenomas) may be further evaluated by examining their washout characteristics after the administration of intravenous contrast. The protocol generally consists of a non-contrast CT of the upper abdomen through the adrenal glands followed by

M.G. Harisinghani, A. Rajesh, *Genitourinary Imaging: A Case Based Approach*, DOI 10.1007/978-1-4471-4772-5_1

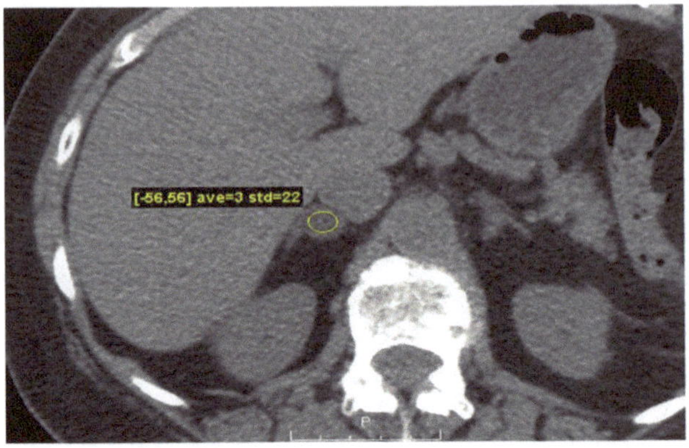

Fig. 1.1 Axial non-contrast CT scan demonstrates a hypodense nodule in the right adrenal gland with attenuation value of 3 Hounsfield units

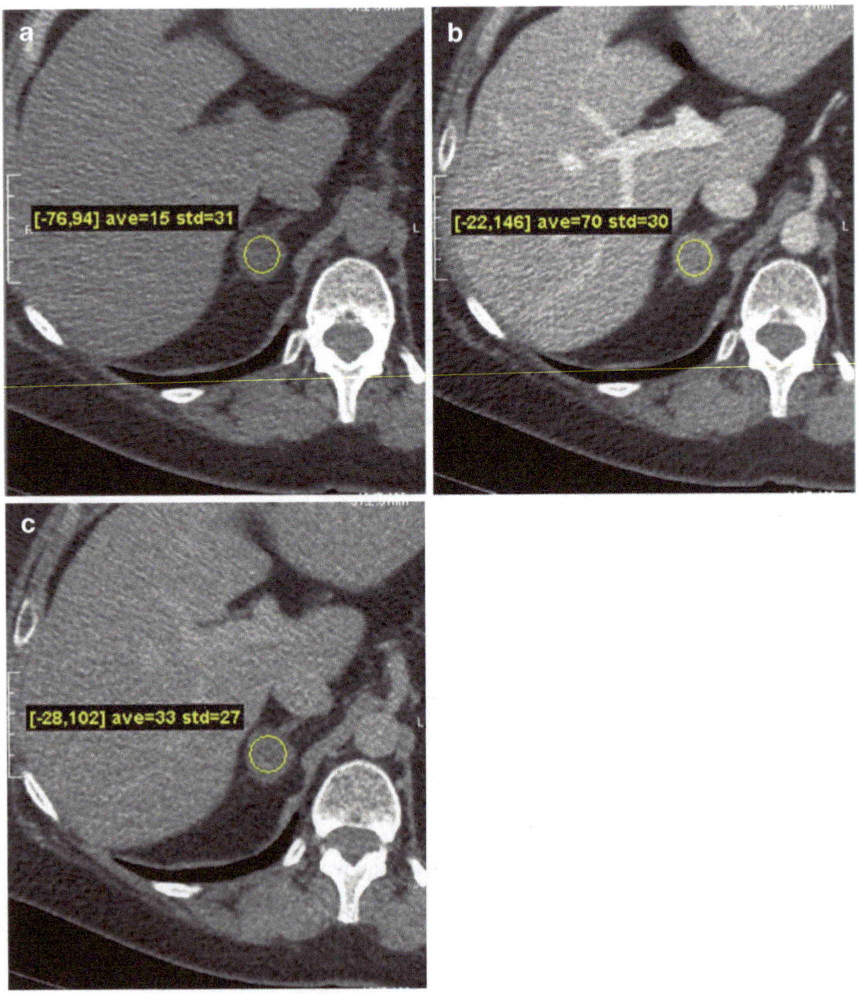

Fig. 1.2 (**a–c**). Axial non-contrast, contrast enhanced images at 1 and 15 min CT images from another patient demonstrate a right adrenal nodule with absolute washout of 67 %

contrast enhanced images at 60 s and delayed images at 15 min. Region of interests are drawn in the adrenal gland on all three phases of the examination and washout calculations are performed. An absolute washout of greater than 60 % or a relative washout of greater than 40 % accurately characterizes an adrenal adenoma. The presence of intracellular lipid in lipid-rich adenomas may be demonstrated on MR imaging evaluating for loss of signal intensity on opposed phase chemical shift imaging.

An incidental adrenal mass greater than or equal to 1 cm which is stable for over 1 year is generally considered to be benign and statistically likely to be an adenoma. Further evaluation with biochemical testing may be considered if there is clinical evidence for adrenal hyperfunction. No specific treatment or imaging follow-up is required for non-functioning adenomas. Surgical evaluation should be considered for functioning neoplasms.

Washout formulas:

1. **Absolute washout**: $$\frac{\text{Enhanced}(60\,\text{s}) - \text{Delayed}(15\,\text{min})}{\text{Enhanced}(60\,\text{s}) - \text{Unenhanced}(\text{non-contrast})}$$
2. **Relative washout**: $$\frac{\text{Enhanced}(60\,\text{s}) - \text{Delayed}(15\,\text{min})}{\text{Enhanced}(60\,\text{s})}$$

Pitfalls Adrenal adenoma can be confidently diagnosed and differentiated using a combination of non-contrast imaging, washout calculations, and chemical shift MRI techniques. However, if non-contrast CT demonstrates an attenuation value of >10 HU, chemical shift MR imaging is unlikely to characterise the lesion further as this is likely to be a lipid poor adenoma. Adrenal cysts are benign non-enhancing lesions that may mimic adenomas on non-contrast imaging. Malignant lesions, such as adrenocortical carcinoma or metastasis are generally more heterogeneous and do not rapidly washout on delayed phase imaging. Pheochromocytomas are generally hypervascular lesions with variable high T2 signal. Washout characteristics are variable and these lesions rarely contain intracellular lipid, mimicking an adrenal adenoma. Clinical and laboratory evaluation of catecholamine excess may be considered, followed by functional imaging using 1–123 or I-131 MIBG imaging.

Teaching Point

1. Adrenal adenomas are benign lesions that can be confidently diagnosed and differentiated using a combination of non-contrast imaging, washout calculations, and chemical shift MRI techniques.
2. Asymptomatic lesions generally require no follow-up, however, adrenal adenomas may be hormonally active with subclinical features. Hormonally active tumors should be surgically evaluated.
3. An incidental adrenal mass ≥1 cm which is stable for over 1 year is generally considered to be benign and statistically likely to be an adenoma. An incidental solid adrenal mass >4 cm without specific benign features (such as macroscopic fat to suggest a myelolipoma) should be surgically evaluated as most benign lesions are smaller in size (<3 cm).

Case 1.2

Brief Case Summary: 55 year old female with abdominal pain

Imaging Findings Coronal CT scan of the abdomen and pelvis with intravenous and oral contrast demonstrates a heterogeneous right suprarenal mass with areas of enhancing soft tissue as well as low attenuating regions compatible with underlying necrosis (Fig. 1.3).

Coronal CT scan of the abdomen and pelvis with intravenous and oral contrast in a different patient demonstrates a heterogeneous right suprarenal mass with extension into the liver parenchyma (Fig. 1.4).

Axial CT scan of the abdomen and pelvis with intravenous and oral contrast in a third patient demonstrates a heterogeneous right retroperitoneal mass with extension into the inferior vena cava (Fig. 1.5).

Differential Diagnosis Adrenal gland neoplasm (metastasis, adrenocortical carcinoma, pheochromocytoma), renal cell carcinoma, primary retroperitoneal neoplasm (such as a leiomyosarcoma).

Diagnosis and Discussion: Adrenocortical carcinoma

Adrenocortical carcinoma (ACC) is a rare and aggressive neoplasm with a bimodal age of distribution, most often occurring before the age of 5, or within the third to fourth decades of life. Smoking and the use of oral contraceptives before the

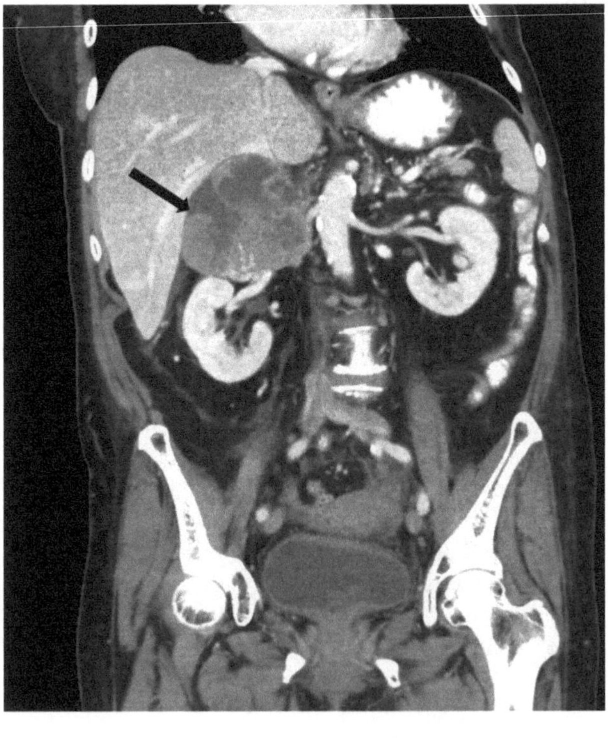

Fig. 1.3 Coronal CT scan of the abdomen and pelvis with intravenous and oral contrast demonstrates a heterogeneous right suprarenal mass (*arrow*) with areas of enhancing soft tissue as well as low attenuating regions compatible with underlying necrosis

age of 25 are risk factors for developing ACC. The majority of ACCs are sporadic though some can be associated with genetic syndromes such as Li-Fraumeni syndrome and Carney complex. Clinically, patients may be asymptomatic or present with non-specific symptoms such as vague abdominal pain and nausea related to mass effect from the tumor. A subset of these tumors are hormonally active, with patients most commonly presenting with signs of Cushing syndrome or rapidly progressive virilization/feminization features.

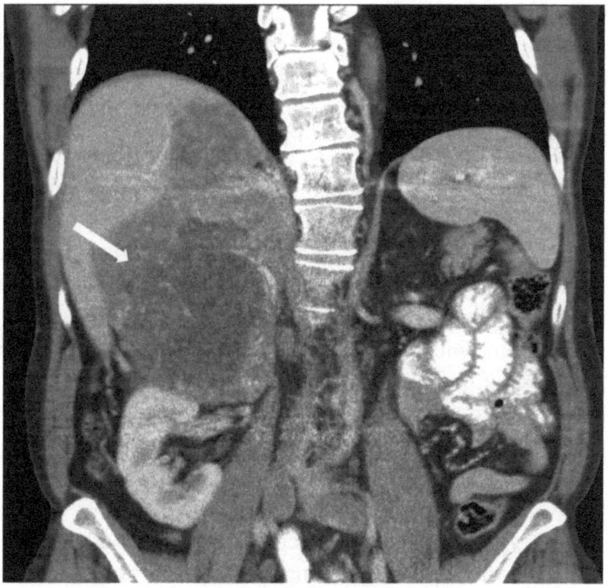

Fig. 1.4 Coronal CT scan of the abdomen and pelvis with intravenous and oral contrast in a different patient demonstrates a heterogeneous right suprarenal mass (*arrow*) with extension into the liver parenchyma

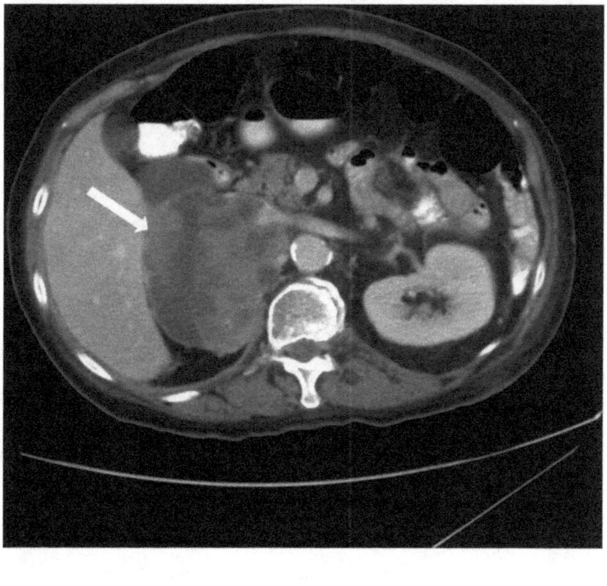

Fig. 1.5 Axial CT scan of the abdomen and pelvis with intravenous and oral contrast in a third patient demonstrates a heterogeneous right retroperitoneal mass (*arrow*) with extension into the inferior vena cava

ACCs are typically large at presentation, with most lesions measuring larger than 6 cm. The mass is heterogeneous with central areas of low attenuation corresponding pathologically to areas of necrosis. Approximately one-third of these tumors will demonstrate calcifications, typically centrally located. Contrast enhancement is often inhomogeneous with frequent retention of intravenous contrast material. Invasion of the inferior vena cava is seen in 9–19 % of patients on presentation. MRI demonstrates a heterogeneous mass with variable areas of T1 signal due to underlying hemorrhage as well as focal regions of high T2 signal related to underlying necrosis.

Open surgical resection of the neoplasm for localized neoplasm offers the best overall prognosis. For locally advanced or metastatic disease, chemotherapy with or without radiation is the standard, though primary debulking surgery of hormonally active neoplasm may be considered to alleviate symptoms. The overall prognosis is poor with 5 year survival rate of 38 %. Local recurrence and metastatic disease are common with one third of patients demonstrating metastatic disease on presentation.

Pitfalls Common mimickers of ACC include adrenal metastases, pheochromocytoma, and adrenal adenoma. Adrenal metastases should be considered if there is a known primary with metastatic disease elsewhere, particularly if there are bilateral adrenal masses. Adrenal adenoma can be distinguished by their attenuation values on non-contrast CT exams and their rapid washout after the administration of contrast. Pheochromocytomas may present with signs of catecholamine excess and will often demonstrate uptake on MIBG scintigraphy. Distinguishing an ACC from a renal cell cancer or primary retroperitoneal sarcoma can be done by observing the mass effect on surrounding structures. Coronal and sagittal reformatted images are often helpful in this regard.

Teaching Points

1. ACCs are large, heterogeneous neoplasms with areas of necrosis and calcifications. Prognosis is poor and complete surgical resection offers the best overall prognosis.
2. IVC invasion is frequent on initial presentation. Although IVC invasion does not preclude surgical resection, accurate reporting of this is imperative for surgical planning.
3. A solid adrenal mass greater than 4 cm, despite benign imaging features, is generally managed as a malignant lesion. In addition, distinguishing an ACC from a non-functioning pheochromocytoma without MIBG uptake may be impossible without surgical resection.

Case 1.3

Brief Case Summary: 34 year old female, incidental adrenal mass on CT scan of the chest.

Imaging Findings A CT scan of the chest performed with intravenous contrast demonstrates an incompletely imaged, low attenuating left adrenal mass with a single peripheral punctate calcification (Fig. 1.6). Gray scale and color images of

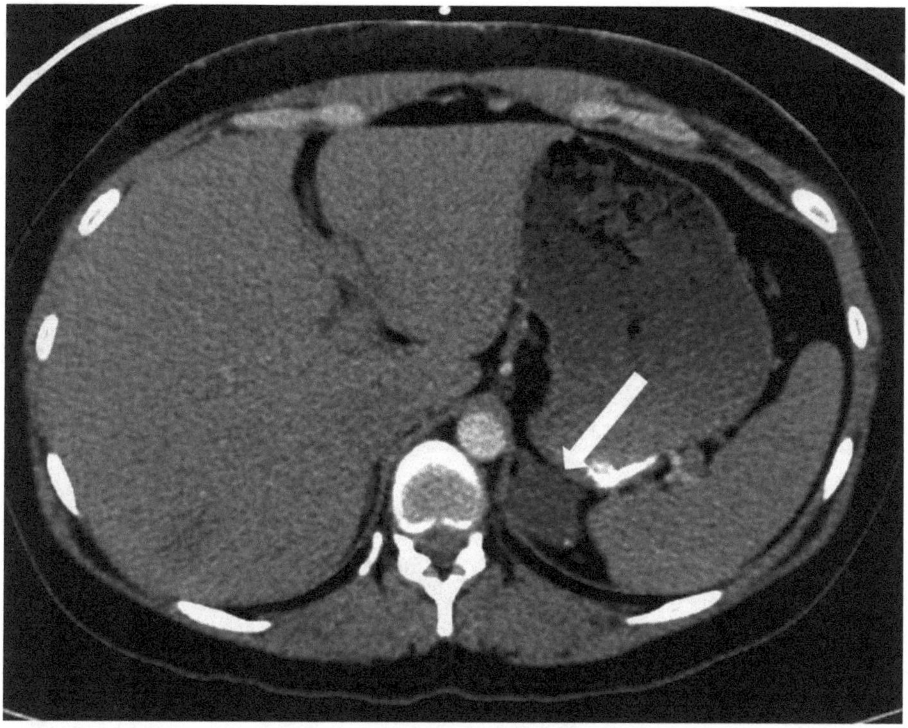

Fig. 1.6 CT scan of the chest performed with intravenous contrast demonstrates an incompletely imaged, low attenuating left adrenal mass (*arrow*) with a single peripheral punctate calcification

the left kidney demonstrate the presence of hypoechoic left adrenal mass (Fig. 1.7a) without detectable flow (Fig. 1.7b). Non-contrast MRI evaluation demonstrates the presence of a T2 hyperintense left adrenal mass (Fig. 1.8) without loss of signal on the opposed phase images (Fig. 1.9).

Differential Diagnosis Pheochromocytoma, adrenal adenoma, adrenal metastases, adrenal cyst

Diagnosis and Discussion: Adrenal cyst (lymphangioma)

Adrenal cysts are uncommon lesions and are histologically classified as endothelial cysts, pseudocysts, epithelial cysts, and parasitic cysts, in decreasing order of frequency. Endothelial cysts include lymphangiomatous (more common) and angiomatous types, while pseudocysts are thought represent the sequelae of hemorrhage related to an underlying mass, trauma, or infection. Adrenal cysts are most often discovered as incidental masses, though they may occasionally grow large enough to cause non-specific symptoms related to mass effect. In addition, adrenal cysts can be associated with a variety of syndromes including polycystic renal disease, Beckwith-Wideman syndrome and Klippel-Trenaunay-Weber syndrome. Cystic metastases or a primary cystic endocrine tumor, are important mimickers of benign adrenal cysts.

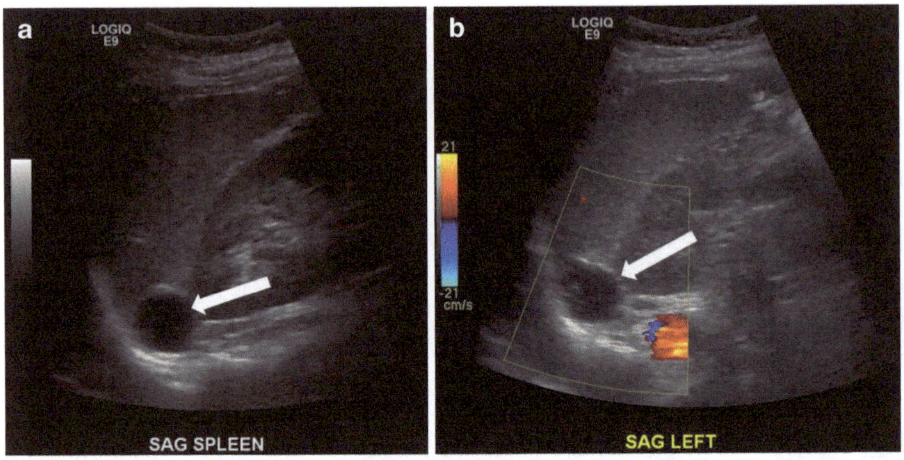

Fig. 1.7 Gray scale and color images of the left kidney demonstrate the presence of hypoechoic left adrenal mass (*arrow*) (**a**) without detectable flow (**b**)

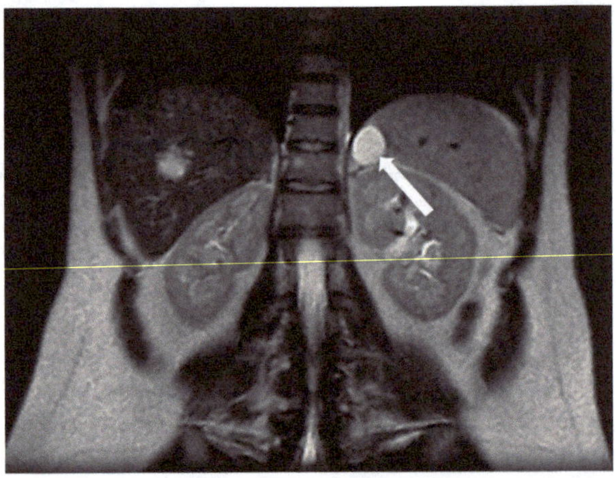

Fig. 1.8 Non-contrast MRI evaluation demonstrates the presence of a T2 hyperintense left adrenal mass (*arrow*)

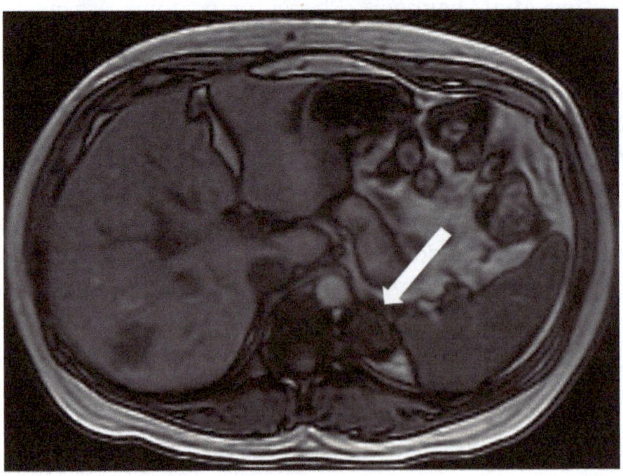

Fig. 1.9 Non-contrast MRI evaluation demonstrates the presence of a left adrenal mass (*arrow*) without loss of signal on the opposed phase images

Radiological differentiation of the subtypes of benign adrenal cysts is challenging. Endothelial cysts are typically non-enhancing masses with thin smooth walls with an internal density value of less than 20 Hounsfield units. A multilocular appearance with thin septations and occasional septal calcifications has also been described. On the other hand, pseudocysts typically manifest as unilocular cystic masses with a variable degree of wall thickness (often up to 5 mm) and mural calcification. Internal hemorrhage within the pseudocyst may give a complex appearance, though evolution of the internal appearance over time due to break down of blood products and the lack of enhancement will be noted. Epithelial cysts manifest as simple appearing cysts on both CT and MR imaging with fluid signal, thin walls, and no enhancement after contrast administration. Parasitic cysts are most often secondary to echinococcus with imaging demonstrating the presence of septal and mural calcifications as well as the presence of internal floating membranes and daughter cysts.

Management of adrenal cysts is controversial. Further evaluation is based on determining the functional status of the mass to exclude a cystic endocrine neoplasm and imaging features to exclude the possibility of a cystic degeneration of solid mass. In addition, some authors advocate the resection of any benign appearing adrenal cyst >5 cm due to the potentially increased risk of hemorrhage and symptoms from adjacent mass effect.

Pitfalls Adrenal cysts with internal hemorrhage can often have a complex CT and sonographic imaging appearance, potentially mimicking an adrenal cortical carcinoma or metastases. MRI is more useful in these circumstances, given the better contrast resolution of soft tissues.

Teaching Point

1. Adrenal cysts are uncommon lesions typically manifesting as uni or multiloculated fluid attenuating masses with thin walls, variable septations and smooth, thin calcifications.
2. Internal hemorrhage may result in a complex imaging appearance on CT or US. MRI is useful in these settings to demonstrate the variable appearance of hemorrhage and the lack of soft tissue enhancement.
3. Patients with adrenal cysts should undergo a hormonal evaluation. Hormonally active cysts, cysts with complex features suggesting the possibility of cystic degeneration of solid mass, and simple cysts larger than 5 cm should be surgically evaluated.

Case 1.4

Brief Case Summary: 66 year old male. History withheld.

Imaging Findings CT scan of the abdomen with intravenous and oral contrast demonstrates the presence of high density fluid in the region of the left adrenal gland (arrow, Fig. 1.10). Small amount of extravasated contrast material is noted within the high atteuenation fluid (dashed arrow, Fig. 1.10). Note the presence of a linear band of decreased attenuation across the medial aspect of the left kidney

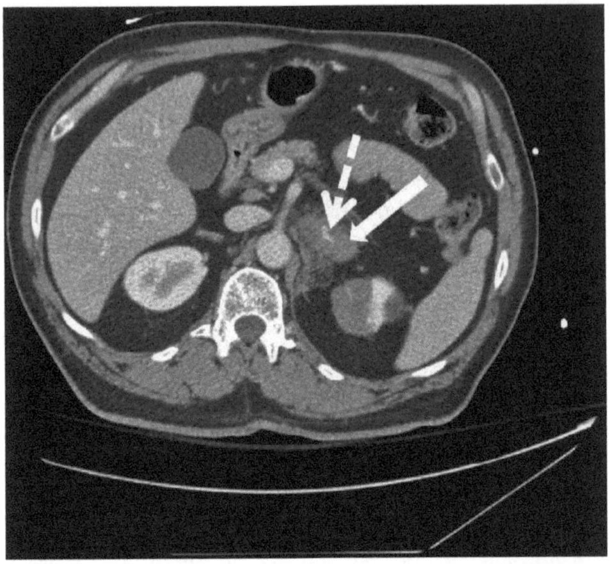

Fig. 1.10 CT scan of the abdomen with intravenous and oral contrast demonstrates the presence of high density fluid in the expected region of the left adrenal gland (*arrow*). Small amount of extravasated contrast material is noted within the high density fluid (*dashed arrow*)

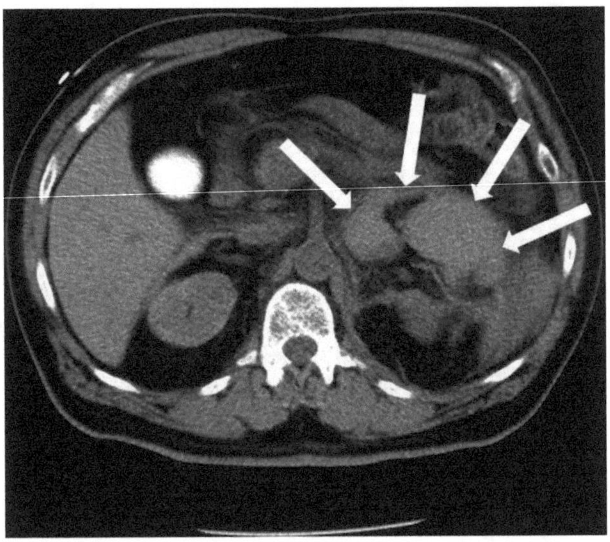

Fig. 1.11 Repeat noncontrast CT scan of the abdomen performed 24 h later due to declining patient condition demonstrates an enlarging left adrenal hematoma and the presence of high density fluid in the perirenal space compatible with hemorrhage (*arrows*)

compatible with an infarct. A repeat noncontrast CT scan of the abdomen performed 24 h later due to patient instability demonstrates an enlarging left adrenal hematoma and the presence of high density fluid in the perirenal space compatible with hemorrhage (arrows, Fig. 1.11). A conventional angiogram was subsequently performed (not shown) and demonstrated no active extravasation.

Differential Diagnosis Adrenal hemorrhage secondary to trauma, iatrogenic injury, anticoagulation, underlying bleeding diathesis or underlying mass.

Diagnosis and Discussion: Adrenal hemorrhage secondary to trauma (motor vehicle collision)

Unilateral adrenal hemorrhage is often asymptomatic and produces no biochemical alterations to suggest the diagnosis. A minority of patients may complain of non-specific symptoms including back or flank pain. The degree of hemorrhage is usually insufficient to cause a significant drop in hematocrit and clinical signs of volume loss, such as orthostatic hypotension, are often absent. Bilateral adrenal hemorrhage, on the other hand, can be a life-threatening condition, which, in the setting of underlying sepsis, can result in a mortality rate of over 90 %. Signs of adrenal insufficiency, including hyponatremia, hypokalemia, and hypoglycemia may be invariably present.

Etiologies of adrenal hemorrhage may be classified as traumatic or atraumatic, with the former typically seen in the setting of severe trauma or iatrogenic injury such as from adrenal vein sampling. Atraumatic causes can be related to anticoagulation use, underlying bleeding diathesis (such as thrombophilia) or severe sepsis classically associated with meningococcemia. In addition, bleeding of both benign and malignant adrenal masses may result in adrenal hematomas.

In its earliest stages, acute adrenal hemorrhage may manifest as thickening of the adrenal glands with preservation of the normal shape. There may be a tram-track appearance with preserved enhancement along the periphery of the gland and no enhancement in the hemorrhagic central portions. Infiltration of hemorrhage into the surrounding fat is almost always present, particularly in the setting of trauma. Over time, the hematoma expands to manifest as a round or oval shape, with non-contrast density values ranging from 50 to 90 Hounsfield units. Active extravasation is uncommon, though it should be recognized as this may require urgent embolization. With continued evolution of hematoma, the hematoma gradually decreases in size to complete resolution of the imaging findings. Chronic hemorrhage may organize to form an adrenal pseudocyst which typically manifests as a unilocular thin-walled cystic mass with a variable amount of mural calcification. Adrenal hematomas demonstrate variable signal intensity on MRI which is dependent on the stage of hemoglobin breakdown. Acute hematoma demonstrates iso- to hypointense signal on T1 weighted images and hypointense signal on T2 weighted images. Over time, hematoma will be hyperintense on both T1 and T2 weighted sequences eventually demonstrating the presence of a hypointense rim due to the presence of hemosiderin.

Patients with adrenal hemorrhage are most often non-operatively managed with supportive care and close attention to hematocrit levels. Embolization may be attempted in cases of persistent bleeding. Bilateral adrenal hemorrhage results in an adrenal crisis is a life-threatening emergency, which requires fluid and electrolyte resuscitation and the use of corticosteroids.

Pitfalls Hemorrhage related to tumors may be difficult to distinguish from the other causes. Comparison to prior imaging to demonstrate the presence or absence of an underlying mass is critical to help make this distinction. MR imaging may be also be useful, allowing the detection of subtle areas of enhancement. Serial imaging with CT or MRI may be required in difficult cases to exclude the presence of an underlying mass.

Teaching Point

1. Adrenal hemorrhage can result from a variety of causes. It is critical to exclude the presence of an underlying hemorrhagic neoplasm. Comparison to prior imaging, MRI and/or serial imaging examination may be required to make this distinction
2. Bilateral adrenal hemorrhage can be a life-threatening emergency.
3. Adrenal hemorrhage can progress from adrenal enlargement to a round or oval mass. Over time, there may be complete resolution or formation of a pseudocyst.

Case 1.5

Brief Case Summary: 67 year old male with lung cancer.

Imaging Findings CT scan of the abdomen with intravenous contrast demonstrates the presence of a normal right adrenal gland (arrow, Fig. 1.12). Subsequent restaging scan performed 6 months later demonstrates the development of a soft tissue mass in the right adrenal gland (arrow, Fig. 1.13a). A small amount of high attenuation fluid is noted along the medial and inferior aspects of the region (Fig. 1.13b), compatible with hemorrhage.

Differential Diagnosis Adrenal metastases, adrenal adenoma, adrenocortical carcinoma, pheochromocytoma

Diagnosis and Discussion: Hemorrhagic adrenal metastases

The adrenal glands are a common site for metastatic disease, with autopsy studies demonstrating the incidence of metastases ranging from 13 to 35 %. Primary

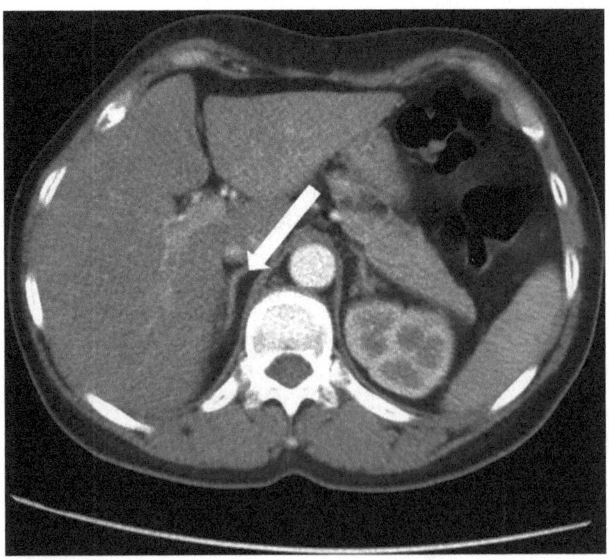

Fig. 1.12 CT scan of the abdomen with intravenous contrast demonstrates the presence of a normal right adrenal gland (*arrow*)

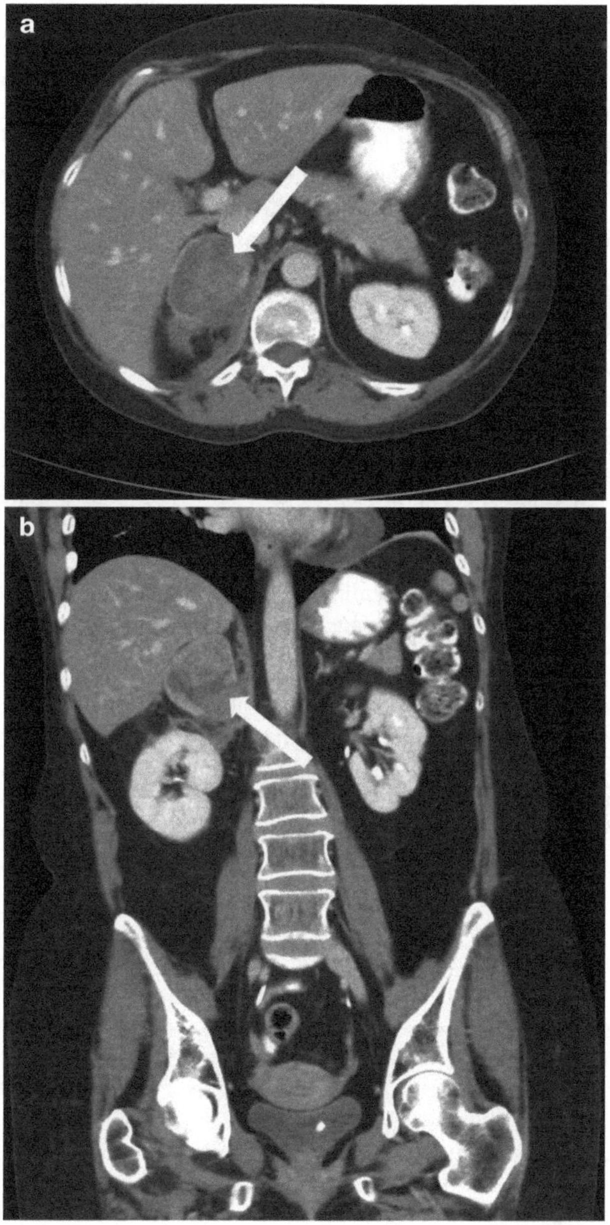

Fig. 1.13 Subsequent restaging scan performed 6 months later demonstrates the development of a soft tissue mass in the right adrenal gland (**a**, *arrow*). A small amount of high attenuation fluid is noted along the medial and inferior aspects of the region (**b**), compatible with hemorrhage

neoplasms that commonly hematogenously metastasize to the adrenal gland include lung, liver, breast, and colon. Contiguous extension from adjacent tumors may be occasionally seen with primary retroperitoneal, renal, and pancreatic neoplasms. Adrenal metastases are generally seen in the context of metastatic disease elsewhere and may be unilateral or bilateral in distribution.

The imaging appearance is non-specific. Small metastatic lesions may appear relatively well-defined and homogenous, while large lesions are usually more heterogeneous in appearance due to internal necrosis and may demonstrate ill-defined or nodular borders. Calcifications are uncommonly seen. Unlike adrenal adenomas, metastatic lesions demonstrate delayed washout on multiphase imaging (less than 60 % using absolute washout calculations) and do not lose signal on opposed phase MR imaging. Metastases may be occasionally complicated by hemorrhage, a finding more often seen with lung and malignant melanoma primary neoplasms. Detection of adrenal metastases on combined PET/CT is dependent on the FDG avidity of the primary neoplasm and size of the adrenal lesion.

An isolated adrenal metastatic lesion has been traditionally treated surgically. Percutaneous ablation may be considered in patients with unresectable lesions or in patients who are poor surgical candidates. Stereotactic body radiation therapy is an emerging alternative treatment that allows the delivery of high doses of radiation to the target lesion, while limiting damage to adjacent organs.

Pitfalls Small adrenal metastases may mimic an adrenal adenoma. An absolute washout value of greater than 60 % and loss of internal signal on opposed phase imaging is suggestive of an adrenal adenoma. Adrenocortical carcinomas or pheochromocytomas may be indistinguishable from an isolated metastatic lesion, although the clinical context as well as laboratory parameters can usually help in this differentiation. If further doubt persists, a biopsy may be needed.

Teaching Points

1. Adrenal metastases are common with an incidence of 13–35 % with lung, liver, breast, and colon malignancies being the most common primary neoplasms. The presence of a new adrenal lesion with a known primary malignancy will almost always represent a metastatic lesion.
2. Small adrenal metastases and adenomas may have similar imaging appearances. Multiphase imaging and/or evaluation on opposed phase MR images can help distinguish these lesions.
3. Isolated adrenal metastatic lesion may be removed surgically. Percutaneous ablation and/or stereotactic body radiation therapy are emerging alternative therapies.

Case 1.6

Brief Case Summary: 78 year old male with abdominal pain

Imaging Findings CT scan of the abdomen with intravenous and oral contrast demonstrates the presence of a predominantly fat containing mass in the right adrenal

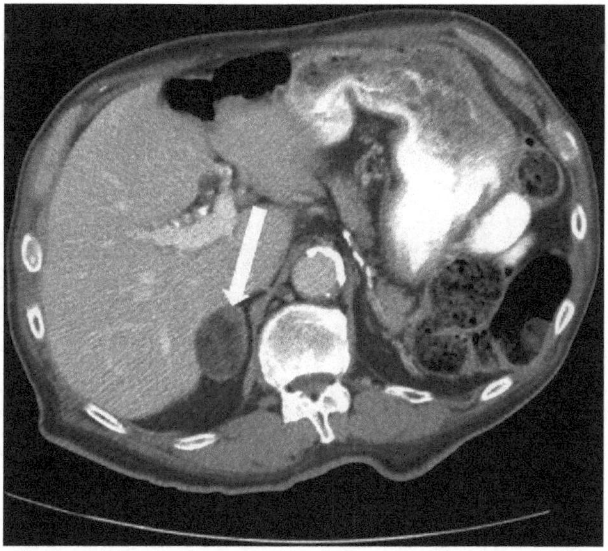

Fig. 1.14 CT scan of the abdomen with intravenous and oral contrast demonstrates the presence of a predominantly fat containing mass in the right adrenal gland (*arrow*)

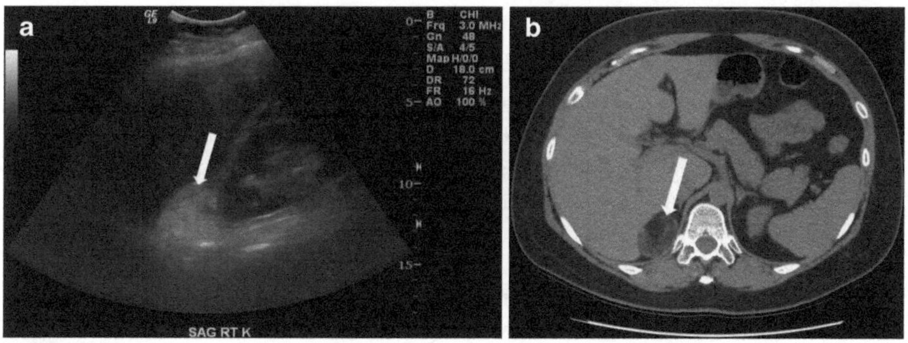

Fig. 1.15 Gray scale ultrasound image in another patient (**a**) demonstrates an echogenic right suprarenal mass (*arrow*) without posterior shadowing. Subsequent noncontrast CT scan of the abdomen demonstrates a predominantly fat containing mass in the right adrenal gland (*arrow*) with small areas of interspersed soft tissue (**b**)

gland (arrow, Fig. 1.14). Close inspection of the mass demonstrates the presence of small, subtle regions of soft tissue density.

Gray scale ultrasound image in another patient (Fig. 1.15a) demonstrates an echogenic right suprarenal mass without posterior shadowing. Subsequent noncontrast CT scan of the abdomen demonstrates a predominantly fat containing mass in the right adrenal gland with small areas of interspersed soft tissue (Fig. 1.15b).

Axial MR images in a third patient demonstrate the presence of a mass in the left adrenal gland. Again, the mass demonstrates several discrete foci of fat on a T1 weighted image (Fig. 1.16a) which lose signal on the T1 post-gadolinium image with fat saturation (Fig. 1.16b). T2 fat saturated image (arrow on Fig. 1.16b).

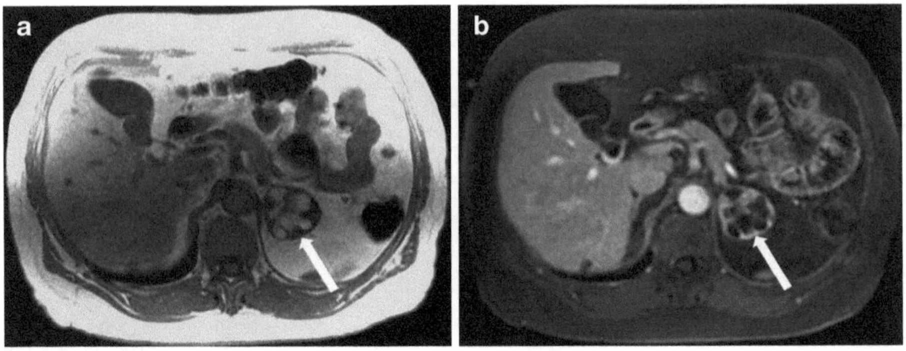

Fig. 1.16 Axial MR images in a third patient demonstrate the presence of a mass in the left adrenal gland (*arrow*). The mass demonstrates several discrete foci of hyperintense fat on a T1 weighted image (**a**) which lose signal on the T1 post-gadolinium image with fat saturation (**b**). T1 fat saturated image (**b**)

Regions of enhancing soft tissue are interspersed within the fat as seen on the T1 post-gadolinium image.

Differential Diagnosis Adrenal myelolipoma, adrenal lipoma, adrenal liposarcoma, adrenal adenoma, retroperitoneal liposarcoma, renal angiomyolipoma

Diagnosis and Discussion: Adrenal myelolipoma.

Adrenal myelolipomas are relatively rare, with an incidence of approximately 3–5 % of all primary adrenal neoplasms. Histologically, these benign tumors are composed of a combination of mature adipose tissue and hematopoietic elements (myeloid and erythroid). The majority are asymptomatic and are typically incidentally discovered, with only case reports of associated hormonal activity. On occasion, large myelolipomas may present with abdominal pain related to compression on adjacent structures or internal hemorrhage.

Imaging findings typically demonstrate the presence of a well-defined mass with evidence of discrete foci of internal fat, interspersed with a variable amount of enhancing soft tissue representing the hematopoietic elements. On ultrasound, these foci of fat are seen as areas of increased echogenicity (Fig. 1.15a), while CT will demonstrate low attenuating tissue with densities ranging from −30 to −100 Hounsfield units. MR imaging will demonstrate the presence of macroscopic fat, with evidence of "India ink" artifact at the interface of the lipid and hematopoietic elements. Approximately 20 % of adrenal myelolipomas will demonstrate the presence of internal calcifications, typically related to prior hemorrhage.

The diagnosis of adrenal myelolipoma can almost always be made from the imaging findings. Fine-needle aspiration (FNA) is a potential alternative if the diagnosis cannot be made on imaging. Small, asymptomatic neoplasms less than 4 cm can be typically managed with observation, with consideration of annual imaging to monitor growth. Larger or symptomatic tumors should warrant a surgical evaluation. Once resected, the overall prognosis is excellent, with reports of recurrence-free survival of up to 12 years.

Pitfalls Adrenal lipomas or liposarcomas are exceedingly rare, such that a macroscopic fat containing neoplasm in the adrenal gland should almost always be assumed to be a myelolipoma. Close attention to the organ of origin should be made to exclude the possibility of a renal angiomyolipoma or a primary retroperitoneal liposarcoma. Adrenal adenomas demonstrate the presence of microscopic lipid elements, with no visible fat on cross sectional imaging, density values less than 10 HU on a non-contrast CT, and internal loss of signal on opposed phase T1 weighted MR images.

Teaching Point

1. A lesion containing macroscopic fat is virtually diagnostic of an adrenal myelolipoma.
2. Asymptomatic lesions less than 4 cm may be observed. Annual imaging may be considered as a subset of these benign neoplasms may grow with a subsequent increased risk of hemorrhage.
3. Symptomatic lesions or lesions greater than 4 cm should warrant a surgical evaluation. Post-resection prognosis is excellent.

Case 1.7

Brief Case Summary: 35 year old female with headaches, palpitations and sweating.

Imaging Findings Axial T2 with fat-saturation image (Fig. 1.17a) demonstrates a T2 hyperintense right suprarenal mass which enhances on the T1 post-gadolinium fat-saturated sequence (Fig. 1.17b). The lesion is isointense to muscle on the T1 in phase image (Fig. 1.17c) with no loss of signal on the T1 opposed phase image (Fig. 1.17d). The mass is noted to have restricted diffusion (Fig. 1.17e, f) and demonstrates avid uptake on 1–123 metaiodobenzylguanidine (I-123 MIBG) SPECT imaging (Fig. 1.17g).

Axial contrast-enhanced CT image in a second patient demonstrates the presence of a low density right suprarenal mass with irregular enhancing septations (Fig. 1.18a). Axial T2 with fat saturation (Fig. 1.18b) and coronal T2 weighted (Fig. 1.18c) MR images confirm the suprarenal location of this mass and demonstrates the presence of an internal fluid level (Fig. 1.18b). Post contrast T1 weighted image with fat saturation demonstrates the presence of irregular enhancing septations (Fig. 1.18d).

Differential Diagnosis Pheochromocytoma, adrenal adenoma, adrenocortical carcinoma, adrenal cyst

Diagnosis and Discussion: Pheochromocytoma

Pheochromocytomas are rare catecholamine-secreting neuroendocrine neoplasms that arise from the chromaffin cells of the adrenal medulla. Approximately

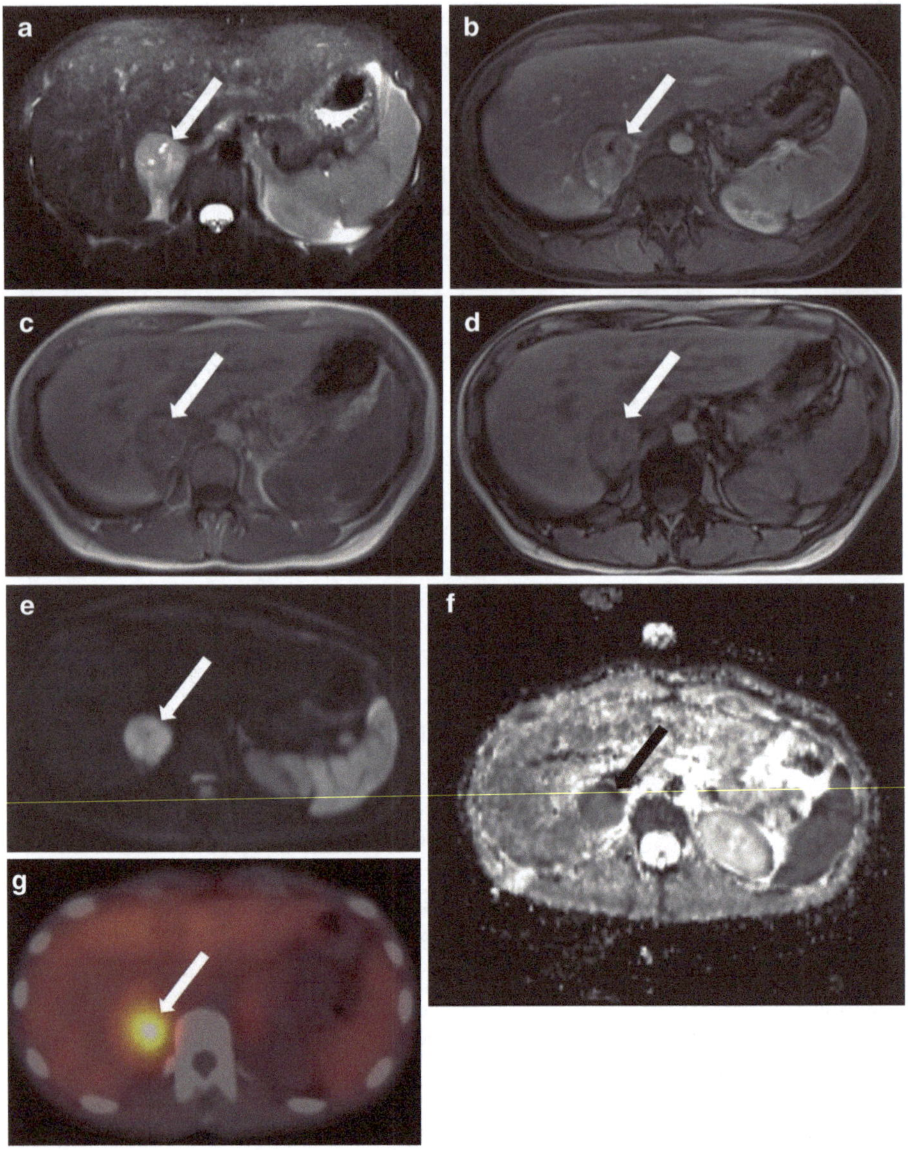

Fig. 1.17 Axial T2 with fat-saturation image (**a**) demonstrates a T2 hyperintense right suprarenal mass (*arrow*) which enhances on the T1 post-gadolinium fat-saturated sequence (**b**). The lesion is isointense to muscle on the T1 in phase image (**c**) with no loss of signal on the T1 opposed phase image (**d**). The mass is noted to have restricted diffusion (**e**, **f**) and demonstrates avid uptake on 1–123 metaiodobenzylguanidine (I-123 MIBG) SPECT imaging (**g**)

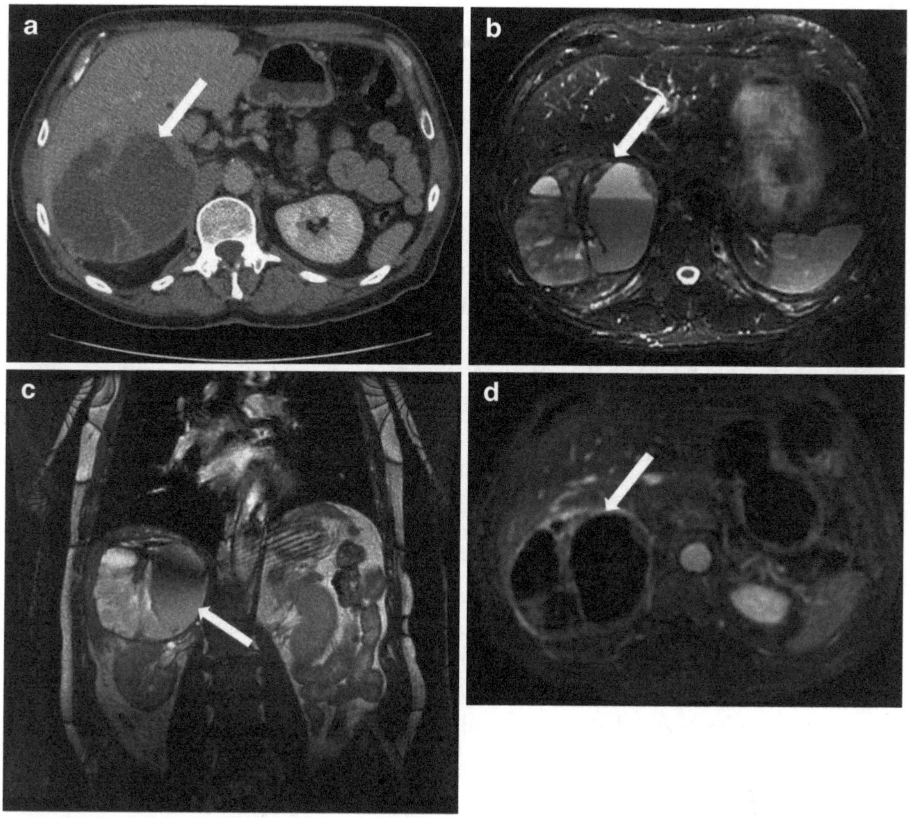

Fig. 1.18 Axial contrast-enhanced CT image in a second patient demonstrates the presence of a low density right suprarenal mass (*arrow*) with irregular enhancing septations (**a**). Axial T2 with fat saturation (**b**) and coronal T2 weighted (**c**) MR images confirm the suprarenal location of this mass and demonstrates the presence of an internal fluid level (**b**). Post contrast T1 weighted image with fat saturation demonstrates the presence of irregular enhancing septations (**d**)

10 % of these tumors arise from chromaffin cells in extra-adrenal paraganglionic tissue (in which case they are referred to as paragangliomas). Sporadic occurrence is most common, though a genetic predisposition should be sought in patients who present at a younger age (particularly before the age of 18) or those who have multifocal or bilateral neoplasms. Multiple endocrine neoplasia (MEN) type II, von-Hippel Lindau (VHL) and neurofibromatosis (NF) type 1 are associated with an increased incidence of pheochromocytomas.

Clinical presentation is variable, although patients classically present with paroxysmal episodes of headaches, palpitations, and sweating. The risk of malignant hypertensive crises, potentially prompted by biopsy or surgical resection, has resulted in the routine administration of alpha adrenergic blockers prior to tumor manipulation. Laboratory evaluation is mandatory in clinically suspected pheochromocytoma, and includes measurements of plasma metanephrines and/or catecholamine and vanillylmandelic acid levels in 24 h urine collections.

Imaging findings are non-specific. Ultrasound may demonstrate a solid, mixed cystic and solid or cystic mass. The majority of pheochromocytomas present as solid masses with a density value of greater than 10 Hounsfield units on non-contrast CT, though approximately one-third will be complex or cystic. In addition, a rare subset of these tumors may have enough intracellular lipid to attain a density of less than 10 Hounsfield units and thus a mimic an adenoma. High density material due to internal areas of hemorrhage and calcifications may be occasionally seen. Pheochromocytomas will typically demonstrate avid enhancement of the soft tissue components with a variable degrees of washout. The classical "light-bulb" bright T2 hyperintense signal intensity on MR imaging is seen across a wide range spanning 11–65 % of tumors. The T1 signal is typically isointense to muscle though this can vary with increasing amount of internal hemorrhage. Avid enhancement of the soft tissue components is noted after the administration of contrast medium. Pheochromocytomas will rarely loose signal on opposed phase images due to the presence of microscopic fat.

Iodine-123 or iodine-131 labeled metaiodobenzylguanidine (MIBG, a norepinephrine analog) is the most commonly used functional technique used in evaluating pheochromocytomas. The combination SPECT/CT technology with MIBG examinations derives the benefits of both anatomic and functional imaging, allowing for accurate localization of primary and metastatic disease.

Apart from the detection of distant metastatic disease, imaging cannot differentiate benign from malignant pheochromocytomas. This differentiation is clinically important, as malignant pheochromocytomas have a worse prognosis. Surgical resection is the mainstay of localized disease. A combination of tumor debulking, chemotherapy and/or treatment with 1–131 MIBG may be attempted for metastatic disease.

Pitfalls Pheochromocytomas may mimic other benign and malignant adrenal neoplasms. Adrenal adenoma will commonly demonstrate a density value of less than 10 Hounsfield units on non-contrast CT, loss of signal on opposed phase MRI imaging and/or rapid washout on multiphase contrast enhanced CT examinations. These findings are only rarely seen with pheochromocytomas. A new adrenal mass in a patient with a known primary malignancy will almost certainly represent a metastatic lesion. Adrenocortical carcinomas are aggressive heterogeneous neoplasms with a propensity for adjacent vessel and organ invasion. Adrenal cysts will not demonstrate soft tissue enhancement after the administration of contrast medium.

Teaching Point

1. Pheochromocytomas have a non-specific imaging appearance and can mimic other benign or malignant neoplasms. Functional imaging with I-123 or I-131 labeled MIBG offers the most specificity.
2. Laboratory workup is mandatory in clinically suspected pheochromocytoma. Premedication with alpha adrenergic blockers should be administered prior to biopsy or other tumor manipulation.
3. An adrenal mass in the context of certain syndromes such as MEN type II, VHL and NF1 should be evaluated as a pheochromocytoma.

Suggested Readings by Case

Case 1.1

Blake MA, Holalkere NS, Boland GW. Imaging techniques for adrenal lesion characterization. Radiol Clin North Am. 2008;46(1):65–78.
Berland LL, Silverman SG, Gore RM, et al. Managing incidental findings on abdominal CT: white paper of the ACR incidental findings committee. J Am Coll Radiol. 2010;7(10):754–73.
Patel J, Davenport MS, Cohan RH, et al. Can established CT attenuation and washout criteria for adrenal adenoma accurately exclude pheochromocytoma? AJR Am J Roentgenol. 2013; 201(1):122–7.

Case 1.2

Bharwani N, Rockall AG, Sahdev A, et al. Adrenocortical carcinoma: the range of appearances on CT and MRI. AJR Am J Roentgenol. 2011;196(6):W706–14.
Blake MA, Cronin CG, Boland GW. Adrenal imaging. AJR Am J Roentgenol. 2010a; 194(6):1450–60.
Fassnacht M, Kroiss M, Allolio B. Update in adrenocortical carcinoma. J Clin Endocrinol Metab. 2013;98(12):4551–64.

Case 1.3

Wedmid A, Palese M. Diagnosis and treatment of the adrenal cyst. Curr Urol Rep. 2010;11(1):44–50.
Sebstiano C, Zhao X, Deng FM, et al. Cystic lesions of the adrenal gland: our experience over the last 20 years. Hum Pathol. 2013;44(9):1797–803.
Taffel M, Haji-Momenian S, Nikolaidis P, et al. Adrenal imaging: a comprehensive review. Radiol Clin North Am. 2012;50(2):219–43.

Case 1.4

Jordan E, Poder L, Courtier J, et al. AJR Am J Roentgenol. 2012;199(1):W91–8.
Sacerdote MG, Johnson PT, Fishman EK. Emerg Radiol. 2012;19(1):53–60.
Simon DR, Palese MA. Clinical update on the management of adrenal hemorrhage. Curr Urol Rep. 2009;10(1):78–83.

Casve 1.5

Blake MA, Cronin CG, Boland GW. Adrenal imaging. AJR Am J Roentgenol. 2010b; 194(6):1450–60.
Dunnick NR, Korobkin M. Imaging of adrenal incidentalomas: current status. AJR Am J Roentgenol. 2002;179(3):559–68.
Eldaya RW, Lo SS, Paulino AC, et al. Diagnosis and treatment options including stereotactic body radiation therapy (SBRT) for adrenal metastases. J Radiat Oncol. 2012;1:43–8.

Case 1.6

Afaq AA, Lefkowitz RA. Imaging of adrenal neoplasms. In: Atlas of genitourinary oncological imaging. New York: Springer; 2013. p. 121–58.

Daneshmand S, Quek ML. Adrenal myelolipoma: diagnosis and management. Urol J. 2006;3(2):71–4.

Johnson PT, Horton KM, Fishman EK. Adrenal mass imaging with multidetector CT: pathologic conditions, pearls, and pitfalls. Radiographics. 2009;29(5):1333–51.

Case 1.7

Blake MA, Cronin CG, Boland GW. Adrenal imaging. AJR Am J Roentgenol. 2010c; 194(6):1450–60.

Blake MA, Kalra MK, Maher MM, et al. Pheochromocytoma: an imaging chameleon. Radiographics. 2004;24(1):S87–99.

Leung K, Stamm M, Raja A, et al. Pheochromocytoma: the range of appearances on ultrasound, CT, and MRI and functional imaging. AJR Am J Roentgenol. 2013;200(2):370–8.

Chapter 2
Kidneys

Case 2.1

Brief Case Summary: 37 year old female with persistent, asymptomatic microscopic hematuria.

Imaging Findings CT scan of the abdomen and pelvis with intravenous and oral contrast demonstrates the absence of a kidney in the expected location of the left renal fossa. A portion of the right kidney is noted (arrow in Fig. 2.1a). Note the flattened appearance of the left adrenal gland (the "lying down") compatible with a congenitally absent left renal fossa. Figure 2.1b demonstrates a displaced left kidney across the midline which is fused with a caudally located right kidney. Figure 2.1c (obtained during a delayed portion of this exam to opacify the collecting system) demonstrates the normal entry zone of both ureters (arrows).

Differential Diagnosis Horseshoe kidney

Diagnosis and Discussion: Crossed Fused Ectopia

Crossed fused renal ectopia is the second most common congenital renal fusion anomaly where both kidneys are on one side of the body and the renal parenchyma fuses. Patient with cross fused renal ectopic are usually asymptomatic and it is usually incidentally diagnosed. However, if symptoms are present, they are usually abdominal and flank pain, hematuria, or urinary tract infection.

Four types of crossed renal ectopia have been described according to the McDonald and McClellan classification. The most common accounts for 85 % of cases and is crossed renal ectopia with fusion. Crossed renal ectopia without fusion accounts for 10 % and solitary crossed renal ectopia and bilaterally crossed renal ectopia account for the minority of crossed renal ectopia types. The most common form is where the upper pole of the inferiorly positioned kidney fuses with the lower pole of the superiorly positioned kidney. The ureter of the ectopic kidney crosses

M.G. Harisinghani, A. Rajesh, *Genitourinary Imaging: A Case Based Approach*, DOI 10.1007/978-1-4471-4772-5_2

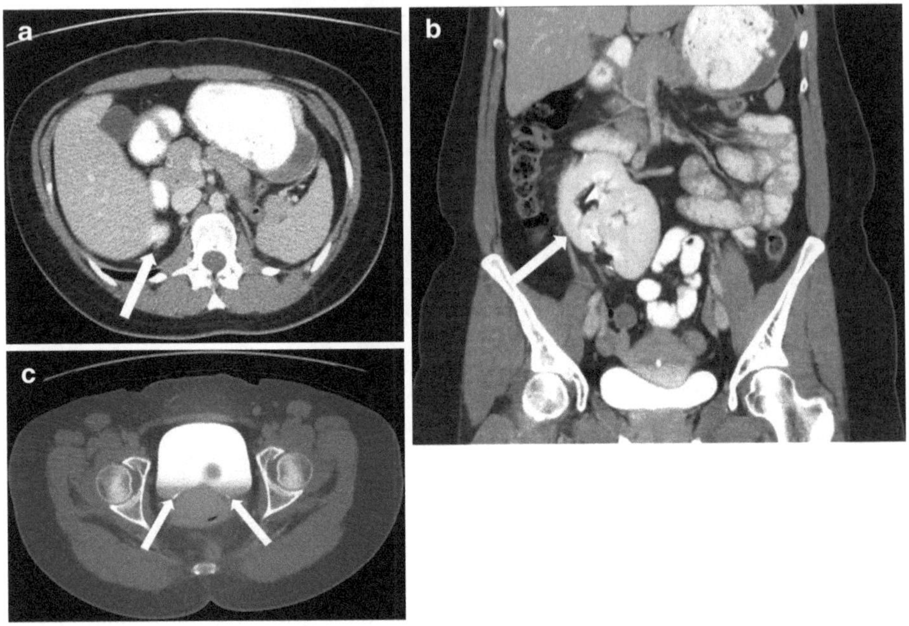

Fig. 2.1 CT scan of the abdomen and pelvis with intravenous and oral contrast demonstrates the absence of a kidney in the expected location of the left renal fossa. A segment of the right kidney is noted (*arrow* in **a**). Note the flattened appearance of the left adrenal gland (the "lying down") compatible with a congenitally absent left renal fossa. (**b**) Demonstrates a displaced left kidney across the midline which is fused with a caudally located right kidney (*arrow*). (**c**) Obtained during a delayed portion of this exam to opacify the collecting system, demonstrates the normal location of both ureters (*arrows*)

midline and enters the bladder in the anatomic position. Most commonly, the left kidney is ectopic and is abnormally located in the right hemiabdomen.

On imaging, CT and MR are the best imaging modalities for diagnosis and classification of the type of crossed renal ectopia. CT and MR can evaluate the blood supply to the kidneys and evaluate for potential urologic complications. The blood supply to the normally-located kidney as well as the ectopic kidney commonly have aberrant vascular anatomy that can be readily evaluated on cross sectional imaging. The ectopic kidney frequently receives some blood supply from the ipsilateral vessels.

Potential complications include urinary reflux, ureteropelvic junction obstruction, and ectopic ureteroceles. The abnormal position of the kidneys predisposes to urinary stasis resulting in hydronephrosis, calculi formation, and recurrent urinary tract infections. In the pediatric population, crossed fused renal ectopia may be associated with other congenital abnormalities involving the cardiovascular, gastrointestinal, and skeletal systems.

Pitfalls Differentiating between crossed fused renal ectopia and horseshoe kidney can be readily done by evaluating whether the kidneys are both on one side of the body in crossed fused renal ectopia or on both sides of the body as in horseshoe kidney.

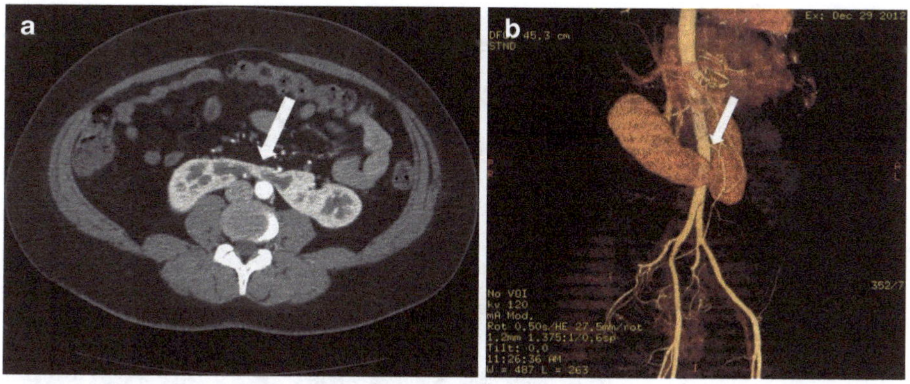

Fig. 2.2 CT scan of the abdomen and pelvis with intravenous and oral contrast demonstrate midline fusion of the lower poles of the kidneys (**a**). Note that the fusion is located below the level of the inferior mesenteric artery as demonstrated on the 3D rendered reconstruction (*arrow* in **b**)

Teaching Point

1. Crossed fused renal ectopia is the second most common congenital renal fusion anomaly, second to horseshoe kidney.
2. Congenital renal fusion anomalies are usually associated with variant renal anatomy and can be associated with other congenital anomalies.
3. The diagnosis, variant arterial anatomy, and complications can be readily assessed with CT and MR.

Case 2.2

Brief Case Summary: 57 year old male with abdominal pain.

Imaging Findings CT scan of the abdomen and pelvis with intravenous and oral contrast demonstrate midline fusion of the lower poles of the kidneys (Fig. 2.2a). Note that the fusion is located below the level of the inferior mesenteric artery as demonstrated on the 3D rendered reconstruction (arrow in Fig. 2.2b). US (Fig. 2.3) demonstrates the sonographic appearance of a horseshoe kidney in a different patient, with the fused segment lying anterior to the abdominal aorta (arrow). Non-contrast CT scan of the abdomen in the same patient as Fig. 2.3 demonstrates the presence of a non-obstructing stone within the lower pole of the left kidney (arrow in Fig. 2.4).

Differential Diagnosis On ultrasound, crossed fused renal ectopia may have a similar appearance. Otherwise, no differential diagnosis.

Diagnosis and Discussion: Horseshoe kidney

Horseshoe kidneys are the most common renal fusion anomaly with an incidence of 1 in 400 births, with males being twice as commonly affected. Patients may be

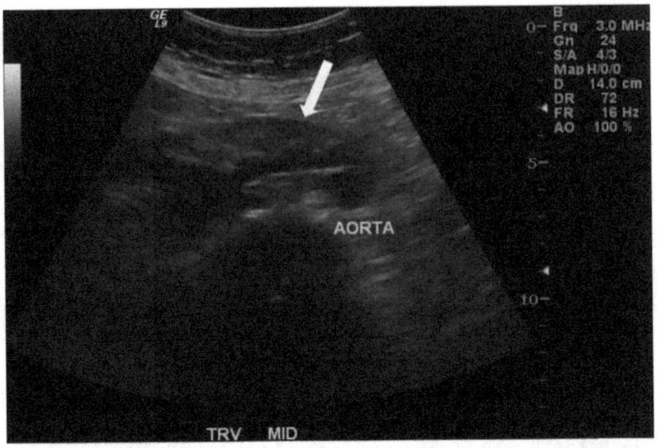

Fig. 2.3 US demonstrates the sonographic appearance of a horseshoe kidney in a different patient, with the fused segment lying anterior to the abdominal aorta (*arrow*)

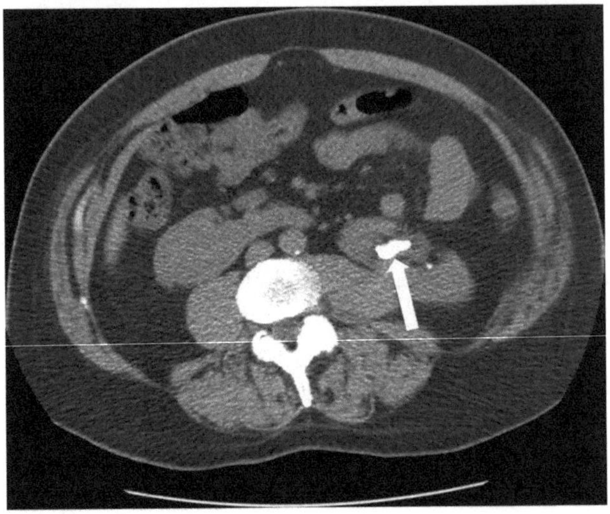

Fig. 2.4 Non-contrast CT scan of the abdomen in the same patient as Fig. 2.3 demonstrates the presence of a non-obstructing stone within the lower pole of the left kidney (*arrow*)

asymptomatic, however, vague abdominal pain with possible radiation to the back is a possible symptom. On physical examination, a palpable abdominal mass in the midline may be noted.

The best imaging diagnostic feature is two kidneys located in the renal fossa on opposite sides of the body with fusion of the lower poles forming an isthmus of tissue crossing the midline. The isthmus crosses anterior to the abdominal aorta. The isthmus in a horseshoe kidney acts as an impediment to normal rotation and upward ascent where the isthmus encounters the inferior mesenteric artery. 90 % of horseshoe kidneys have midline or symmetrical fusion, whereas the remaining 10 % of cases have a lateral or asymmetrical fusion.

On radiography, the kidneys are close to the spine with the lower poles being the medial most portions of the kidneys. CT examination allows for assessment of the degree and type of fusion, evaluation of renal parenchymal and collecting system changes, delineation of variant renal arterial supply, and diagnosing complications. The benefit of CT includes the ability to perform multiplanar reformats and 3-D reconstructions. MR may also be performed to show fusion of the lower poles of the kidneys which crosses midline and the low position of the kidneys which are located caudal to the inferior mesenteric artery.

Other congenital anomalies that are associated with horseshoe kidneys include vertebral, esophageal, anorectal, and tracheal malformations as well as chromosomal and hematologic abnormalities.

Complications of horseshoe kidneys are not uncommon and include traumatic injury, ureteropelvic junction obstruction, recurrent infections, calculi formation, and increased risk of renal cell carcinoma. The isthmus's location immediately anterior to the abdominal aorta and vertebral bodies predisposes the horseshoe kidney to traumatic injury, particularly due to the absence of protection by the overlying ribs. The abnormal position of the kidneys may lead to poor outflow and urinary stasis which predisposes to hydronephrosis, recurrent infection, and calculi formation.

Pitfalls The main differential consideration for a horseshoe kidney is renal ectopia where the kidneys are congenitally located in an abnormal position. In crossed fused ectopia, the kidneys are located on the same side of the body and typically the ureter crosses midline to insert into the bladder in the normal anatomic position.

Teaching Point

1. Horseshoe kidney is the most common renal fusion anomaly where the kidneys remain in anatomic location with fusion of the lower poles across midline forming an isthmus, located anterior to the abdominal aorta and vertebral bodies.
2. Anomalous renal vasculature and complications including predisposition to traumatic injury, calculi formation, and recurrent infections are important associations of horseshoe kidneys.
3. CT allows for evaluation of the degree and type of fusion in addition to associated complications, particularly with the multiplanar reformats and 3D rendered reconstruction.

Case 2.3

Brief Case Summary: 40 years old male, asymptomatic

Imaging Findings Coronal reconstructed T1-weighted MIP MRI image shows enlarged calyces (white arrows) with normal size renal pelvis of left kidney (Fig. 2.5). Also note associated megaureter (arrow head).

Differential Diagnosis Hydronephrosis, Polycalycosis, Intermittent hydronephrosis and Infundibular stenosis

Diagnosis and Discussion Congenital megacalycosis

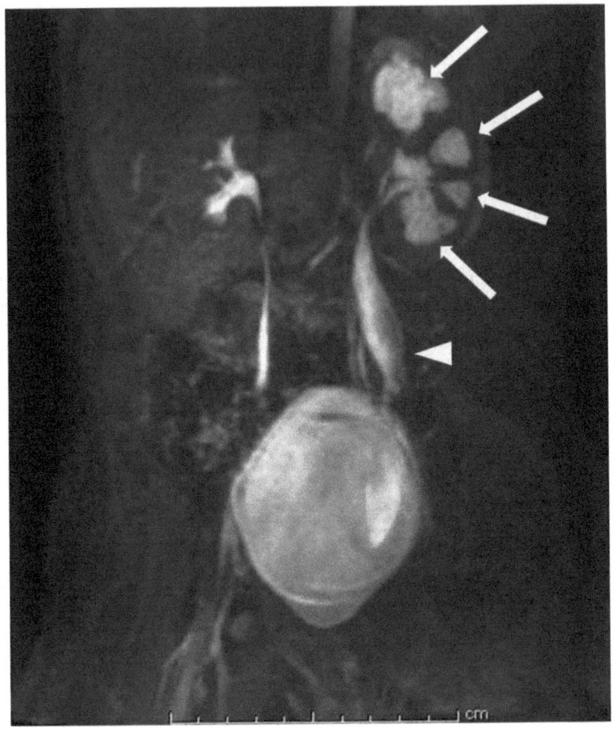

Fig. 2.5 Coronal reformatted T1-weighted MIP MRI image shows enlarged calyces (*white arrows*) with normal size renal pelvis of left kidney. Also note associated megaureter (*arrow head*)

Congenital megacalycosis (CM), also called megacalyces or Puigvert's disease, is a rare renal disorder first reported in 1963, which presence caliceal dilatation and hypoplasia of the pyramids of Malpighi without evidences of renal pelvic or ureteral obstruction and impaired renal function. This disease commonly involves unilateral kidney and occurs in male. This abnormality may be caused by a transient delay in the recanalization of the upper ureter after the ureteral bud connects to the metanephros or the underdevelopment of the pyramids with lack of projection of the papillae into the calyces. The calyces commonly increase to 12–20 in number and have a rounded appearance. The pyramids have a semilunar configuration, instead of the normal triangular or cone shape, and the tip of each papilla is flat. The disease is usually diagnosed by accident or by its complications such as renal calculi and urinary tract infections. It also can accompany with other urogenital malformations, such as mega-ureter or multicystic dysplastic kidney, or with other congenital disorders, such as Schinzel–Giedion syndrome.

The imaging diagnosis of CM is first established by ultrasound and intravenous urography (IVU). CM may appear as an enlarged kidney with caliectasis. IVU can display not only the morphological abnormalities, including increased renal size, decreased thickness of the parenchyma and ectatic, polygonal and outnumbered calyces, but also the functional change as delayed enhancement of the pelvicaliceal system. Both pelvises and ureters appear normal and obstructive signs are absent. This point is important when distinguishing with obstructive hydronephrosis. CT urography (CTU) and MR urography (MRU) can further demonstrate these findings, moreover, providing more details on shapes of calyces and pyramids and associated complications. Micturating cystourethrography and ascending urography excluded vesicoureteral reflux or obstruction. Scintigraphies with 99 m-dimercaptosuccinic acid (Tc99mDMSA) and Technetium 99 m-diethylenetri aminepentaacetic acid (Tc99mDTPA) usually present normal.

Pitfalls Megacalycosis should be carefully discriminated with obstructed hydronephrosis because the former does not cause the renal function damage and thus no surgical intervention need. CM can be differentiated from obstructive hydronephrosis by imaging methods, based on the normal-sized pelvis and ureter on IVU, CTU and MRU, normal excretory function on IVU, normal display on scintigraphies with Tc99mDMSA and Tc99mDTPA. However, sometimes the findings of CM on these imaging methods also can be abnormal, which adds a little confusion on differential diagnosis. For example, CM may show a delay in visualization of the collecting system due to the large volume of the calyces. The results of scintigraphies may be abnormal due to the accompanying urinary tract infections. Renal function and radiographic appearances have remained stable in cases followed over several years.

Teaching Point

1. The increased number and dilatation of calyces with undilated pelvis and ureter and normal renal function are the key points to distinguishing CM from obstructive hydronephrosis.
2. IVU is the preferred diagnostic tool for CM for it combines the morphological and functional features.
3. The complications of CM, such as urinary tract infections and renal calculi, sometimes may alter the imaging manifestations and influence the diagnosis.

Case 2.4

Brief Case Summary None. Middle aged patient complaining of non specific abdominal pain

Imaging Findings Axial contrast-enhanced CT scans demonstrate a simple renal cyst at right renal sinus displacing contrast-filled right renal pelvis (arrows in Fig. 2.6a, b).

Differential Diagnosis Hydronephrosis

Diagnosis and Discussion: Parapelvic Cysts

Parapelvic renal cysts are lymphocytic in origin or may develop from embryologic rests and do not communicate with the collecting system. Parapelvic cysts are clinically important as they can be confused with hydronephrosis or an extrarenal pelvis. Parapelvic cysts may also compress the collecting system resulting in hypertension, hematuria, or can become secondarily infected.

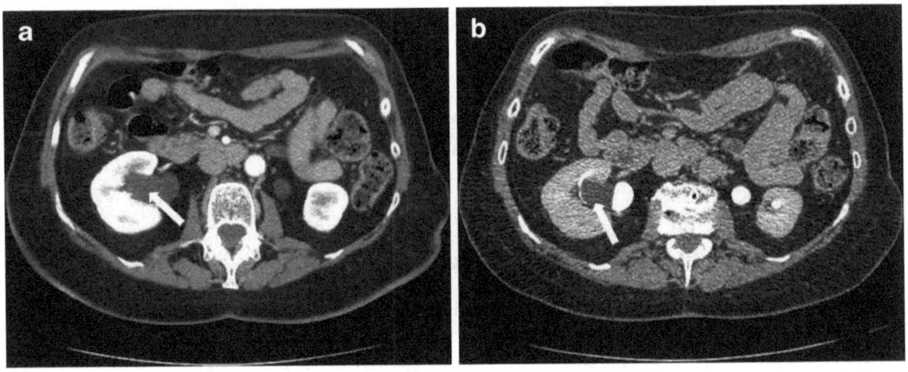

Fig. 2.6 Axial contrast-enhanced CT scans demonstrate a parapelvic cyst in the right renal sinus displacing contrast-filled right renal pelvis (*arrows* in **a**, **b**)

On CT, parapelvic cysts are thin walled with a homogeneous appearance and attenuation of water. The parapelvic cysts are smoothly marginated and often have lobulated margins. A parapelvic cyst can also mimic a dilated renal pelvis or an extra renal pelvis on CT. After injection of intravenous contrast and imaging in an excretory phase of contrast, the normal collecting system partially or completely opacifies with contrast material and in contradistinction, a parapelvic cyst will remain unchanged in the excretory phase.

Treatment is usually not needed unless compression of the renal collecting system causing symptoms is present.

Pitfalls Differentiating parapelvic cysts from a dilated renal pelvis, hydronephrosis, and extrarenal pelvis is clinically important as a misdiagnosis may lead to additional imaging studies or subsequent treatment, particularly for treatment of hydronephrosis.

Teaching Point

1. Parapelvic cysts are not true cysts and are likely lymphatic in origin or may result from embryologic rests.
2. There is no communication with the collecting system which allows for accurate differentiation from hydronephrosis on an excretory or urographic phase of a contrast enhanced CT.
3. Accurate differentiation of parapelvic cysts from hydronephrosis will prevent additional workup and treatment.

Case 2.5

Brief Case Summary: 64 year-old male with end-stage renal disease

Imaging Findings Non contrast CT image (Fig. 2.7a) of the patient 1 year prior shows atrophic kidneys and ascites from renal failure. Contrast enhanced current

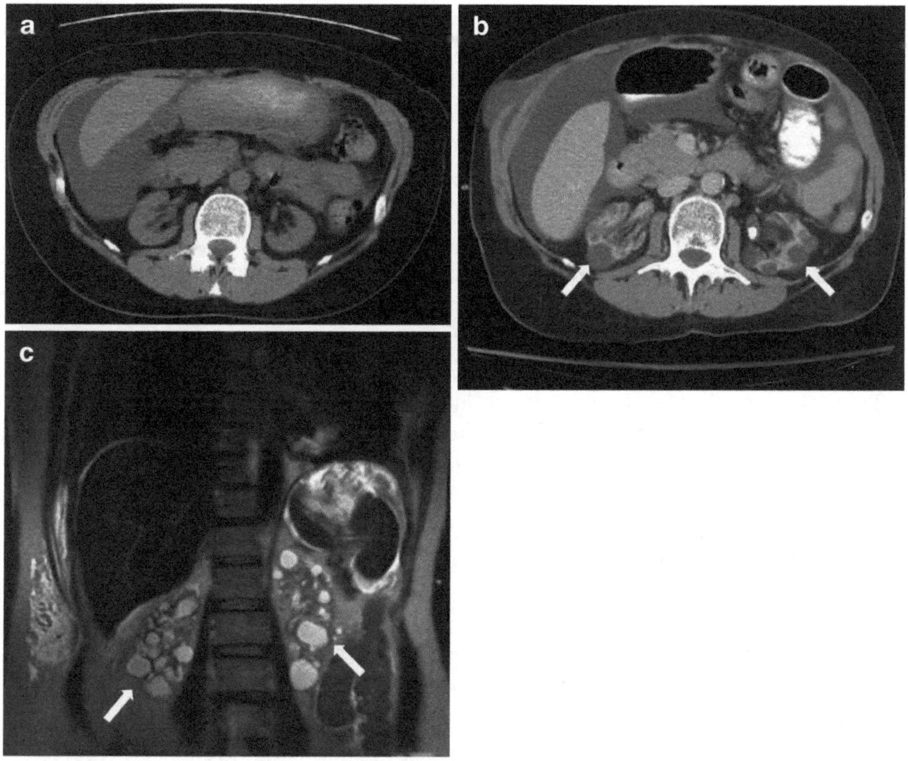

Fig. 2.7 Non contrast CT image (**a**) of the patient 1 year prior shows atrophic kidneys and ascites from renal failure. Contrast enhanced current axial CT image (**b**) shows bilateral renal cysts of varying sizes with non-obstructing left renal pelvic stone and ascites. Coronal T2-weighted image (**c**) shows the bilateral cysts within kidneys along with ascites

axial CT image (Fig. 2.7b) shows bilateral renal cysts of varying sizes with non obstructing left renal pelvic stone and ascites. Coronal T2-weighted image (Fig. 2.7c) shows the bilateral cysts within kidneys along with ascites.

Differential Diagnosis

Multiple simple renal cysts
Tuberous sclerosis
Medullary cystic disease
Von Hippel-Lindau disease

Diagnosis and Discussion Acquired cystic kidney disease

Patients with end-stage renal disease undergo a proliferative process in their kidneys and are at increased risk for renal cyst formation and malignancy. Acquired cystic kidney disease (ACKD) develops in patients with end-stage renal disease (ESRD), particularly in patients receiving dialysis, where multiple bilateral renal cysts develop progressively over time. The number, size, and prevalence of cysts increase with the duration of dialysis with nearly 100 % of ESRD patients treated for 10 or more years. ACKD occurs in patients treated with peritoneal dialysis and hemodialysis.

On imaging, multiple, small <1 cm, fluid-filled renal cysts are seen in atrophic to normal-sized kidneys. The cysts involve predominantly the renal cortex but may also involve the medulla. On US, multiple anechoic cysts are visualized with small to normal-sized kidneys with increased parenchymal echogenicity and loss of the corticomedullary differentiation. Hemorrhagic cysts appear as hypoechoic lesions with internal echoes with increased posterior acoustic enhancement. On CT, bilateral cysts are seen and hemorrhagic cysts are hyperdense, making accurate differentiation from malignancy difficult. MR allows for improved soft tissue characterization with <1 cm simple cysts manifesting as nonenhancing T1 hypointense, T2 hyperintense lesions. Complicated cysts have variable T1 and T2 signal depending on the proteinaceous and hemorrhagic contents. MR is helpful in assessing for soft tissue enhancement which accurately differentiates enhancing renal cell carcinoma from complicated cysts, particularly with the use of subtraction imaging.

Hemorrhage within cysts, perinephric hemorrhage, and development of renal cell carcinoma are important potential complications of ACKD. Risk factors for developing renal cell carcinoma in patients on dialysis include male sex, prolonged dialysis, and ACKD. Other potential complications include infection of the cysts, microhematuria, and calculi formation.

The average life-expectancy in patients on dialysis is lower than that of the general population with the life-expectancy ranging from 1.5 to 10 years after initiation of dialysis. Treatment for ESRD is renal transplantation and if renal cell carcinoma is detected, the treatment is surgical excision.

Pitfalls Differentiating ACKD from other renal cyst forming diseases is based on clinical history and occurs in patients with ESRD on dialysis. Imaging features such as multiple small cysts <1 cm in size in atrophic kidneys is also helpful in making the diagnosis. Other differential considerations include cysts seen in syndromes such as tuberous sclerosis and Von Hippel Lindau disease, however, other organs are typically affected. Autosomal dominant polycystic kidney disease typically have multiple cysts of varying sizes in enlarged kidneys. Medullary sponge kidney manifests as renal cysts in the medulla of kidneys in young patients with progressive renal failure.

Teaching Points

1. Acquired cystic kidney disease occurs in patients with end stage renal disease on dialysis and the number, size, and prevalence of cysts increase with the duration of dialysis.
2. ACKD manifests as multiple small <1 cm bilateral cysts in atrophic to normal size kidneys in patients with end stage renal disease.
3. These patients are at increased risk for associated complications and renal cell carcinoma and MR is an important imaging modality used to detect renal cell carcinoma.

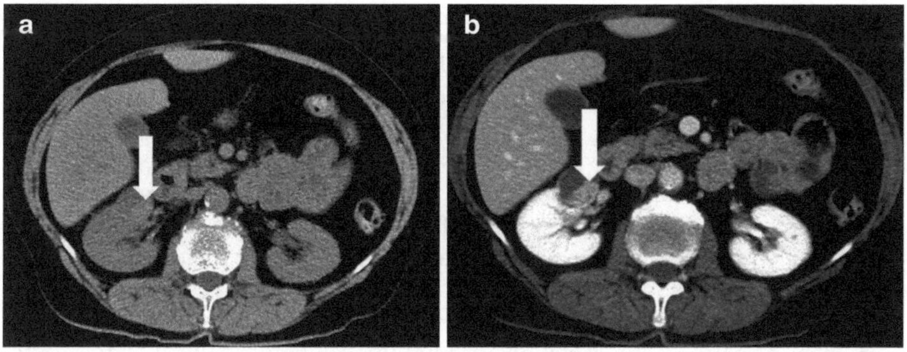

Fig. 2.8 CT scan of the abdomen performed with and without the administration of intravenous contrast demonstrates the presence of an exophytic cystic mass in the interpolar region of the right kidney with the presence of an enhancing soft tissue nodule (*arrows*, **a**, **b**)

Case 2.6

Brief Case Summary: 54 year old male with hematuria

Imaging Findings CT scan of the abdomen performed with and without the administration of intravenous contrast demonstrates the presence of a cystic mass in the interpolar region of the right kidney with the presence of an enhancing soft tissue nodule (arrows, Figs. 2.8a, b and 2.8).

Differential Diagnosis Cystic renal cell carcinoma (Bosniak category IV).

Diagnosis and Discussion Renal cysts are common and occur in 20–30 % of middle-aged adults and the incidence increases with age. Simple, uncomplicated renal cysts are easy to diagnose, however, renal cell carcinoma can manifest as a cystic lesion, therefore, complicated renal cysts pose a diagnostic challenge. In 1986, the Bosniak classification of renal cysts was developed to evaluate cystic renal masses, generate interobserver agreement, and decide clinical management. The Bosniak classification system is based on CT criteria but the classification system can be used with MR imaging.

Evaluation of renal masses with MR has continued to increase due to the superior contrast resolution and soft tissue characterization. The detection of enhancement is superior with MR particularly with the use of subtraction techniques to assess for enhancement. The Bosniak classification system has been applied to MR imaging with the caveat that MR can exaggerate some imaging findings. Internal septations tend to appear thicker and enhancement septations is more readily apparent thus experience in MR imaging interpretation is imperative. Additionally the quality of MR images varies by institution and MR is susceptible to more artifacts including patient motion.

The Bosniak classification system is as follows:

Category I: simple benign cysts with hairline-thin walls. The cysts do not contain septations, calcifications, or solid components. No enhancing soft tissue components are seen.

Category II: benign cystic lesions. The cysts may have hairline-thin septations with fine calcifications in the walls. Minimal enhancement of the hairline-thin smooth wall may be seen. No enhancing soft tissue components are present. Non-enhancing high-attenuation cysts less than 3 cm in size are included.

Category IIF: Complex cysts requiring follow-up imaging. These cysts are more complex and cannot fit into either category II or III. These cysts have an increased number of hairline-thin septations or mild thickening of the wall and/or septations. No enhancing soft tissue components are present.

Category III: Indeterminate masses. The cystic lesions are thickened walls and septations that are irregular. The cyst walls or septations demonstrate enhancement.

Category IV: Malignant cystic masses. Thick and irregular walls and septations may be present but enhancing soft tissue components are seen, independent of wall or septal enhancement.

Categories I and II are considered leave-alone lesions which do not require further follow-up imaging. Category IIF lesions should be follow-up imaging, however, the exact duration of follow-up imaging is uncertain. Some have proposed a minimum duration of follow-up imaging of 1–2 years. Category III lesions carry a risk of malignancy between 31 and 100 % should undergo renal biopsy and radiologic follow-up to avoid unnecessary surgery in patients with nonmalignant lesions. Category IV lesions have an incidence of malignancy between 67 and 100 % and surgical resection is the treatment of choice.

Pitfalls Simple renal cysts are common and are benign, however, renal cell carcinoma may repsent as a cystic mass. Careful attention to the cyst walls and septations and accurate detection of enhancing soft tissue components

Teaching Point

1. Renal cysts are common and are usually benign, but renal cell carcinoma can present as a cystic mass. Accurate characterization of cystic renal lesions is important to avoid unnecessary surgery in patients with nonmalignant lesions.
2. The Bosniak classification system of cystic renal masses helps categorize masses based on imaging findings to assess the risk of malignancy and for evaluation of clinical treatment.
3. Bosniak category IV cystic masses have a 67–100 % risk of malignancy and surgical resection is the preferred treatment.

Case 2.7

Brief Case Summary: 45 year old man with hematuria

Imaging Findings Plain radiograph of the abdomen demonstrates the presence of multiple bilateral peripherally calcified masses overlying the abdomen (arrows in

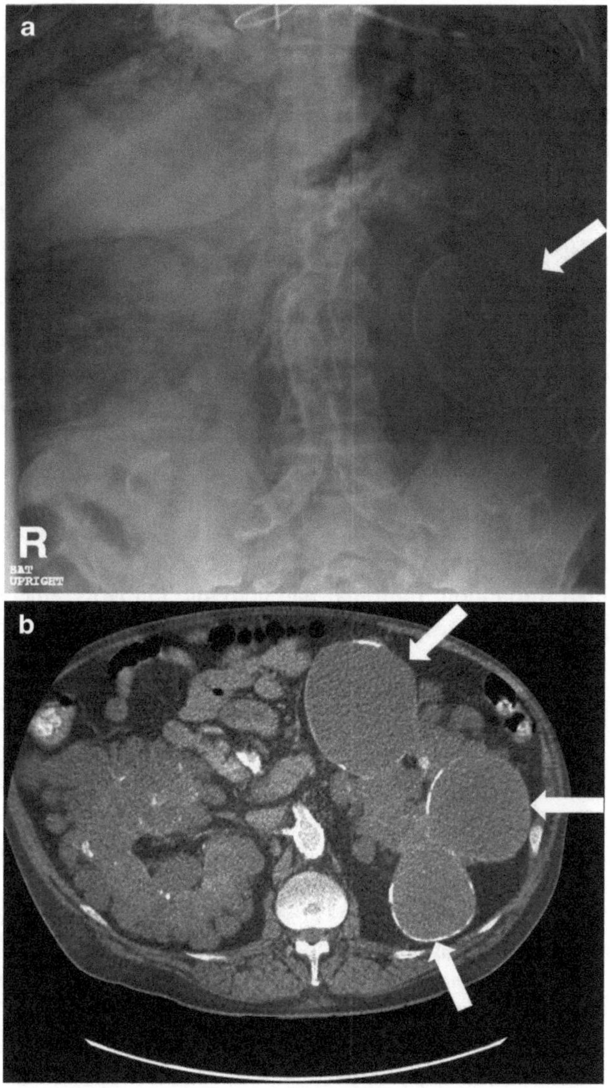

Fig. 2.9 Plain radiograph of the abdomen demonstrates the presence of multiple bilateral peripherally calcified masses overlying the abdomen (*arrows* in **a**). Non-contrast CT scan (**b**) demonstrates the presence of bilateral renal cysts, some of which have thin, mural calcifications. Both the right and left kidney are enlarged (left renal parenchyma not clearly shown on the provided CT images)

Fig. 2.9a). Non-contrast CT scan (Fig. 2.9b) demonstrates the presence of bilateral renal cysts, some of which have thin, mural calcifications. Both the right and left kidney are enlarged (left renal parenchyma not clearly shown on the provided CT images).

Differential Diagnosis

Autosomal dominant polycystic kidney disease
Multiple simple cysts
Von Hippel Lindau disease
Tuberous sclerosis
Medullary sponge kidney
Acquired cystic kidney disease

Diagnosis and Discussion: Autosomal dominant polycystic kidney disease (ADPKD) is the most common hereditary cystic disease characterized by autosomal dominant inheritance but can also occur with spontaneous mutation. Patients are symptomatic and present in adulthood, between ages 30–50, with renal failure or hypertension. Renal parenchyma is normal at birth but is gradually replaced by cysts.

Patients with ADPKD can also demonstrate extrarenal cysts, most commonly in the pancreas and liver, and less commonly in the spleen, ovaries and testes. Other associated abnormalities include intracranial aneurysms, aortic and mitral valve abnormalities, colonic diverticula, aortic aneurysms and dissections. 45 % of ADPKD patients will develop end stage renal disease, the most common cause of morbidity and mortality. ADPKD patients are not at increased risk for renal cell carcinoma.

The disease is characterized by bilaterally enlarged kidneys which are replaced by multiple expansile renal cysts which may have varying attenuation, indicative of prior infection or hemorrhage. Imaging is important for diagnosis as well as the management of ADPKD with assessing complications, disease progression, and response to treatment. On CT, the kidneys are enlarged bilaterally with innumerable cysts of varying sizes. The cysts are typically large, >3 cm or larger, and are distributed throughout the renal parenchyma. On MRI, uncomplicated cysts are nonenhancing and are typically T1 hypointense and T2 hyperintense. Complicated cysts may have varying T1 and T2 signal depending on protein/hemorrhagic content. Patients with family history of cystic renal disease can be screened with ultrasound.

Patients with multiple renal cysts may have a similar appearance, however, these patients typically do not present with hypertension and/or renal failure. Family history and cysts in other organs also suggests ADPKD.

Von Hippel Lindau disease is also autosomal dominant and presents with cysts in the kidneys and may also have cysts in the other organs. However, these patients tend to have fewer cysts. These patients may also present with multiple and bilateral renal cell carcinomas which occur at a young age. Other associated lesions include retinal angiomas, cerebellar hemangiomas, adrenal pheochromocytomas and serous cystadenomas.

Tuberous sclerosis also has an autosomal dominant inheritance pattern. Patients present with multiple renal cysts in association with renal angiomyolipomas, hamartomas in the skin, brain and retina.

Medullary sponge kidney may be associated with renal failure at a young age. Cysts are typically too small to be seen. When visible, cysts occur in the renal medulla in contrast to ADPKD where cysts can appear in both medulla and cortex.

Acquired cystic kidney disease occurs in patients with chronic renal failure receiving long-term hemodialysis or peritoneal dialysis. Cysts typically occur in the cortex and rarely exceed 2 cm.

Pitfalls Without appropriate clinical history ADPKD can be easily mistaken for other cystic renal diseases. Family history of ADPKD, hypertension and renal failure supports the diagnosis. History of chronic renal failure and long-term hemodialysis suggests uremic cystic disease.

Teaching Point

1. ADPKD is the most common hereditary cause of renal cystic disease characterized by numerous cysts of varying sizes in bilaterally enlarged kidneys.
2. Approximately 45 % of patients develop end stage renal disease which is the most common cause of morbidity and mortality, however, these patients are not at increased risk for renal cell carcinoma.
3. In addition to renal cysts, ADPKD patients have extrarenal manifestations including cysts in the liver, spleen, and pancreas, intracranial aneurysms, and aortic aneurysm and dissections.

Case 2.8

Brief Case Summary: 50 year old female with systemic lupus erythematosus (SLE).

Imaging Findings Patient is status post right nephrectomy. Axial T2 weighted MRI demonstrates a thin band of signal void along the periphery of left kidney (Fig. 2.10a). Axial non contrast CT at the corresponding slice position reveals diffuse cortical calcification extending towards the columns of Bertini with sparing of the medulla (Fig. 2.10b).

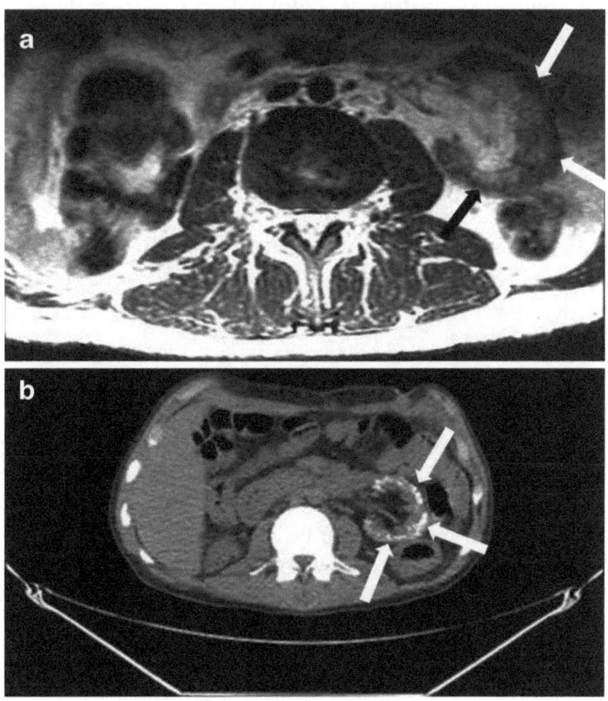

Fig. 2.10 Axial T2 weighted MRI demonstrates a thin band of signal void along the periphery of left kidney (*arrow*) (**a**). Axial non contrast CT at the corresponding slice position reveals diffuse cortical calcification (*arrows*) extending towards the columns of Bertini with sparing of the medulla (**b**)

Differential Diagnosis Medullary nephrocalcinosis, renal tuberculosis, cortical nephrocalcinosis

Diagnosis and Discussion: Cortical nephrocalcinosis

Nephrocalcinosis refers to deposition of calcium salts within the renal parenchyma. It may involve the cortex or medulla.

Cortical nephrocalcinosis results from diffuse cortical disease. The three most common causes include chronic glomerulonephritis, acute cortical necrosis and transplant rejection. Less common causes include chronic hypercalcemia, ethylene glycol poisoning, primary oxalosis, acquired immunodeficiency syndrome (AIDS) associated infections and sickle cell disease. In the above patient, the etiology was believed to be chronic glomerulonephritis in the setting of SLE.

On imaging, cortical nephrocalcinosis most often presents as bilateral fine renal calcifications. While these findings may be seen on plain radiographs, they are best depicted on non contrast abdominal CT. On ultrasound, it presents as increased peripheral echogenicity. On MRI, calcifications typically present as signal voids on T1 and T2 weighted images owing to susceptibility.
Three patterns of calcification have been described in cortical nephrocalcinosis:

1. A thin peripheral band or rim of calcification beneath the capsule, which may extend into the columns of Bertini.
2. Two parallel lines of cortical calcification known as tram track appearance.
3. Randomly distributed punctate calcifications, likely related to calcium deposition in necrotic glomeruli.

The natural history and clinical presentation depend essentially on the underlying etiology. When detected incidentally in asymptomatic patients, further work up should be undertaken to elucidate the primary etiology, and attention directed towards treating underlying metabolic derangement.

Pitfalls The distribution of calcification typically allows cortical nephrocalcinosis to be readily differentiated from other potential mimickers. Medullary nephrocalcinosis demonstrates calcium deposition in the medulla, while renal tuberculosis is typically unilateral and often presents with globular calcifications and/or infundibular strictures. Note that cortical nephrocalcinosis may be difficult to detect on MRI where the thin band of peripheral subcapsular signal void may be overlooked.

Teaching Points

1. Cortical nephrocalcinosis refers to calcification within the renal cortex.
2. Commonly causes include acute cortical necrosis, chronic glomerulonephritis and transplant rejection.
3. Non contrast CT is the best imaging test for diagnosis. It typically reveals fine bilateral calcification, which may present as a hyperdense subcapsular band, two parallel lines of calcification within the cortex (tram track) or scattered punctuate calcifications.

Case 2.9

Brief Case Summary: 45 year old female with abdominal pain

Imaging Findings Plain radiograph of the abdomen demonstrates the presence of bilateral calcifications overlying the region of the renal medulla (arrows, Fig. 2.11a). Gray scale ultrasound images of both kidneys demonstrate the presence of increased echogenicity in the region of the renal medulla (Fig. 2.11b, c). Coronal reformatted image of the abdomen and pelvis without intravenous contrast demonstrates the presence of bilateral renal stones distributed in the region of the renal medulla (arrows, Fig. 2.11d).

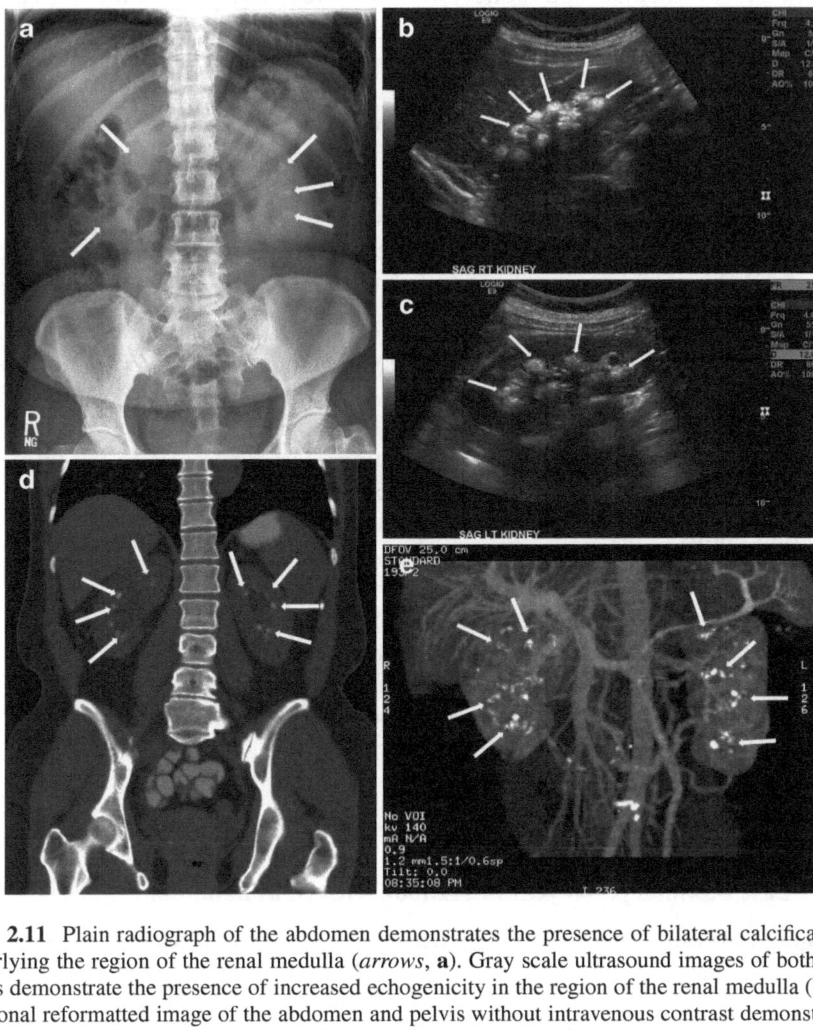

Fig. 2.11 Plain radiograph of the abdomen demonstrates the presence of bilateral calcifications overlying the region of the renal medulla (*arrows*, **a**). Gray scale ultrasound images of both kidneys demonstrate the presence of increased echogenicity in the region of the renal medulla (**b**, **c**). Coronal reformatted image of the abdomen and pelvis without intravenous contrast demonstrates the presence of bilateral renal stones distributed in the region of the renal medulla (*arrows*, **d**). Three-dimensional reformatted image in another patient demonstrates the presence of bilateral renal stones in the region of the renal medullar (**e**)

Three-dimensional reformatted image in another patient demonstrates the presence of bilateral renal stones in the region of the renal medulla (Fig. 2.11e)

Differential Diagnosis Medullary nephrocalcinosis, cortical nephrocalcinosis, papillary necrosis, renal tuberculosis

Diagnosis and Discussion: Medullary nephrocalcinosis

The most common causes of medullary nephrocalcinosis include primary hyperparathyroidism, medullary sponge kidney disease and distal renal tubular acidosis (RTA). There are two mechanisms of calcification; metastatic calcium deposition secondary to underlying metabolic derangement (as seen in hyperparathyroidism) or the precipitation of calcium salts due to urinary stasis within ecstatic distal tubules and collecting ducts (as seen in medullary sponge kidney).

Imaging findings typically demonstrate fine or coarse calcifications within the medullary pyramids. Medullary nephrocalcinosis in the setting of underling metabolic derangements is often bilateral and symmetrical while asymmetric medullary calcifications may be seen with medullary sponge kidney.

CT is very sensitive in demonstrating these calcifications which may be distributed diffusely through the pyramids (diffuse type) or along the periphery of the pyramids (rim type). On ultrasound, calcifications appear as multiple bright echogenic foci with or without distal acoustic shadowing.

Pitfalls The distribution of calcification typically allows medullary nephrocalcinosis to be readily differentiated from other potential mimickers. Cortical nephrocalcinosis demonstrates calcium deposition in the cortex, while renal tuberculosis is typically unilateral and often presents with globular calcifications and/or infundibular strictures. Note that medullary calcifications occurring close to the tip of the pyramids may be difficult to differentiate from tiny calculi in the fornices.

Teaching Points

1. Medullary nephrocalcinosis refers to calcification within the renal medulla.
2. The most common causes include primary hyperparathyroidism, medullary sponge kidney disease and distal renal tubular acidosis (RTA).
3. Imaging studies typically demonstrate calcifications within the medullary pyramids which could be diffuse or involve the periphery of the pyramids (rim type).

Case 2.10

Brief Case Summary: 48 year old female with right flank pain

Imaging Findings Scout radiograph from a non-contrast CT scan of the abdomen and pelvis demonstrates a high density overlying the right kidney, the shape of which conforms to the right collecting system and renal pelvis (arrow, Fig. 2.12a). Non-contrast CT scan of the abdomen demonstrates the presence of a renal stone conforming to the right renal pelvis (arrow, Fig. 2.12b)

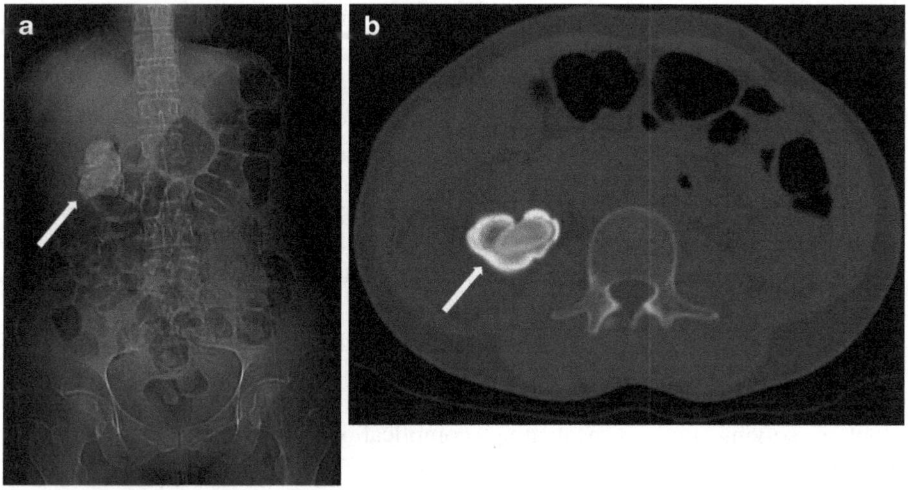

Fig. 2.12 Scout radiograph from a non-contrast CT scan of the abdomen and pelvis demonstrates a high density overlying the right kidney, the shape of which conforms to the right collecting system and renal pelvis (*arrow*, **a**). Non-contrast CT scan of the abdomen demonstrates the presence of a renal stone conforming to the right renal pelvis (*arrow*, **b**)

Differential Diagnosis Staghorn calculus, opaque collecting system after contrast administration

Diagnosis and Discussion: Staghorn Calculus

Staghorn calculi are branching calculi which occupy the renal pelvis and collecting system forming a cast and hence their characteristic name. They are divided into partial (involving a part of collecting system) and complete staghorn (involving almost entire collecting system). They are the result of recurrent infection and affect females more than males with predisposing factors being renal tract anomalies, VUR, neurogenic bladder or ileal ureteral diversion.

70 % of the staghorn calculi are composed of struvite (magnesium ammonium phosphate) and/or calcium carbonate apatite. Infection by urease producing bacteria (proteus, klebsiella) cause an alkaline environment in urine by breaking down urea into ammonia and hydroxide. This along with the presence of magnesium and phosphate create an environment conducive for growth of staghorn calculi. Uric acid and cystine make up for the minority of these calculi.

Imaging modalities include plain X ray KUB, ultrasound and CT.

Plain X ray KUB shows radiopaque branching laminated calcific densities in the region of renal outline. Although no consensus exists regarding definition of stag horn calculi, they are traditionally defined as partial if the renal pelvic stone extended into at least two calyceal groups or complete if at least 80 % of the collecting system is filled

The vast majority of staghorn calculi are radiopaque and appear as branching calcific densities overlying the renal outline and may mimic an excretory phase IVP. Lamination within the stone is common.

Ultrasound shows dense calcific mass filling the collecting system producing intense posterior acoustic shadowing with or without hydronephrosis.

CT shows a large branching calcific density conforming to the shape of the dilated collecting system. Their laminated appearance is best visualized on bone window which shows alternating bands of magnesium ammonium phosphate and calcium phosphate. Three dimensional images for accurate anatomical localization can be obtained which help in deciding the management. CT urography is extremely useful in delineating anatomic abnormalities of collecting system that may predispose patients to stone formation or alter therapy and for assessing complications such as pyelonephritis and urinoma due to calculus.

Recently dual source CT with advanced post acquisition processing is being used to assess the stone composition.

Although MRI holds no place in evaluation of renal calculi, it may be a useful problem solving tool in evaluating complications of calculus especially in pregnancy.

Pitfalls An easily differentiable fallacy is presence of contrast within an opacified collecting system which may simulate the appearance of a stag horn calculus.

Teaching Point

1. Infection by urease producing bacteria are causative organisms for formation of staghorn calculus.
2. CT with CT urography is the modality of choice for detecting calculi and their underlying cause.
3. Dual source CT is useful in assessing stone composition.

Case 2.11

Brief Case Summary: A 45-year-old woman with fever and right flank pain.

Imaging Findings Contrast enhanced CT showing focal enlargement of the right kidney with striated nephrogram. Perinephric fat stranding is noted (Fig. 2.13).

Differential Diagnosis Pyelonephritis, infarction, nephritis caused by granulomatous diseases, acute obstruction, infiltrative neoplasm.

Diagnosis and Discussion Acute pyelonephritis.

Acute pyelonephritis (APN) is the result of infection of renal parenchyma and pelvis which usually spreads in a retrograde fashion from lower urinary tract. Rarely it may also be caused by hematogenous spread and in these cases it is usually due to S. Aureus. Vesicoureteric reflux and underlying renal conditions like calculus disease are predisposing factors.

Not all patients suspected of APN warrant imaging. Indications of imaging include high risk patients prone for complications of acute pyelonephritis like diabetics, immunocompromised patients and in presence of obstructive calculus disease.

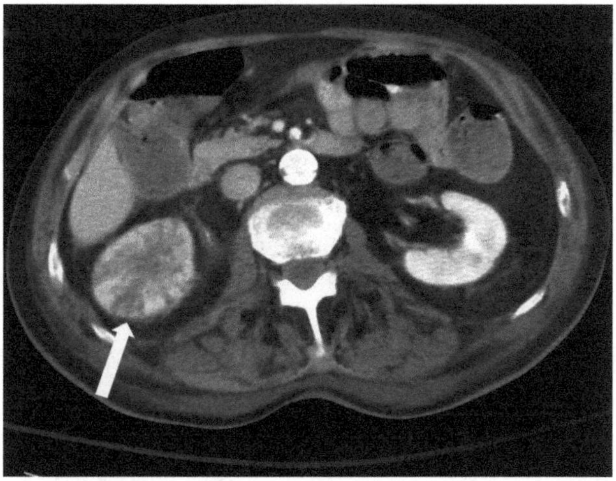

Fig. 2.13 Contrast enhanced CT showing focal enlargement of the right kidney with striated nephrogram (*arrow*). Perinephric fat stranding is noted

Ultrasound shows renal enlargement with diffuse or focal altered echogenicity – hypoechoic (edema) or hyperechogenicity (hemorrhage). Focal changes may simulate a mass. Other findings include hydronephrosis, loss of renal sinus fat and loss of corticomedullary differentiation. Local complications like presence of gas (emphysematous pyelonephritis), formation of abscess or infarct may be noted. Presence of echoes or particulate matter may be seen in the collecting system suggestive of pus or cells in urine. Doppler study shows hypoperfusion of affected segment.

CT is the modality of choice for imaging APN. The findings are best appreciated in the nephrographic phase of contrast (50–90 s after injection). If a noncontrast series is also performed it may show predisposing factors such as obstructive calculi or complications such as foci of air. Contrast CT shows wedge shaped areas in kidney, extending from renal papilla unto the cortex with focal enlargement and subtle reduction or differential contrast enhancement in corticomedullary phase as compared to the rest of the parenchyma. The periphery/cortex is also involved as opposed to renal infarct where there is sparing of the cortical rim. Focal hypodense rounded lesions may be seen. The classic sign on CT is a striated appearance with alternate areas of hypodense and normal enhancing parenchyma. Delayed phase (3–6 h post contrast) if taken shows persistent nephrogram in affected regions due to slow flow of contrast through the tubules.

CT is helpful for imaging of complications of APN as well which include renal abscess, infarction and perinephric changes of fluid, thickening of renal fascia and fat stranding.

MRI for APN is useful in patients in whom contrast material and radiation is contraindicated (e.g. contrast sensitivity and iodinated pregnancy). Imaging features are similar to CT. Gadolinium enhances conspicuity of focal lesions which remain hypointense relative to the rest of the enhancing kidney. MRI, however, lacks in detection of calcification/gas in renal parenchyma owing to unpredictable characterization.

Pitfalls The main differential of APN is acute renal infarct and this condition can be differentiated from acute pyelonephritis by the "cortical rim sign" which signifies sparing of renal cortex vascular supply.

Teaching Point

- Imaging is necessary only in high risk patients and where obstruction is suspected.
- Other causes of interstitial nephritis being less common, characteristic findings in proper clinical setting point to diagnosis of bacterial pyelonephritis.

Case 2.12

Brief Case Summary: 50 year old diabetic with prior renal transplant, now complaining of acute onset right lower quadrant pain.

Imaging Findings Ultrasound of the right lower quadrant shows the transplant kidney showing normal contour, the pelvicaliceal system displays echogenic contents with reverberation and ring down artefacts ("dirty shadowing") suggesting gas pockets (arrows in Fig. 2.14a).

Axial and coronal CT scan images (Fig. 2.14b, c) confirms these findings of locules of gas within the collecting system of the transplant kidney (arrow), in addition it demonstrates gas within renal parenchyma as well. A perinephric collection is also shown to contain gas pockets.

Differential Diagnosis Emphysematous pyelonephritis, Emphysematous pyelitis.

Diagnosis and Discussion: Emphysematous pyelonephritis.

Emphysematous pyelonephritis is a necrotizing infection of the renal parenchyma or its surrounding tissues with resultant gas formation. The common causative organisms are Ecoli, Klebsiella and proteus organisms. Majority of cases occur in diabetics, if non- diabetic; the patients are usually immunocompromised or have urinary tract obstruction. Recognition of this condition is important as without treatment it is commonly fatal.

Ultrasound is usually the first modality used, it shows numerous echogenic foci representing gas pockets with reverberation artefacts also termed as "dirty shadowing". The modality of choice however is CT. A CT scan usually demonstrates varying amounts of gas in and around the kidney; pathognomonic for the condition in the appropriate clinical setting. Associated findings such as perinephric stranding or collections, calculi, renal enlargement may be seen.
Classification:

- class 1 – gas restricted to collecting system
- class 2 – gas restricted to renal parenchyma (no extrarenal extension)

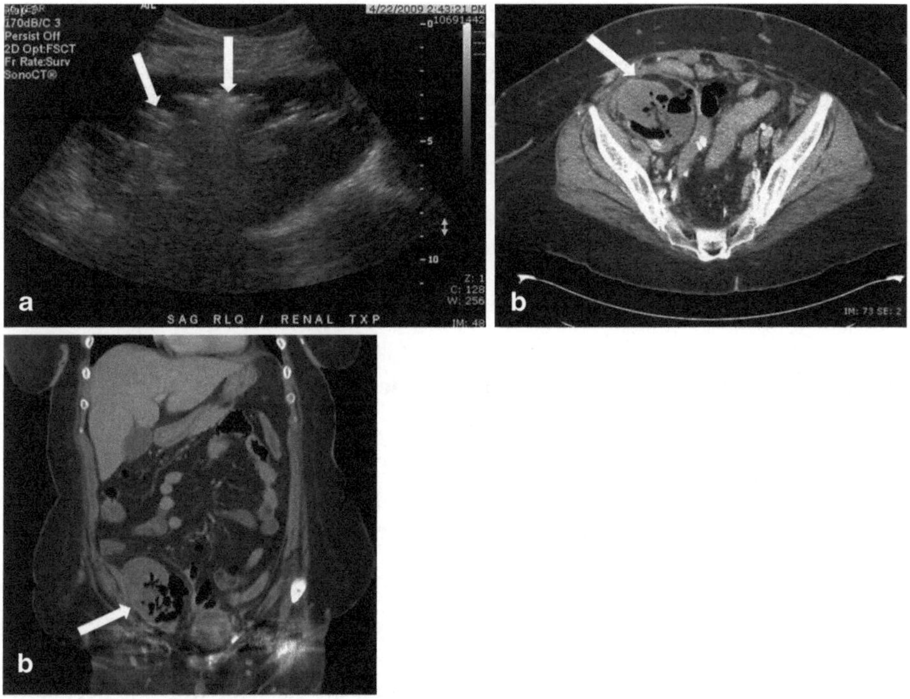

Fig. 2.14 Ultrasound of the right lower quadrant shows the transplant kidney showing normal contour, the pelvicaliceal system displays echogenic contents with reverberation and ring down artefacts ("dirty shadowing") suggesting gas pockets (*arrows* in **a**). Axial and coronal CT scan images (**b**, **c**) confirms these findings of locules of gas within the collecting system of the transplant kidney (*arrow*), in addition, it demonstrates gas within renal parenchyma as well. A perinephric collection is also shown to contain gas pockets

- class 3
  - class 3a – extension of gas or abscess to perinephric space
  - class 3b – extension of gas or abscess to pararenal space
- class 4 – bilateral emphysematous pyelonephritis or solitary kidney with emphysematous pyelonephritis

Medical management may be tried but surgical treatment with nephrectomy is needed (especially for extensive i.e. class 3 or 4 disease)

Pitfalls the main differential diagnosis is emphysematous pyelitis- this is a less severe form of urinary tract infection with gas only in the collecting system it usually occurs in the setting of urinary tract obstruction and differentiation from pyelonephritis is important as emphysematous pyelitis shows lower mortality and good response to medical management.

Teaching Points

1. Emphysematous pyelonephritis should be suspected in all patients who are diabetic or immunosuppressed and present with urinary tract infections.
2. Most common causative organisms are E.coli, klebsiella and proteus sp.
3. CT is the most sensitive method to demonstrate gas within the collecting system and renal parenchyma.

Case 2.13

Brief Case Summary: 54 year old male patient with abdominal pain.

Imaging Findings Axial enhanced CT image shows the presence of a large calcified left renal pelvic stone (Fig. 2.15, arrow). The kidney parenchyma is replaced with multiple hypoattenuating areas. Incidental note is made of stone in right renal pelvis along with peripheral hypoattenuating areas.

Differential Diagnosis Xanthogranulomatous Pyelonephritis (XGP), renal Tuberculosis, long standing hydronephrosis.

Diagnosis and Discussion: XGP

XGP is a rare chronic granulomatous condition the cause of which is debatable, but may result from an incomplete immune response to a subacute bacterial infection, most commonly in association with renal pelvic calculi. While renal function and destruction of renal parenchyma can be caused by obstructive hydronephrosis from the calculi, most destruction occurs secondary to extensive persistent inflammation. Typically, *P* Mirabilis and *E Coli* are the most common causative bacteria, but various others can incite the same response. Histologically, the renal parenchyma is ultimately

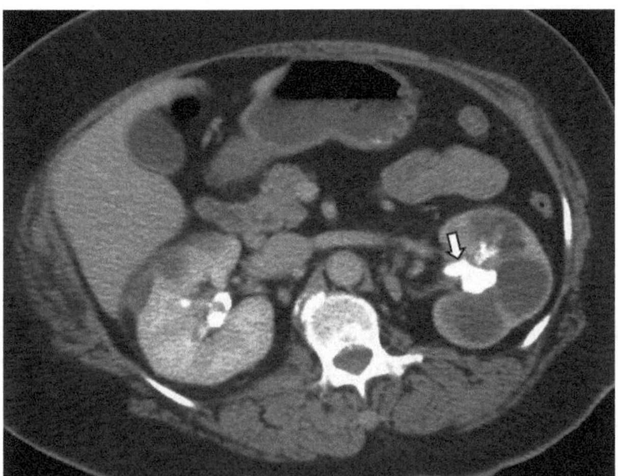

Fig. 2.15 Axial enhanced CT image shows the presence of a large calcified left renal pelvic stone (*arrow*). The kidney parenchyma is replaced with multiple hypoattenuating areas. Incidental note is made of stone in right renal pelvis along with peripheral hypoattenuating areas

replaced by lipid-laden (foamy) macrophages and the ulcerated calyceal mucosa is replaced with numerous inflammatory cells and adjacent granulation tissue.

CT imaging is most useful and helps with surgical planning, allowing a confident diagnosis. The combination of a nonfunctioning enlarged kidney, central calculus within a contracted renal pelvis, calyceal expansion, and perinephric inflammatory changes are virtually diagnostic. US typically demonstrates an enlarged kidney with disturbed renal architecture and an amorphous central echogenicity that corresponds to a renal pelvis staghorn. On radiograph, visualization of a large staghorn calculi is not typically associated with the extensive inflammation of XGP. MRI is more variable, but generally shows T1 hypointense, T2 hyperintense cavitary fluid (with T2 intracavitary fluid-fluid levels reflecting varied content) with strong rim enhancement of the cavity borders and T1 hypointense, T2 hypointense perirenal stranding (thick fibrinous exudate). The condition may be complicated by psoas abscess and fistula formation.

Less commonly, XGP can be focal (10 %, also called tumefactive type) and may have imaging findings similar to the diffuse form or mimic a bacterial abscess or RCC.

XGP is surgically managed with either nephrectomy or rarely partial nephrectomy, and annual imaging of the contralateral urinary tract is suggested. Elimination or control of the underlying cause is important.

Pitfalls Rarely, XGP can present with atrophy instead of enlargement. Occasionally (10 %) calculi are absent. Sometimes staghorn calculi formation can be secondary to stasis from an underlying mass lesion such as transitional cell carcinoma (TCC). Close attention to the renal pelvis to exclude TCC, and the rarer mucinous adenocarcinoma, is advised.

Teaching Point

1. CT is the test of choice to confirm XGP with the characteristic findings listed above.
2. Extrarenal manifestations are uncommon, but should be looked for, along with underlying salient tumor.
3. Careful attention should be paid to the focal type, as it has similar appearances to a bacterial abscess and RCC.

Case 2.14

Brief Case Summary: Young male immunocompromised patient with abdominal pain.

Imaging Findings Grey scale US of right and left kidneys demonstrated enlargement of both kidneys with increase cortical echogenicity (Fig. 2.16a, b). Axial and coronal CT scans showed bilateral renal enlargement and diffuse decreased parenchymal enhancement (Fig. 2.16c, d).

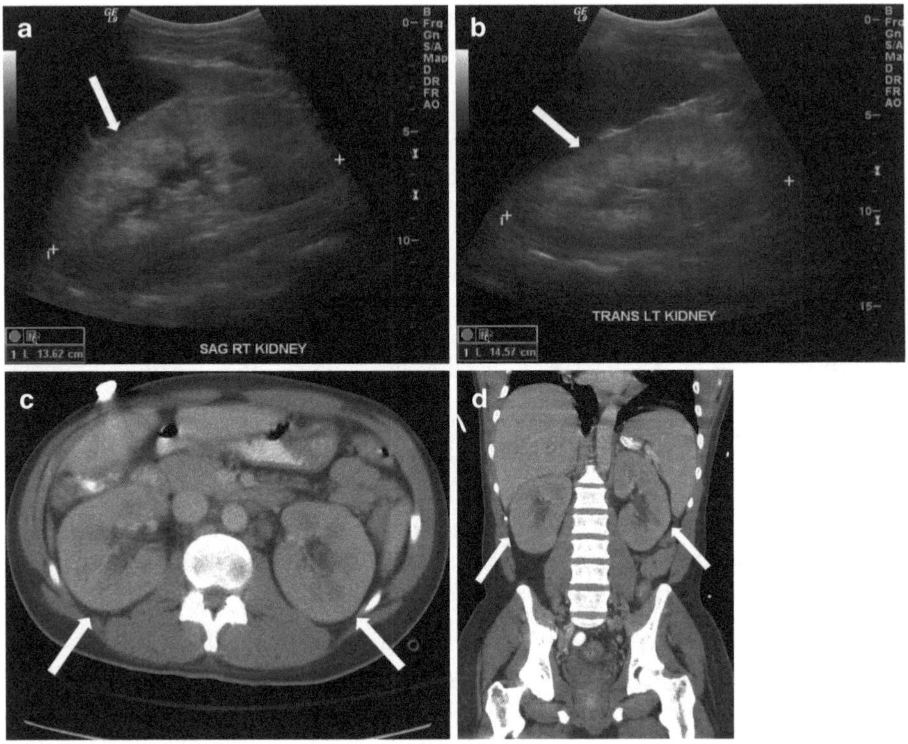

Fig. 2.16 Grey scale US of right and left kidneys demonstrated enlargement of both kidneys (*arrow*) with increase cortical echogenicity (**a**, **b**). Axial and coronal CT scans showed bilateral renal enlargement and diffuse decreased parenchymal enhancement (*arrows*) (**c**, **d**)

Differential Diagnosis Nonspecific medical renal disease, acute tubular necrosis (ATN), and Renal Pneumocystis carinii

Diagnosis and Discussion: HIV Nephropathy

With the advent of antiretroviral therapy (HAART) to treat human immunodeficiency virus (HIV) infection, patient survival has increased, resulting in an increased frequency of HIV-associated renal disease in this population subset. Whilst a low CD4 count (<200) has a higher incidence of HIV-nephropathy, it can still present in earlier stages of HIV infection, sometimes as the first manifestation of disease. HIV nephropathy is the most common cause of renal failure in HIV-positive patients (40 %), and is only diagnosed definitively by biopsy.

Histologically, collapsing glomerulopathy (collapsed glomerular tufts) is seen, possibly a result of injury to the renal epithelial cells by the virus, HIV gene products, or cytokine release by infected renal lymphocytes.

Ultrasound is the most common imaging modality used to suggest the diagnosis, followed by CT. Enlarged or normal-sized echogenic kidneys with loss of renal sinus fat (from edema of the fat, not actual loss) and pelvicaliceal thickening are the most common findings. True increased cortical echogenicity is the most characteristic feature, appearing more echogenic than the liver and equal to the renal sinus. With progression of disease, decreased corticomedullary differentiation and parenchymal heterogeneity have been described. On CT, enlarged kidneys and striated nephrogram (dilated protein-filled tubules) may be seen. There are no MR specific imaging features described.

Pitfalls When comparing echogenicity, make sure the liver does not inherently have fatty infiltration. The degree of glomerulopathy does not correlate with the scope of imaging findings.

Teaching Point

1. HAART increases patient survival and slows the progression of HIV nephropathy – early detection is key to avoid future morbidity.
2. Echogenic, globular kidneys with loss of renal sinus fat are some of the most common findings. More commonly, the renal size is normal, but the kidneys may also be enlarged.

Case 2.15

Brief Case Summary: A 35-year-old woman with fever and abdominal pain.

Imaging Findings Grey scale ultrasound showed a well-defined hypoechoic lesion in the interpolar region of the right kidney (arrow in Fig. 2.17a) which showed no color flow on color Doppler image (arrow in Fig. 2.17b). Axial contrast enhanced CT (Fig. 2.17c) showed well defined lesion with subtle wall enhancement and revealed additional abscess in the left kidney which was not appreciated on the ultrasound.

Differential Diagnosis Cystic /Necrotic Renal cell carcinoma, infected renal cyst.

Diagnosis and Discussion Renal Abscess

Renal abscess is a common complication of inadequately treated or neglected pyelonephritis. The corticomedullary abscesses occur as a result of ascending spread of infection from the lower urinary tract due to E.coli. The cortical abscesses occur due to hematogenous spread, Staphylococcus aureus being the most common etiological agent. Vesicoureteric reflux, renal calculi, immunocompromised states are also associated with higher incidence of UTI and subsequent renal abscess formation. Acute onset flank pain, dysuria, fever with chills and rigors are the usual presenting features.

Ultrasonography typically shows a hypoechoic area with low-amplitude internal echoes and disruption of the corticomedullary junction in an enlarged inflamed kidney. The interface with normal renal parenchyma may be ill or well defined depending on the presence of pseudocapsule. The lack of vascularity on Doppler imaging helps to distinguish a complex abscess from necrotic malignancy. Although ultrasound may be sufficient in appropriate clinical context, CT is the imaging modality of choice for confirmation and accurate delineation of spread of

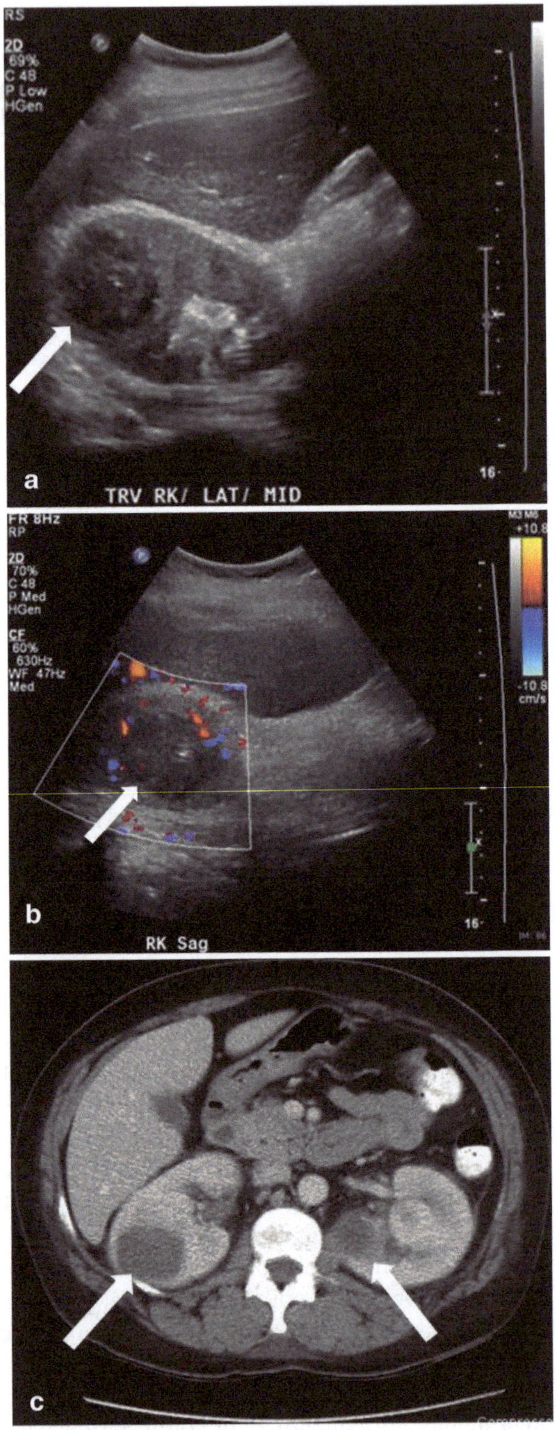

Fig. 2.17 Grey scale ultrasound showed a well-defined hypoechoic lesion in the interpolar region of the right kidney (*arrow* in **a**) which showed no color flow on color Doppler image (*arrow* in **b**). Axial contrast enhanced CT (**c**) showed well defined lesion with wall enhancement and revealed additional abscess in the left kidney which was not appreciated on the ultrasound

abscess. CT shows a peripherally enhancing hypodense lesion with perinephric fat stranding and adjacent fascial thickening. Presence of gas within the hypodense peripherally enhancing lesion is virtually diagnostic. During the nephrographic phase there may be diminished enhancement surrounding the abscess (halo sign). CT also demonstrates the extent of abscess and if it has ruptured into the perinephric space. MRI especially diffusion weighted (DWI) sequences offer a distinct advantage in coexistent renal failure when iodinated contrast is contraindicated. Significantly low ADC values are seen in nephritic areas and within the abscess, however the values are lowest within the abscess. Imaging studies not only help in confirmation of diagnosis but also serve as a guide for percutaneous drainage.

Pitfalls Necrotic RCC can be differentiated from abscess by the presence of enhancing mural nodule however differentiation may be difficult when typical findings of infection are not present and needle aspiration may be required for confirmation of abscess. Infected cysts cannot be reliably differentiated from abscesses.

Teaching Points

1. Well defined peripherally enhancing hypodense lesion in kidney with no internal vascularity is diagnostic of abscess.
2. CT forms the cornerstone in delineation of extent of abscess and differentiation from cystic or necrotic RCC.
3. MRI with DWI may be useful when CT is contraindicated due to impaired renal function.

Case 2.16

Brief Case Summary

1. 58 year old Asian immigrant with incidentally detected left renal calcified lesion.
2. 45 year old HIV positive patient with abdominal pain.

Imaging Findings Patient 1. Coronal reformatted image from a non-contrast CT scan of the abdomen and pelvis demonstrates the presence of an atrophic left kidney containing multiple dystrophic calcifications (Fig. 2.18).

Patient 2. Coronal reformatted image from a non-contrast CT scan of the abdomen and pelvis demonstrates calcifications lining the left collecting system as well as multiple small calcifications in the spleen. Calcified lymph nodes were also noted in the mesentery (not shown). The constellation of findings reflect the effect of prior granulomatous disease (Fig. 2.19).

Differential Diagnosis Renal Tuberculosis; Chronic pyelonephritis; xanthogranulomatous pyelonephritis; medullary sponge kidney.

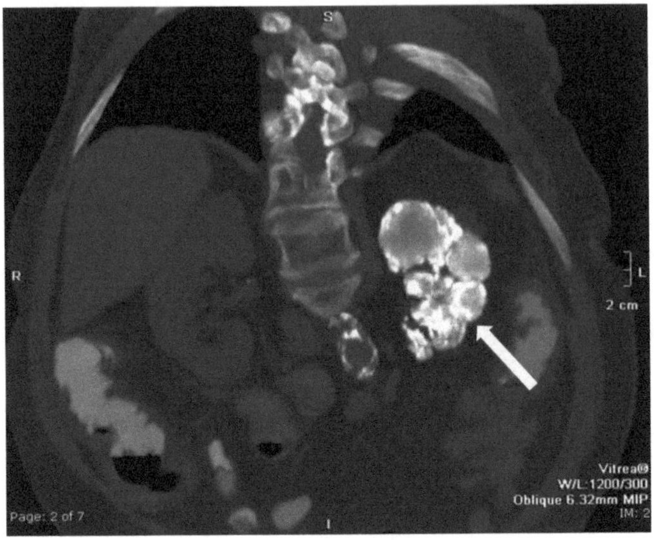

Fig. 2.18 Patient 1. Coronal reformatted image from a non-contrast CT scan of the abdomen and pelvis demonstrates the presence of an atrophic left kidney containing multiple dystrophic calcifications (*arrow*)

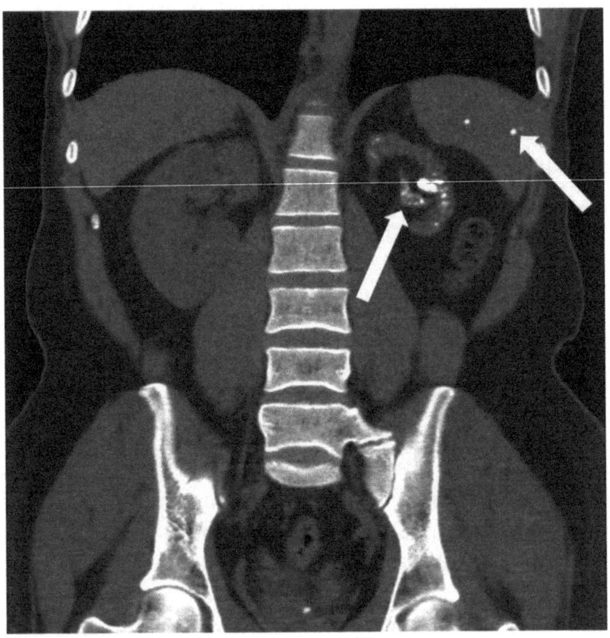

Fig. 2.19 Patient 2. Coronal reformatted image from a non-contrast CT scan of the abdomen and pelvis demonstrates calcifications lining the left collecting system (*arrows*) as well as multiple small calcifications in the spleen. Calcified lymph nodes were also noted in the mesentery (not shown). The constellation of findings reflect the effect of prior granulomatous disease

Diagnosis and Discussion

1. "Putty kidney" – renal tuberculosis
2. Stigmata of genitourinary tuberculosis with calcified granulomas in the spleen.

The genitourinary tract is the most common site of extra pulmonary involvement of tuberculosis with increase in incidence seen commensurate to the spread of acquired immunodeficiency syndrome (AIDS) and HIV. Mycobacterium tuberculosis (MTB) is the commonest pathogen with Mycobacterium avium intracellulare (MAI) and Mycobacterium bovis as other organisms causing disease in the immunocompromised population. The bacilli are known to involve the kidneys, prostate and seminal vesicles primarily via hematogenous spread with secondary involvement of the ureter and bladder once the bacilli are shed in the urine. The range of imaging findings is closely related to the stage of involvement as well the pathophysiology of the disease. There could be uni- or bilateral renal involvement. With hematogenous spread, the bacilli are trapped in the capillaries located adjacent to the glomeruli in the cortex where they form caseating granulomas and eventually extend into the renal pyramids. From here they spread into the pelvicaliceal system with seeding of the ureteric and bladder urothelium as they spread downstream.

Various imaging modalities have been used to demonstrate the findings seen with renal involvement of tuberculosis. Plain radiographs are useful in demonstration of various patterns of calcification caused as a result of caseating granulomas that have been described including coarse calcification within the parenchyma; curvilinear rim calcification in a lobar distribution, ring like calcification associated with papillary necrosis or blotchy amorphous calcification of the so called "putty kidney". Intravenous Urography used in the earlier days has now become obsolete as an imaging modality.

Computed tomography with and without intravenous contrast scores over plain radiographs in demonstrating the various sites and degree of involvement. Renal parenchymal granulomas are visualized as small millimeter sized hypoattenuating foci within the cortex. Papillary necrosis with distortion of the renal papillae can be demonstrated on the coronal and sagittal reformatted images on CT. Infundibular strictures and focal caliectasis may be an associated finding. Conglomerated granulomas can present as a multilobulated mass resembling hydronephrosis or a multiloculated cystic tumor. Renal and perinephric abscesses are another form of presentation which in the late phase of the disease can calcify giving rise to the calcified non-functioning "putty kidney".

Computed tomography is also helpful in depiction of extrarenal findings such as involvement of other solid organs, lymph nodal involvement, presence of ascites, omental disease or formation of various types of fistulae.

Ultrasound and MRI have not been used as screening imaging tools for this disease entity. Ultrasound may help guide interventional procedures such as percutaneous drainage of large abscesses or biopsy of unsuspected tuberculous pseudomass like lesions.

Teaching Point

- High index of suspicion in the relevant patient population can enhance early imaging diagnosis of renal involvement by tuberculous disease.
- The appropriate conglomeration of imaging findings however needs to be correlated with urine culture and blood tests such as PCR (polymerase chain reaction) to confirm presence of the organism. Imaging thus plays a major role in detection and follow up of renal TB

Case 2.17

Brief Case Summary: 70 year old with right flank pain

Imaging Findings Gray scale and Color Doppler US images of the right kidney demonstrate the presence of an avascular crescentic lesion in the right perinephric space indenting the interpolar region of the right kidney (arrows in Fig. 2.20a, b). A MAG3 study performed on the same day (arrow in Fig. 2.20c) shows mass effect over the right kidney. Non-contrast CT scan of the abdomen demonstrates a crescent shaped high attenuation perinephric lesion conforming to the outer contour of the right kidney (arrow in Fig. 2.20d).

Differential Diagnosis Perinephric hematoma, perinephric lymphoma, amyloidosis, retroperitoneal fiboris.

Diagnosis and Discussion Perinephric hematoma, in this patient caused by spontaneous hemorrhage related to anticoagulants.

Accumulation of blood in the perinephric space between the renal capsule and Gerota's fascia can result from a multitude of traumatic and non traumatic etiologies. Traumatic etiologies include motor vehicle accidents; penetrating injuries such as gun shot wounds; blunt trauma caused by contact sports or falls. Injuries induced by this mechanism often involve multiple other compartments of the retroperitoneum and may have associated renal injuries. Non traumatic etiologies on the other hand may be confined to a single side and can be induced by bleeding from underlying tumors such as a renal cell carcinoma or an angiomyolipoma; ruptured renal artery aneurysm; ruptured cyst; spontaneous hemorrhage related to anticoagulation.

Imaging plays a key role in the diagnosis and in some cases treatment of this condition. Although ultrasound is an easily available screening tool to assess the perinephric space, computed tomography (CT) is the most sensitive imaging modality to diagnose the extent of involvement as well as to assess any underlying source of bleeding. On a non intravenous contrast enhanced CT, hemorrhage confined to the perinephric space presents as a crescentic hyperattenuating lesion with mass effect on the adjacent renal parenchyma. A search for any underlying mass lesion in the adjacent renal parenchyma including presence of macroscopic fat in an angiomyolipoma should be made on the non contrast CT. Intravenous contrast plays a role in demonstration of active extravasation from a bleeding vessel; grading any associated renal injury as well as in evaluation of delayed contrast extravasation as a marker of injury to the renal collecting system. Although MRI can also help in the diagnosis of this condition, it plays a less significant role in the acute setting. MRI may be useful in detecting underlying parenchymal lesion once the hematoma has resolved.

Imaging can guide management depending upon the extent of mass effect and underlying etiology causing the bleed. When there is active ongoing bleeding, angiography with embolization of the bleeding arteries is a therapeutic interventional radiology option. The perinephric space being expandable, blood often tracks to the inferior retroperitoneal space. Occasionally, mass effect is seen to

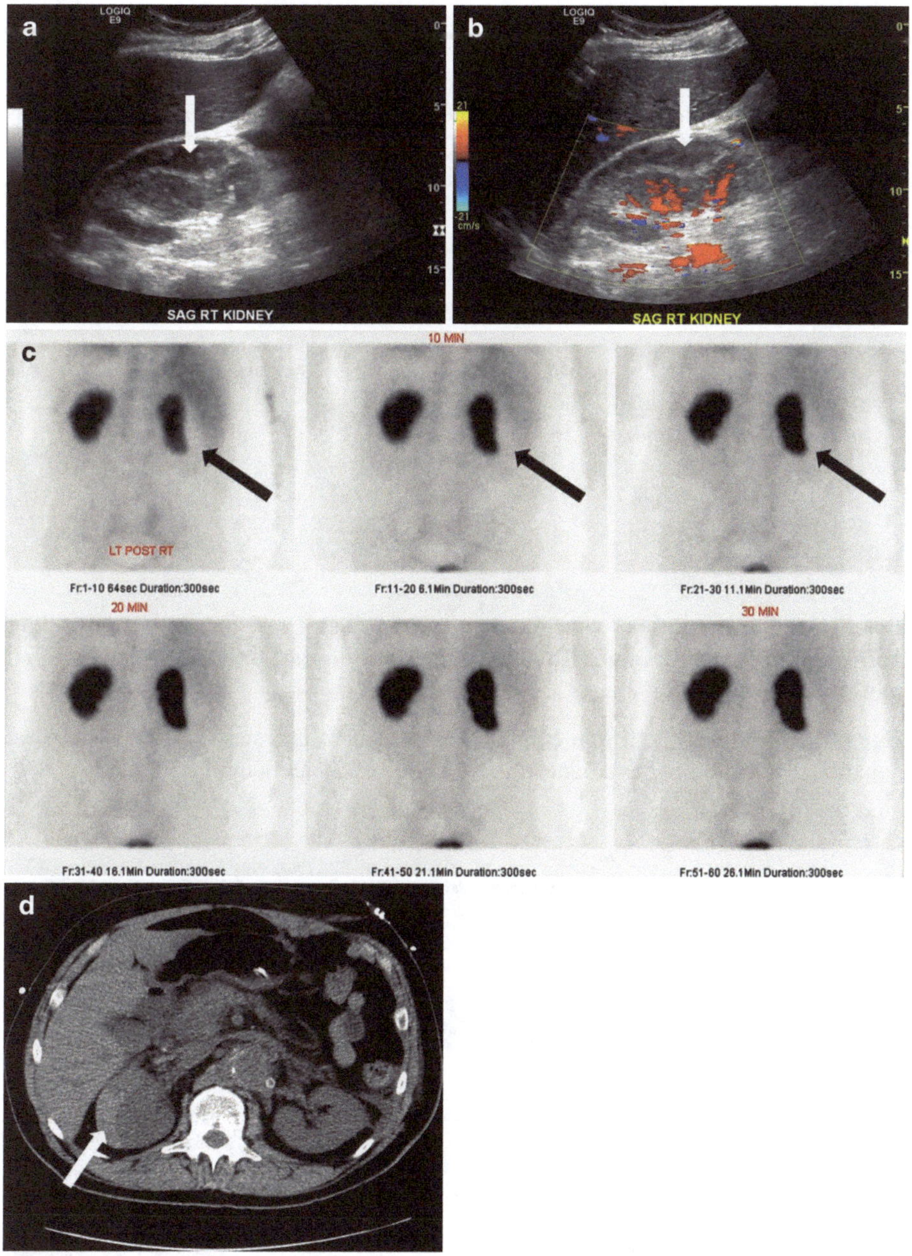

Fig. 2.20 Gray scale and Color Doppler US images of the right kidney demonstrate the presence of an avascular crescentic lesion in the right perinephric space indenting the interpolar region of the right kidney (*arrows* in **a, b**). A MAG3 study performed on the same day (*arrow* in **c**) shows mass effect over the right kidney. Non-contrast CT scan of the abdomen demonstrates a crescent shaped high attenuation perinephric lesion conforming to the outer contour of the right kidney (*arrow* in **d**)

induce hypertension secondary to renal parenchymal compression, a condition called the Page kidney. Minimally invasive options such as image guided percutaneous catheter drainage are available to decrease the tamponade effect in an effort to improve renal function. Patients with perinephric hematomas extending into the adjacent retroperitoneum especially when caused by coagulopathies, may be managed conservatively. In these patients, serial follow up imaging plays an important role in assessment till resolution.

Teaching Point

- Early diagnosis of perinephric hematomas is important for preservation of renal function.
- Computed tomography without and with intravenous contrast plays a major role in detection of extent and underlying cause.
- Interventional options exist in management in the acute setting.

Case 2.18

Brief Case Summary: 62 year old male with a history of coronary stenting on anticoagulants presenting with acute onset abdominal pain and uncontrolled hypertension.

Imaging Findings Axial non-contrast CT scan demonstrates a large perinephric hematoma compressing and distorting the right renal parenchyma (Fig. 2.21)

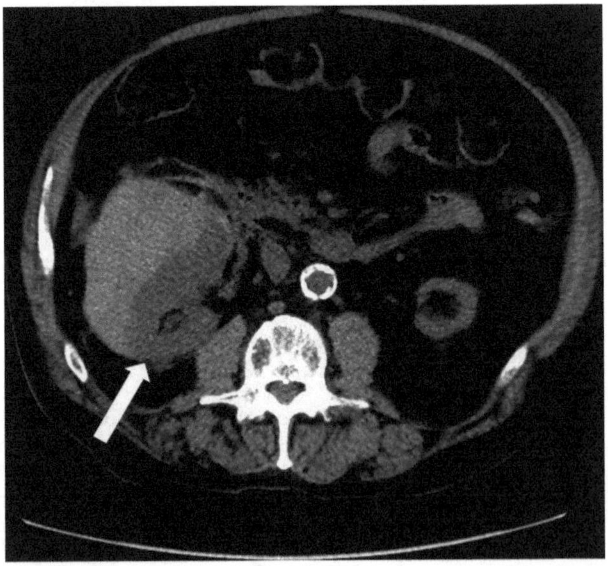

Fig. 2.21 Axial non-contrast CT scan demonstrates a large perinephric hematoma compressing and distorting the right renal parenchyma (*arrow*)

Differential Diagnosis Perinephric hematoma secondary to spontaneous retroperitoneal hemorrhage or tumor bleed.

Diagnosis and Discussion Page kidney – related to spontaneous hemorrhage in a patient on anticoagulants.

Page kidney refers arterial hypertension induced by stimulation of the renin-angiotensin -aldosterone system presumably caused by ischemia induced by mechanical compression of the renal parenchyma. This mechanical compression can result from traumatic and non traumatic causes. Traumatic causes include sports related injuries; motor vehicle accidents or blunt trauma caused by any other mechanism. Non traumatic etiologies include iatrogenic injuries such as hemorrhagic complications following renal biopsy (either of the native kidney or a transplanted kidney); post lithotripsy or following any surgery of the renal system. Any condition causing spontaneous renal /perinephric hemorrhage including ruptured aneurysms; tumoral bleed; bleeding from an angiomyolipoma; cyst rupture; bleeding arteriovenous malformations; vasculitides; glomerulonephritis or bleeding related to anticoagulation therapy. Non acute conditions such as a lymphocele related to renal transplant are also known to be one of the causes.

This phenomenon was originally described by Page in 1939 where hypertension was induced by wrapping dog kidneys in cellophane. Thereafter, in 1955, it was described in a young athlete who sustained a sports related injury causing a subcapsular renal hematoma leading to hypertension. Various case reports and retrospective studies have published the range of findings leading to this condition. Depending upon the underlying cause, this can be seen in all age groups and has no gender predilection. Traumatic causes were commonly observed in young males while non traumatic causes were seen in elderly or patients with renal transplant following an iatrogenic injury.

Compression of a single native kidney by any of the aforementioned causes manifests less dramatically when compared to compression of a single renal transplant kidney. Hence the importance of this phenomenon lies in early detection at a stage when renal function can be potentially salvaged in the early stages.

Computed tomography (CT) with or without intravenous contrast remains the modality of choice for both detection of compression as well as to diagnose the associated underlying condition. Non intravenous contrast enhanced scans help determine presence of hyperattenuating blood of HU ranging from 40–60. Administration of IV contrast can demonstrate presence of underlying tumors, arteriovenous malformations or other conditions in the absence of known trauma.

Management has come a long way from nephrectomy to minimally invasive procedures such as image guided percutaneous interventions including drainage of compressive collections and angiographic embolization of bleeding vessels to control recurrent hemorrhage. Thus imaging plays a very important role not only in diagnosing causes of but also treating conditions leading to Page phenomenon.

Pitfalls Delay in diagnosis of this treatable cause of secondary hypertension may cause irreversible loss of renal function.

Teaching Point Early screening with computed tomography to assess presence of renal parenchymal compression paves the way for intervention based on underlying cause.

Case 2.19

Brief case History: 50 year old male with obstructive calculus disease.

Imaging Findings Axial contrast enhanced CT scan demonstrates fluid density in the perinephric region surrounding the right kidney (arrow in Fig. 2.22a) which on excretory phase CT shows leakage of contrast (arrow in Fig. 2.22b).

Differential Diagnosis Perinephric urinoma, perinephric hematoma; lymphangioma; perinephric abscess, lymphangiectasia

Diagnosis and Discussion Perinephric urinoma

Urinoma occurs when urine extravasates from the kidney, ureter, bladder, or urethra into the retroperitoneal space due to raised intrapelvic pressures and subsequent rupture of caliceal fornices. Lipolysis ensues with resultant encapsulation of urine. Urinomas may result due to obstructive or non-obstructive causes. Obstructive causes include intrinsic causes such as calculi and extrinsic compression due to pelvic masses or post-radiation scarring. Non-obstructive causes include external trauma to the kidneys, pelvicaliceal system and ureters or iatrogenic injury during surgery. Complications include secondary infection and abscess formation, peritonitis, sepsis, and damage to the urinary tract by fibrosis and granuloma formation.

Ultrasonography shows perinephric fluid accumulation with or without fine septations. Urinomas on CT appear as fluid density collections commonly in perirenal and subcapsular space. On delayed excretory phase, urine leakage may be directly

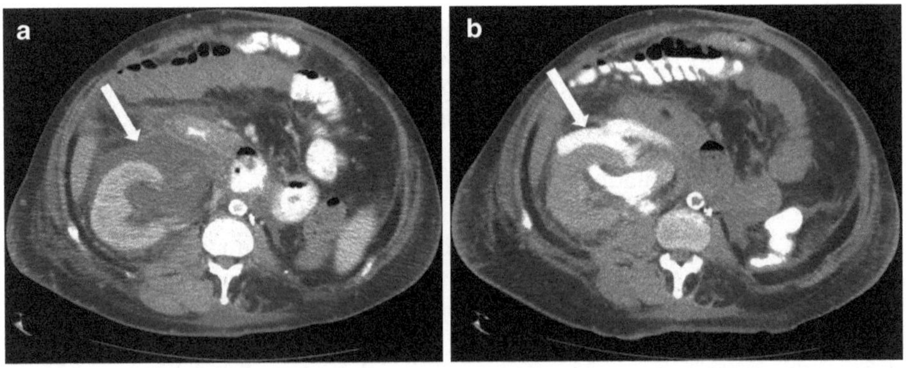

Fig. 2.22 Axial contrast enhanced CT scan demonstrates fluid density in the perinephric region surrounding the right kidney (*arrow* in **a**) which on excretory phase CT shows leakage of contrast (*arrow* in **b**)

demonstrated by extravasation of contrast from the pelvicaliceal system or ureter into the collection. On MRI, the collections follow fluid intensity appearing uniformly low signal intensity on T1-weighted imaging, and very high signal intensity on T2-weighted imaging. Excreted radiotracer outside the genitourinary tract at renal scintigraphy may also allow a diagnosis of a urine leak.

Imaging also serves as guidance for percutaneous drainage of large symptomatic urinomas. Percutaneous nephrostomy with or without ureteral stent placement may be required when urinomas do not resolve. Fluid analysis shows a significantly higher creatinine level and a lower glucose concentration compared to serum.

Small urinomas are treated conservatively.

Pitfalls Renal lymphangiomatosis characterized by dilated lymphatic structures is seen as septated cystic areas in perirenal, intrarenal and parapelvic region. Absence of contrast extravasation into the fluid on delayed excretory scans and presence of chyle within the fluid helps differentiating it from urinomas. Perirenal hematoma due to underlying renal tumoral bleed is more heterogenous and may appear hyperdense.

Teaching Points

1. Urinomas occur due to leakage of urine into the perinephric space which are a result of pyelosinus back flow due to raised intrapelvic pressures.
2. Fluid attenuation collections seen in perinephric space with contrast extravasation into it is diagnostic for urinomas.
3. Fluid aspiration and analysis confirms high creatinine levels.
4. Imaging should also be aimed at detecting the underlying cause of urinoma.

Case 2.20

Brief Case Summary: 45 year old female with right flank pain

Imaging Findings CT scan of the abdomen at the level of the kidneys (Fig. 2.23) demonstrates an intraaortic balloon pump. The right kidney (arrow) and wedge shaped areas of the left kidney show no enhancement. Also note presence of peripheral gas in the liver consistent with portal venous air from bowel ischemia.

In a different patient (Fig. 2.24), axial contrast enhanced CT shows the presence of an abnormal region of low attenuation involving the right kidney with a thin rim of enhancement seen (cortical rim sign) surrounding the periphery of the right kidney.

Differential Diagnosis Renal artery infarct, pyelonephritis, lymphoma.

Diagnosis and Discussion: Renal artery infarct

Renal artery infarction is a relatively rare entity that is commonly misdiagnosed initially due to its nonspecific clinical presentation (sudden onset abdominal/flank pain, nausea, and vomiting). Renal infarction occurs from either interruption of the

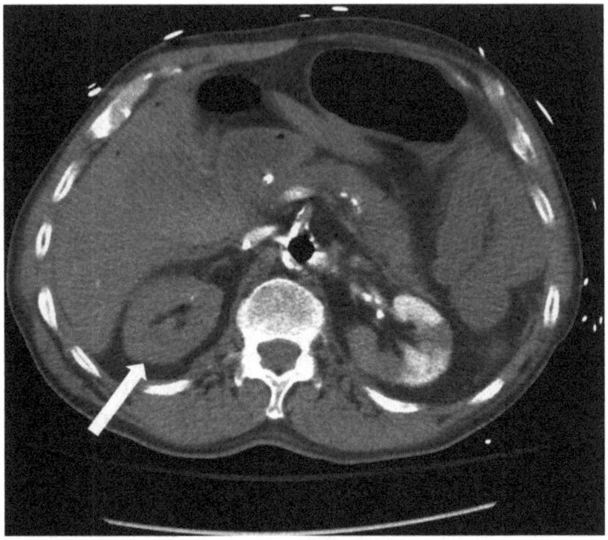

Fig. 2.23 CT scan of the abdomen at the level of the kidneys demonstrates an intraaortic balloon pump. The right kidney (*arrow*) and wedge shaped areas of the left kidney show no enhancement. Also note presence of peripheral gas in the liver consistent with portal venous air from bowel ischemia

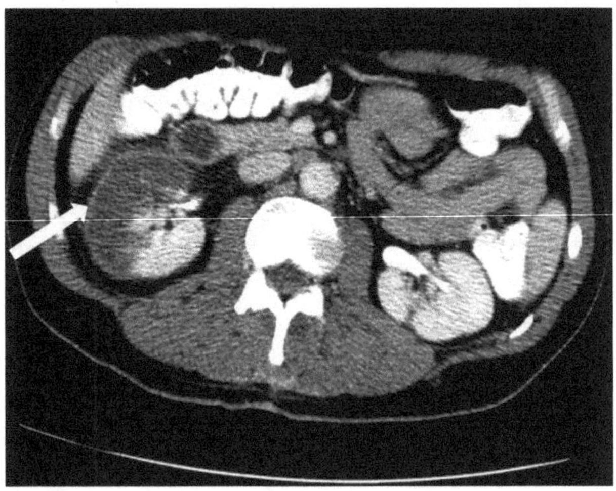

Fig. 2.24 Axial contrast enhanced CT in a different person shows the presence of an abnormal region of low attenuation involving the right kidney with a thin rim of enhancement seen (cortical rim sign) (*arrow*) surrounding the periphery of the right kidney

normal arterial blood supply or from blockage of venous drainage. By far the most common cause of arterial infarct is thromboembolic disease, of either cardiac or aortic source. Other possible etiologies include trauma, renal artery dissection, stenosis, vasculitis, and iatrogenic injury.

CT angiograms may directly visualize the occluded vessel. The parenchymal CT or MR appearance depends on the size of the embolus, the location of the arterial occlusion, and its age. Contrast-enhanced CT readily demonstrates absence of enhancement in the affected renal tissue. Acute infarcts typically appear as wedge-shaped areas of decreased attenuation within an otherwise normal-appearing kidney. When large areas of the kidney are involved, an increase in the size of the kidney due to edema can be seen. In global infarction, the entire kidney is enlarged and its reniform configuration remains preserved. The "cortical rim" sign usually appears several days after onset of the infarction and is due to commonly preserved cortical blood supply via the renal capsular artery, an early branch of the renal artery. On ultrasound examination acute infarct will appear as absence of perfusion on color/Doppler imaging, complete when the entire kidney is affected, or patchy when segmental arteries are involved.

Revascularization of the kidney is the goal of therapy, which can be achieved by anticoagulation, intra-arterial thrombolytic therapy, angioplasty or surgical revascularization depending on the etiology. In cases where infarcts are segmental only supportive management is required, and the cause of infarction investigated.

Pitfalls The main differential is parenchymal hypoenhancement or hypoperfusion due to infection (pyelonephritis or lobar nephronia). However, the "cortical rim" sign is absent and the clinical presentation is often informative with predominantly infectious/inflammatory symptoms and laboratory findings.

Teaching Points

1. Renal artery infarction is a commonly misdiagnosed condition due to its nonspecific clinical presentation.
2. The most common cause of arterial infarct is thromboembolic disease, of either cardiac or aortic source.
3. Imaging is critical for establishing the diagnosis. Typical imaging findings include wedge shaped regions of parenchymal hypoenhancement or hypoperfusion.
4. Presence of "cortical rim" sign increases diagnostic confidence by eliminating infection as the main differential.

Case 2.21

Brief Case Summary: 24 year old female with left flank pain

Imaging Findings CT scan of the abdomen at the level of the kidneys without contrast demonstrates asymmetric enlargement of the left kidney. In addition, there a subtle curvilinear region of increased attenuation within a tubular structure in the left renal hilum (arrow, Fig. 2.25a). Contrast enhanced CT scan at the same level shows the presence of an enlarged left kidney with the presence of a delayed nephrogram. The tubular structure in the left renal hilum does not enhance (arrow, Fig. 2.25b).

Differential Diagnosis Renal vein thrombosis, renal artery thrombosis, transitional cell carcinoma

Diagnosis and Discussion: Renal vein thrombosis

Renal vein thrombosis has numerous etiologies, but most commonly occurs in patients with nephrotic syndrome which is responsible for a hypercoagulable state. Other causes include neoplasms (renal cell and adrenal cortical carcinoma), trauma,

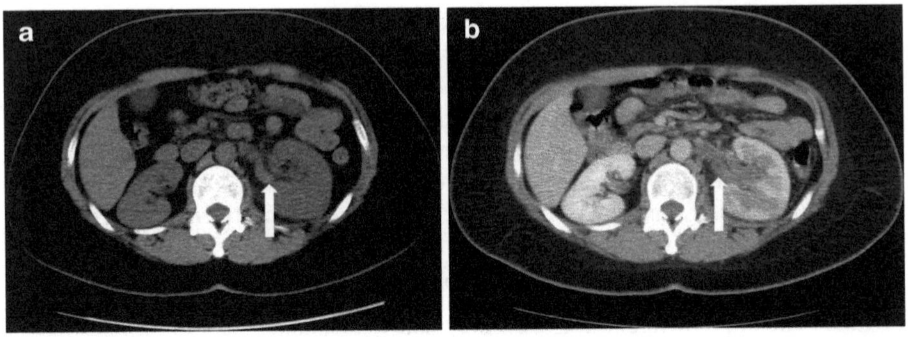

Fig. 2.25 CT scan of the abdomen at the level of the kidneys without contrast demonstrates asymmetric enlargement of the left kidney. Note subtle curvilinear region of increased attenuation within a tubular structure in the left renal hilum (*arrow*, **a**). Contrast enhanced CT scan at the same level shows the presence of an enlarged left kidney with the presence of a delayed nephrogram. The tubular structure in the left renal hilum does not enhance (*arrow*, **b**)

pregnancy, oral contraceptives, collagen vascular disease, diabetes, and glomerulonephritis in adults; dehydration, sepsis, and Wilm's tumor in children.

The clinical manifestations of renal vein thrombosis depend on the age of the patient, the specific disease process, and the speed with which it occurs. A classic acute presentation includes gross hematuria, flank pain, and loss of renal function. Renal vein thrombosis is more common on the left side, presumably because of the longer left renal vein.

Ultrasonography is usually used as an initial study for evaluation of patients with suspected renal vein thrombosis. Common grey scale findings include renal enlargement with hypoechoic cortex secondary to edema during the early phase and decreasing size and increased echogenicity during the late phase. Doppler findings include reversal of arterial diastolic flow, absent venous flow, visualization of thrombus within the lumen, and high resistance in the renal artery.

Contrast-enhanced CT or MRI shows thrombus in a thick-walled renal vein with or without extension into the IVC. In the chronic phase of renal vein thrombosis, the affected renal vein becomes attenuated due to retraction of the clot along with development of extensive collateral vessels along the proximal to middle ureter and around the kidney. The presence of inhomogeneous enhancement in the thrombus is indicative of tumor involvement. Enlargement of the kidney, edema in the renal sinus and perinephric space, and the coarse striations of a diminished nephrogram may be present. An enhancing mass of soft-tissue attenuation in the kidney or renal pelvis may be found as a neoplastic cause of renal vein thrombosis.

In general, anticoagulation therapy is the treatment of choice for renal vein thrombosis. Thrombolytic therapy is warranted in special cases, such as bilateral renal vein thrombosis with acute renal failure, extension into the IVC, massive clot, increased risk of pulmonary emboli, severe flank pain, and failed anticoagulation therapy. Placement of a suprarenal IVC filter may be considered in selected patients.

Pitfalls While renal artery thrombosis and/or ureteral neoplasm (such as transitional cell carcinoma) may also present as tubular masses in the renal hilum, these findings can be anatomically differentiated from renal vein thrombosis. Renal vein thrombosis is a well-recognized but often clinically silent condition. Promptly establishing the correct diagnosis is essential because of serious complications, such as pulmonary embolism and progressive renal impairment related to vascular compromise, and because of the risks of subjecting patients without the disorder to potentially harmful treatment (anticoagulation or thrombolysis).

Teaching Points

1. Renal vein thrombosis is an uncommon disorder that has numerous etiologies, the most common of which is nephrotic syndrome in adults and dehydration in kids.
2. A classic acute presentation includes gross hematuria, flank pain, and loss of renal function.
3. Imaging findings include renal vein thrombus with associated renal enlargement and delayed function.
4. Anticoagulation is the mainstay of therapy with thrombolytic therapy reserved for special circumstances (bilateral renal thrombosis, extension into the IVC, pulmonary emboli, etc.)

Case 2.22

Brief Case Summary: 34 year old female with history of childhood seizures presents with abdominal pain.

Imaging Findings CT scan of the abdomen with intravenous contrast demonstrates the presence of bilateral fat containing masses in both kidneys with the dominant mass in the right kidney (arrow, Fig. 2.26a). Digital subtraction angiogram of the right kidney (Fig. 2.26b) in the same patient demonstrates a blush of vessels within the mass. Note the presence of small aneurysms (arrow, Fig. 2.26b).

Similar lesions in different patients:

- Gray scale US in a different patient shows a well-defined hyperechoic mass at left kidney (arrow in Fig. 2.26c).
- Axial in-phase MR image in another patient shows a hyper intense signal intensity mass at left kidney (arrow in Fig. 2.26d) which shows signal drop off in opposed-phase image (arrow in Fig. 2.26e), confirming presence of intracellular fat within the lesion.

Differential Diagnosis Angiomyolipoma, liposarcoma, renal cell carcinoma

Diagnosis and Discussion: Renal Angiomyolipomas

- Angiomyolipomas (AMLs) are hamartomas containing varying proportions of fat, smooth muscle, and thick-walled blood vessels and can occur as isolated, sporadic entities in 80 % of cases, most commonly manifesting in middle-aged

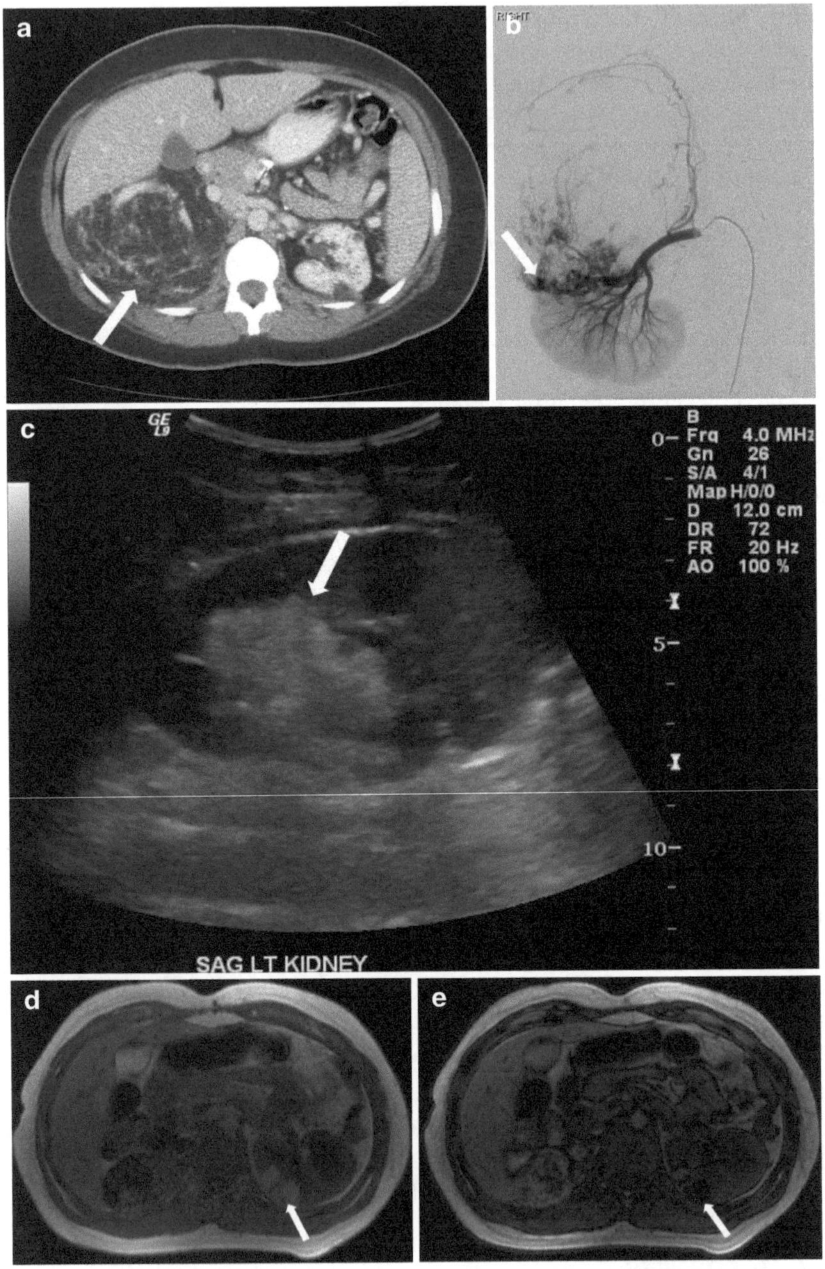

Fig. 2.26 CT scan of the abdomen with intravenous contrast demonstrates the presence of bilateral fat containing masses in both kidneys with the dominant mass in the right kidney (*arrow*, **a**). Digital subtraction angiogram of the right kidney (**b**) in the same patient demonstrates a blush of vessels within the mass. Note the presence of small aneurysms (*arrow*, **b**). Gray scale US in a different patient shows a well-defined hyperechoic mass at left kidney (*arrow* in **c**). Axial T1 weighted gradient echo in-phase MR image in another patient shows a hyper intense signal intensity mass at left kidney (*arrow* in **d**) which shows signal drop off in opposed-phase image (*arrow* in **e**), confirming presence of intracellular fat within the lesion

women. The other 20 % of AMLs develop in association with tuberous sclerosis. AMLs that occur in association with tuberous sclerosis manifest at a younger age are likely to be larger and bilateral.

- AMLs greater than 4 cm carry an increased risk for potentially life-threatening hemorrhage.
- A reliable diagnosis of AMLs can be made when fat is unequivocally demonstrated in a renal mass.
- On ultrasound, AMLs are well-defined hyperechoic masses regardless of the relative fat component.
- The CT appearances of AMLs on nonenhanced CT scans do not have a specific HU threshold. Many publications mention a threshold of −10 HU with use of a 3-pixel ROI size was accurate and effective for the diagnosis of AML.
- AMLs with a predominant fatty component are isointense relative to fat with all MR imaging sequences. The use of in-phase and opposed-phase imaging is also helpful in the diagnosis of AML. Making the diagnosis of AML at MR imaging is virtually impossible in the absence of detectable macroscopic fat. Clear cell RCC should be included in the differential diagnosis when only intracellular fat is visualized.

Pitfalls Angiomyolipoma commonly appear hyperechoic on ultrasound and signal decreasing on opposed-phase image due fat content. Unfortunately, 8–47 % of small renal cell carcinomas are also hyperechoic and clear cell RCC also displays signal change between in- and opposed-phase images. In addition, although majority of AMLs are benign, some subtypes such as epithelioid angiomyolipoma and sarcomatous degeneration could be associated with local invasion and metastasis making it difficult to distinguish from RCC, especially in the patients associated with tuberous sclerosis.

Teaching Point

1. AML larger than 4 cm are prone to risk of life threatening hemorrhage.
2. AMLs with microscopic fat should be carefully distinguished with RCC with intracellular fat;
3. Comparing with CT, in- and opposite-phase MR images are more valuable in detecting microscopic fat in AML.

Case 2.23

Brief Case Summary: 43 year old female with left flank pain.

Imaging Findings CT scan of the abdomen performed with and without intravenous contrast demonstrates the presence of a complex cystic mass in the left kidney with multiple enhancing septations (Fig. 2.27a, b). The mass appears to herniate within the left renal pelvis, as seen on the reformatted coronal images obtained in the delayed excretory phase (Fig. 2.27c). Axial T2 weighted fat saturated image

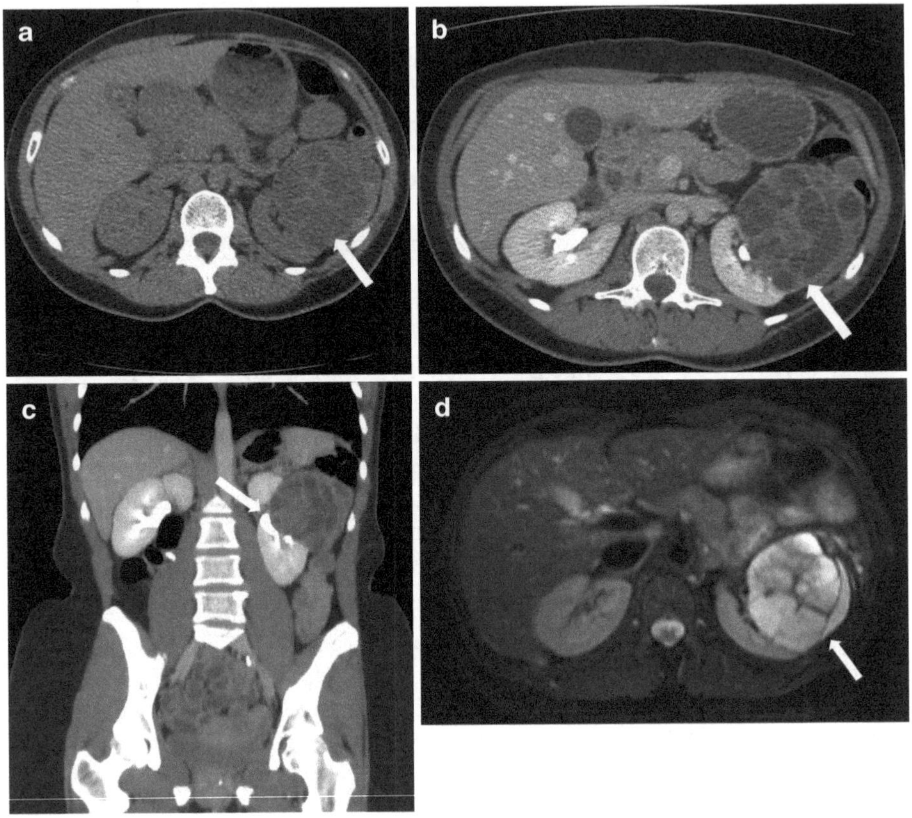

Fig. 2.27 CT scan of the abdomen performed with and without intravenous contrast demonstrates the presence of a complex cystic mass in the left kidney with multiple enhancing septations (**a**, **b**). The mass appears to herniate within the left renal pelvis, as seen on the reformatted coronal images obtained in the delayed excretory phase (**c**). Axial T2 weighted fat saturated image re demonstrates the multicystic nature of the mass (**d**). Note that the intervening septations are T2 hypointense

re demonstrates the multicystic nature of the mass (Fig. 2.27d). Note that the intervening septations are T2 hypointense.

Differential Diagnosis Cystic renal cell carcinoma, cystic nephroma, renal abscess

Diagnosis and Discussion: Cystic nephroma

Cystic nephroma is an uncommon renal cell neoplasm with a bimodal age and sex distribution, typically seen in boys between the ages of 3 months and 4 years, as well as women between the ages of 40 and 60. The nomenclature and histological classification of this neoplasm has undergone significant changes, with the previous terminology referring to this tumor as multilocular cystic nephroma. Furthermore, it is now thought that cystic nephromas occurring in the pediatric and adult population represent different entities, with tumors in the pediatric population now classified as cystic partially differentiated nephroblastoma (CPDN). In adults, there is a histological spectrum ranging from cystic nephroma to *mixed epithelial and stromal tumor of the kidney (MEST)*. Cystic nephroma cannot be differentiated from MEST on imaging. *Clinical manifestations are non-specific* and include abdominal pain and hematuria.

Imaging findings demonstrate the presence of a well-circumscribed cystic mass containing multiple variably enhancing septa. Extension of the mass into the renal pelvis is often found. The cysts may demonstrate higher density than simple fluid due to the presence of hemorrhagic or proteinaceous debris. MRI demonstrates similar findings with a high T2 signal cysts with variable T1 signal intensity due to internal debris and thin enhancing septations. The capsule and thing septations are typically T2 hypointense presumably related to the fibrous content of these structures.

The inability to reliably differentiate cystic nephroma from a cystic renal cell carcinoma on imaging or percutaneous biopsy necessitates surgical excision of these masses.

Pitfalls Multiple cystic locules and the herniation into the renal pelvis are findings not typically seen a renal abscess. Furthermore, renal abscesses typically develop in the setting of a urinary tract infection or pyelonephritis or may be the result of contiguous spread of infection. As mentioned earlier, it is difficult to differentiate a cystic renal cell neoplasm from a cystic nephroma, although the presence of an enhancing mural nodule (Bosniak category IV) is pathognomonic for the former.

Teaching Point

1. The nomenclature and histological classification of cystic nephroma has undergone significant changes, such that the pediatric and adult tumors are thought to represent different entities. Previously this neoplasm was referred to as multilocular cystic nephroma.
2. In adults, this neoplasm is seen in women aged 40–60. Imaging appearances are relatively consistent demonstrating the presence of a multiloculated cystic mass with thin enhancing septations and herniation into the renal pelvis.
3. Adult cystic nephroma cannot be reliably differentiated from cystic renal cell carcinoma on imaging or biopsy. Surgical excision is the treatment of choice.

Case 2.24

Brief Case Summary: 52 years old female with incidental finding on ultrasound.

Imaging Findings Axial contrast-enhanced CT scans in corticomedullary and nephrographic phase (Fig. 2.28a, b) shows a well-defined enhancing mass in the lower pole of right kidney. Note the central hypodense area representing a central scar.

Axial contrast-enhanced MRI in another 54 year old man showing heterogenously enhancing mass in the left interpolar region (Fig. 2.28c) with central scar (Fig. 2.28d).

Differential Diagnosis Renal Cell Carcinoma (RCC), metastases

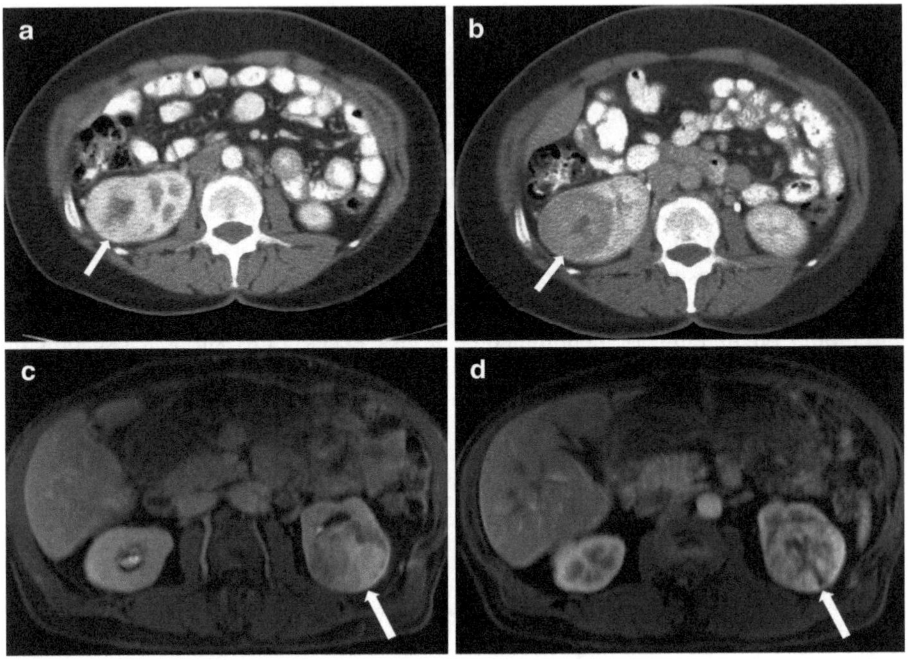

Fig. 2.28 Axial contrast-enhanced CT scans in corticomedullary and nephrographic phase (**a, b**) shows a well-defined enhancing mass in the lower pole of right kidney. Note the central hypodense area representing a central scar. Axial contrast-enhanced MRI in another 54 year old man showing heterogenously enhancing mass in the left interpolar region (**c**) with central scar (**d**)

Diagnosis and Discussion Renal oncocytoma

Renal oncocytoma is an uncommon benign tumor of the renal parenchyma arising from the intercalated cells of the proximal convoluted tubule. The tumor is well encapsulated and usually small in size. Patients are asymptomatic until the lesion becomes large.

Ultrasound depicts the lesion as an isoechoic mass distorting the normal renal contour. The mass may show "spoke wheel" pattern of vascularity on power Doppler.

CT scans show the mass to be isodense to the renal parenchyma. The corticomedullary phase is best suited to assess lesion vascularity, oncocytoma may show a central non enhancing scar. The nephrographic phase provides the best renal to lesion contrast. Oncoytoma's typically appear as hypodense to parenchyma in this phase.

MRI shows the lesion to be hypointense on T1 and hyperintense on T2. The scar if present is hypointense on T1 and T2 (unlike necrosis of RCC that shows a bright signal on T2)- this feature is non specific however. The contrast characteristics mirror those found on CT with the nephrographic phase providing best delineation of the mass.

Angiography though rarely done nowadays depicts a tumor blush and may show the "spoke wheel" vascular pattern of vessels radiating from the center of the lesion. Absence of tumor "neovascularity" helps to differentiate it from RCC.

As differentiation from renal cell carcinoma (especially the chromophobe type) is difficult, surgical resection is preferred by most urologists. Although considered a benign tumor, metastases from oncocytoma have been reported, these lesions are now thought to be misdiagnosed chromophobe Renal Cell carcinoma.

A unique histopathological entity is that of renal oncocytosis, it is characterized by multiple renal oncocytoma, as expected multiple usually bilateral renal nodules are present with one dominant lesion. Histopathological analyses most commonly (in 57 % of cases) reveals hybrid oncocytic and chromophobe RCC components. The association is with that of Birt-Hogg-Dubé syndrome characterized by- trichodiscoma of skin, pulmonary bullae with spontaneous pneumothorax and multiple renal oncocytoma.

As with solitary oncocytoma; the clinical course is benign, most patients have associated renal failure.

Pitfalls Chromophobe RCC in particular has many common imaging features with oncocytoma, this isn't surprising considering that both have a common progenitor cell. The presence of metastases, invasion of surrounding organs/vasculature and tumor vascularity characterize RCC.

Teaching Points

1. Oncocytoma is a small well encapsulated, benign tumor arising from proximal convoluted tubules.
2. Differentiation from RCC based on imaging characteristics alone is unreliable.
3. Timing of the scan protocol is paramount as best lesion delineation is obtained in the nephrographic phase. Vascularity is best assessed in the corticomedullary phase.
4. Most urologists prefer surgical excision by way of nephron sparing surgery or nephrectomy, even on histopathology the diagnosis may be prove to be challenging as RCC can show oncocytic elements.

Case 2.25

Brief Case Summary: 66-year-old male with incidentally discovered renal mass.

Imaging Findings Axial non-contrast and contrast-enhanced CT scans demonstrate a well-defined, solid enhancing cortical mass with necrosis in the interpolar region of right kidney (arrows in Fig. 2.29a, b)

Additional imaging findings within similar lesion in different patients:

Axial T2W image shows high signal intensity right renal mass extending to right renal vein, suggested renal vein invasion (arrow in Fig. 2.29c).

Axial contrast enhanced CT scan in another patient shows a large necrotic enhancing right renal mass (arrow head in Fig. 2.29d) with associated multiple enhancing lymph nodes (white arrows in Fig. 2.29d)

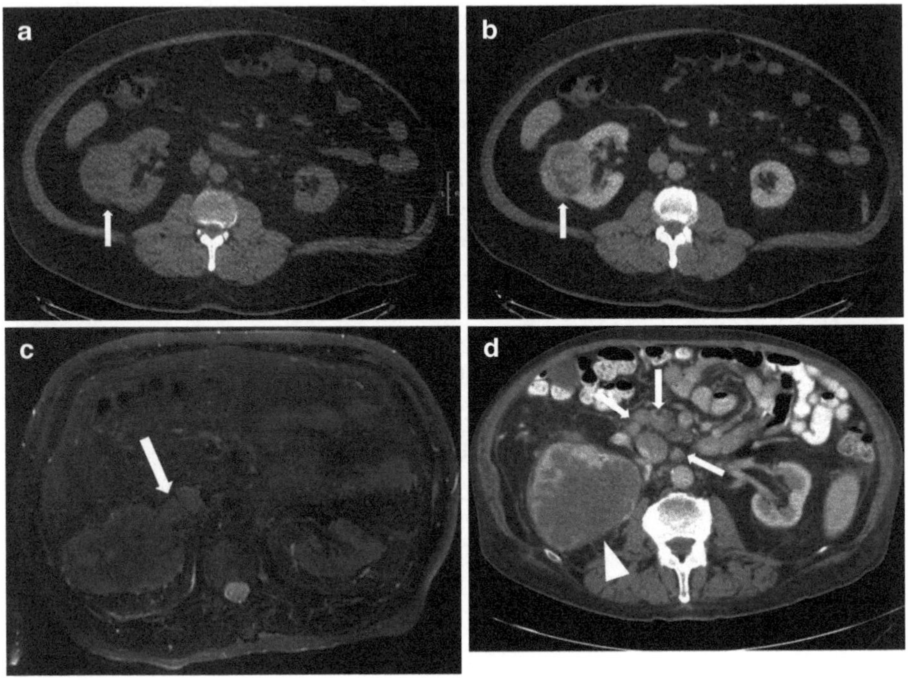

Fig. 2.29 Axial non-contrast and contrast-enhanced CT scans demonstrate a well-defined, solid enhancing cortical mass with necrosis in the interpolar region of right kidney (*arrows* in **a**, **b**). Axial T2W image shows high signal intensity right renal mass extending to right renal vein, suggested renal vein invasion (*arrow* in **c**). Axial contrast enhanced CT scan in another patient shows a large necrotic enhancing right renal mass (*arrow head* in **d**) with associated multiple enhancing lymph nodes (*white arrows* in **d**)

Differential Diagnosis Oncocytoma, lipid poor angiomyolipoma, renal TCC.

Diagnosis and Discussion Renal cell carcinoma

Renal cell carcinoma (RCC) is the most common malignant tumor of kidney and accounts for 90 % of all renal masses. There is a 1.5:1 predominance of men over women, with patients typically presenting in the fifth to seventh decade. Long term dialysis and smoking have been identified as risk factors. Genetic factors are also implicated with VHL being the commonest association with RCC. The classic triad of presentation of flank pain, painless hematuria, and palpable mass is rare. Most cases are asymptomatic and discovered incidentally. 30 % of symptomatic RCC may be associated with paraneoplastic syndromes. The various types of RCC in descending order are as follows: clear cell (70 %), papillary (10–15 %), granular cell (7 %), chromophobe (5 %), collecting duct (1 %), and sarcomatoid (1 %).

CT imaging includes evaluation in corticomedullary, nephrographic, and excretory phases. Imaging aims at localization of the tumor, assessment of the extent of extrarenal spread, involvement of renal vein and extent of IVC thrombus, evaluation of regional lymphadenopathy and distant metastasis, and mapping of renal vessels prior to surgery. Evaluating the morphology and function of the contralateral kidney is also important. MRI is used when CT cannot be performed due to allergy to iodinated contrast or in pregnancy.

Imaging features of RCC depend upon the histological subtype with the most common being the clear cell type. Clear cell RCC is commonly seen as a hypervascular expansile solid mass that arises from the renal cortex and is heterogenous due to presence of hemorrhage, necrosis, and cysts. Multilocular cystic type of RCC is multicystic with thick asymmetric septations and calcifications in the wall in approximately 20 % of cases. The papillary subtype as opposed to clear cell type is hypovascular, homogenous and may be multifocal or bilateral. The third most common variety is the chromophobe type which presents as a homogenously enhancing hypovascular mass. Collecting duct carcinoma shows an infiltrating type of growth with its epicenter in the medulla/pelvicaliceal system and manifest as heterogenous and hypovascular masses on CT. Medullary carcinomas are also infiltrative medullary masses typically associated with caliectasis and are seen in patients with sickle cell trait.

On MRI, RCC is usually hypointense on T1 and have variable signal on T2 due to presence of hemorrhage and necrosis. Sonography plays an important role as a screening modality in that US can detect and characterize septations in renal cysts and can differentiate solid hypovascular masses from cysts.

Surgical resection is the treatment of choice for RCC. However radiofrequency ablation can be performed in small tumors less than 3 cm when surgery is contraindicated.

Pitfalls Oncocytomas cannot be reliably differentiated from RCC, however, the presence of a central scar and a spoke wheel pattern of vascularity favor an oncocytoma. Angiomyolipoma when devoid of macroscopic fat may be indistinguishable on CT but signal drop out on opposed phase MRI is a helpful findings in differentiating the two entities.

Teaching Points

1. RCC is the most common malignant tumor of the kidney with many histological subtypes, the most common is the clear cell type. Papillary and chromophobe RCC are usually hypovascular masses and are lower stage at presentation with better prognosis. Collecting duct and medullary carcinomas are extremely rare central infiltrating masses.
2. RCC are typically hypervascular, heterogenous, and expansile solid masses arising from the renal cortex.
3. RCC may be indistinguishable from oncocytoma and can have a similar imaging appearance to central TCC.

Case 2.26

Brief Case Summary: 74 year old male with hematuria

Imaging Findings Axial contrast-enhanced CT in portal and delayed phases demonstrate a solid minimally enhancing mass centered in right renal pelvis with a preserved renal outline (arrows in Fig. 2.30a, b).

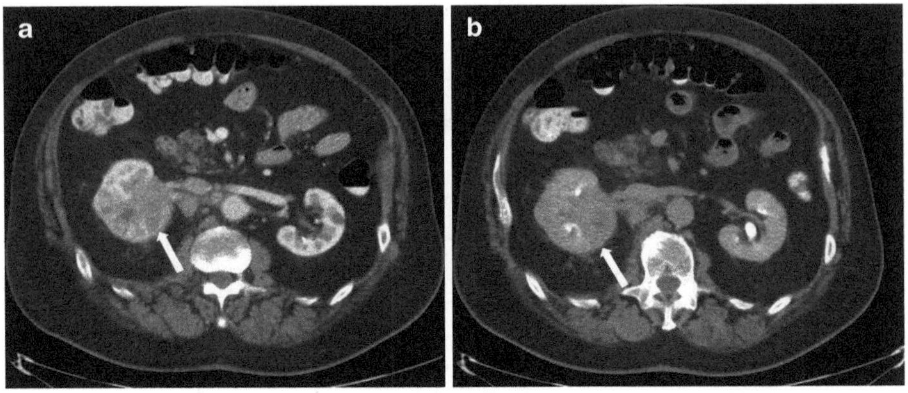

Fig. 2.30 Axial contrast-enhanced CT in portal and delayed phases demonstrate a solid minimally enhancing mass centered in right renal pelvis with a preserved renal outline (*arrows* in **a** and **b**)

Differential Diagnosis Renal cell carcinoma, lymphoma, metastases, xanthogranulomatous pyelonephritis

Diagnosis and Discussion: Transitional cell carcinoma

Transitional cell carcinoma is typically found in the bladder, however, 5 % arise from the ureter or the renal pelvis. Renal TCC accounts for about 10 % of renal malignancies whereas renal cell carcinoma accounts for 90 % of renal malignancies. TCC occurs in patients of between the sixth and seventh decades with a male to female ratio of about 3:1. Presence of synchronous/metachronous bilateral tumours is a common finding; synchronous bilateral TCC occur in 1–2 % of renal lesions and 2–9 % of ureteral lesions. Importantly, 50 % of patients with an upper tract TCC will develop metachronous bladder TCC. Risk factors include smoking, chemical carcinogens, chemotherapeutic agents, and congenital renal anomalies such as horseshoe kidneys.

Renal TCC most frequently arises in the extrarenal part of the pelvis, followed by the infundibulocaliceal region. Renal TCC occurs between the right and left kidneys in an equal distribution and 2–4 % of cases occur bilaterally. Morphologically renal TCC is similar to bladder TCC and can be divided into two types- papillary neoplasms (accounting for 85 % of upper tract TCC) which appears broad base and frondlike morphology and pedunculated or diffusely infiltrating (accounting for 15 % of upper tract TCC)

Multiphasic CT urography is the most sensitive tool for detection of tumors allowing for a thorough investigation of the entire urothelium. TCC presents as a central infiltrating mass with only mild to moderate enhancement and appears hypodense compared to normal enhancing renal parenchyma. They are relatively homogenous masses with hemorrhage and necrosis rarely seen. The larger tumors may infiltrate the renal sinus fat resulting in a "faceless kidney". Invasion into renal vein or IVC may be seen rarely. The large tumors may also show necrosis however the reniform shape of kidney is maintained. In the excretory phase they typically manifest as a centrally located filling defect within the pelvicaliceal system extending towards the ureteropelvic junction (UPJ). Obstruction and dilatation proximal to the tumor is commonly seen. The tumor may distend the calyx or may prevent filling with contrast called as phantom calyx. Metastatic nodules may be seen in the lower urinary tract in the form of mucosal thickening/strictures. Retrograde pyelography may help demonstrate the tumors in a non functioning kidney.

MR with MR urography is useful tool when iodinated contrast CT is contraindicated. TCC is seen as an isointense filling defect in a dilated collecting system. Diffusion weighted imaging may help in detection of metastatic nodules in the urinary tract.

Pitfalls Centrally located RCC may simulate a TCC however a few imaging findings can be helpful in differentiating the two. Renal TCC are located within the collecting system and may extend into the ureteropelvic junction and there is usually preservation of the reniform shape of kidney with renal TCC compared to RCC. Lymphoma may also present as centrally infiltrative hypovascular masses associated with bulky lymphadenopathy however they rarely cause pelvicaliceal obstruction.

Teaching Points

1. Transitional cell carcinoma is typically found in the bladder but a minority (5 %) of TCC occur in the ureter or renal pelvis.
2. Multiphasic CT urography is the imaging modality of choice which allows for a thorough assessment of the entire urothelial tract given the multifocality and metachronous nature of TCC.
3. Multicentric TCC is common and synchronous and metachronous TCC in the contralateral collecting system and bladder is common, necessitating vigilant radiologic and urologic follow-up.

Case 2.27

Brief Case Summary: 61 year old male with hematuria

Imaging Findings Ultrasound images of the right kidney demonstrate the presence of hypoechoic perinephric masses (arrows, Fig. 2.31a, b), with no detectable flow on color Doppler (Fig. 2.31a). Subsequent CT scan of the abdomen and pelvis with intravenous contrast demonstrates the presence of corresponding perinephric soft tissue (arrow- Fig. 2.31c) surrounding the right kidney. CT scan of the abdomen and pelvis with intravenous and oral contrast in another patient (Fig. 2.31d), demonstrates the presence of an infiltrative soft tissue mass in the left kidney (curved arrow, Fig. 2.31d) with retroperitoneal lymphadenopathy (straight arrows, Fig. 2.31d).

Differential Diagnosis Metastases, pyelonephritis, renal abscess, renal cell carcinoma, transitional cell carcinoma.

Diagnosis and Discussion Primary renal lymphoma

Primary renal lymphoma is very rare, accounting for approximately 3 % of all cases. In majority of cases renal lymphoma is secondary to hematogenous spread or direct extension from the retroperitoneum. The genitourinary system is the second

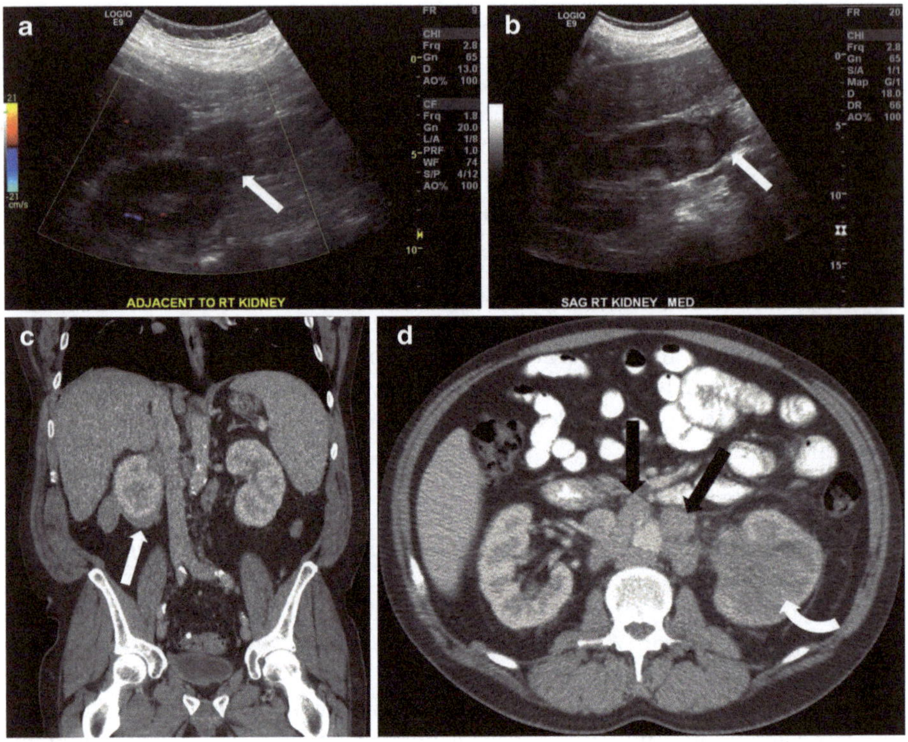

Fig. 2.31 Ultrasound images of the right kidney demonstrate the presence of hypoechoic perinephric masses (*arrows*, **a**, **b**), with no detectable flow on color Doppler (**a**). Subsequent CT scan of the abdomen and pelvis with intravenous contrast demonstrates the presence of corresponding perinephric soft tissue (*arrow*, C) surrounding the right kidney. CT scan of the abdomen and pelvis with intravenous and oral contrast in another patient (**d**), demonstrates the presence of an infiltrative soft tissue mass in the left kidney (*curved arrow*, **d**) with retroperitoneal lymphadenopathy (*straight arrows*, **d**)

most common site of extranodal lymphoma involvement, next to the hematopoietic and reticuloendothelial organs, and the kidneys are most commonly involved. Clinical features include nonspecific symptoms and signs such as flank pain, fever, and night sweats to frank or microscopic hematuria. Renal lymphoma is usually seen as part of multisystem lymphoma, most commonly in widespread non- Hodgkin lymphoma. It is also associated with immunodeficiency states such as HIV and post-transplantation due to unrestricted B lymphocyte proliferation due to infection by Epstein-Barr virus.

Although CT and MR are superior to US in detection of lymphadenopathy, US may be the initial imaging study performed and familiarity with typical sonographic findings is important. US is a useful imaging modality for percutaneous biopsies. On US, hypoechoic, homogeneous renal masses with minimal vascularity on color or power Doppler are seen. Displacement of normal renal vasculature due to mass effect may be visualized. When there is renal parenchymal infiltration, enlarged globular kidneys are seen with loss of the echogenic renal sinus fat.

MDCT is the imaging modality of choice for diagnosis, staging, and monitoring of treatment. On CT, renal lymphoma manifests as unilateral or bilateral, enhancing, non-calcified, homogenous soft tissue renal masses of slightly higher attenuation than surrounding renal parenchyma which may or may not distort the renal contour. There may be extension into the perinephric space and associated retroperitoneal lymphadenopathy. The corticomedullary phase delineates renal vessels and helps to differentiate lymphoma from primary renal tumors. The nephrographic phase is useful in detecting medullary masses and smaller lesions which may be missed on early phases. Centrally located masses affecting the collecting system are better delineated on the excretory phase.

On MR, lymphoma shows lower signal intensity than normal renal cortex with T1-weighted sequences. They are relatively iso- or hypointense with T2-weighted sequences. Lymphoma enhances less than the renal parenchyma following intravenous administration of gadolinium-based contrast material.

Renal lymphoma is intensely FDG avid and PET/CT increases the sensitivity and specificity of detection. PET/CT is very useful for staging and follow up of renal lymphoma cases after treatment.

Pitfalls MDCT is the imaging modality of choice for initial diagnosis in patients with suspected lymphoma. CT allows for detection of lesions but also depicts extension of disease into adjacent structures thereby detecting systemic disease. Multiphase CT is helpful in the accurate assessment and detection of renal lymphoma and can help in accurately diagnosing a renal lymphoma from other primary renal neoplasms.

Teaching Points

1. Primary renal lymphoma is rare, accounting for approximately 3 % of cases, whereas a majority of cases result from hematogenous spread or direct extension from the retroperitoneum.
2. MDCT is the imaging modality of choice for diagnosis, assessment of systemic disease, and response to treatment.
3. The administration of intravenous contrast and the utility of multiphase acquisition on CT after are helpful in detecting renal masses but also in accurately diagnosing lesions.

Suggested Readings by Case

Case 2.1

Bauer SB. Anomalies of the upper urinary tract. In: Walsh PC, Retik AB, Vaughan ED, Wein AJ, editors. Campbell's urology. 8th ed. Philadelphia: WB Saunders; 2002. p. 1898–906.

Rubinstein ZJ, Hertz M, Shahin N, et al. Crossed renal ectopia: angiographic findings in six cases. AJR Am J Roentgenol. 1976;126(5):1035–8.

Turkvatan A, Olcer T, Cumhur T. Multidetector CT urography of renal fusion anomalies. Diagn Interv Radiol. 2009;15:127–34.

Case 2.2

Dyer RB, Chen MY, Zagoria RJ. Classic signs in uroradiology. Radiographics. 2004a; 24:S247–80.
Majidpour HS, Yousefinejad V. Percutaneous management of urinary calculi in horseshoe kidneys. Urol J. 2008;5(3):188–91.
Nino-Murcia M. deVries PA, Friedland GW. Congenital anomalies of the kidney. In: Pollack HM, McClennan BL, editors. Clinical urography. 2nd ed. Philadelphia: Saunders; 2000. p. 690–763.

Case 2.3

Gittes RF, Talner LB. Congenital megacalices versus obstructive hydronephrosis. J Urol. 1972;108:833–6.
Sethi R, Yang DC, Mittal P, et al. Congenital megacalyces. Studies with different imaging modalities. Clin Nucl Med. 1997;22(9):653–5.
Talner LB, Gittes RF. Megacalyces. Clin Radiol. 1972;23(3):55–61.

Case 2.4

Hidalgo H, Dunnick NR, Rosenberg ER, et al. Parapelvic cysts: appearance on CT and sonography. AJR Am J Roentgenol. 1982;138:667–71.
Lee FTJ, Thornbury JR. The Urinary Tract. In: Juhl JH, Crummy AB, Kuhlman JE, editors. Paul and Juhl's Essentials of Radiologic Imaging, vol. 7. Philadelphia: Lippincott Williams & Wilkins; 1998. p. 683.

Case 2.5

Katabathina VS, Kota G, Dasyam AK, et al. Adult renal cystic disease: a genetic, biological, and developmental primer. Radiographics. 2010a;30:1509–23.
Levine E, Slusher SL, Grantham JJ, et al. Natural history of acquired renal cystic disease in dialysis patients: a prospective longitudinal CT study. AJR Am J Roentgenol. 1991;156(3): 501–6.
Miller LR, Soffer O, Nassar VH, et al. Acquired renal cystic disease in end-stage renal disease: an autopsy study of 155 cases. Am J Nephrol. 1989;9(4):322–8.

Case 2.6

Bosniak MA. The Bosniak renal cyst classification: 25 years later. Radiology. 2012;262(3): 781–5.
Harisinghani MG, Maher MM, Gervais DA, et al. Incidence of malignancy in complex cystic renal masses (Bosniak Category III): should imaging-guided biopsy precede surgery? AJR Am J Roentgenol. 2003;180:755–8.
Israel GM, Hindman N, Bosniak MA. Evaluation of cysic renal masses: comparison of CT and MR imaging by using the Bosniak classification system. Radiology. 2004; 231:365–71.

Case 2.7

Katabathina VS, Kota G, Dasyam AK, et al. Adult renal cystic disease: a genetic, biological, and developmental primer. Radiographics. 2010b;30:1509–23.
Parfrey PS, Bear JC, Morgan J, et al. The diagnosis and prognosis of autosomal dominant polycystic kidney disease. N Engl J Med. 1990;323(16):1085–90.
Perrone RD. Extrarenal manifestations of ADPKD. Kidney Int. 1997;51(6):2022–36.

Case 2.8

Dyer RB, Chen MY, Zagoria RJ. Classic signs in uroradiology 1. Radiographics. 2004b;24 suppl 1:S247–80.
Schepens D, Verswijvel G, Kuypers D, Vanrenterghem Y. Renal cortical nephrocalcinosis. Nephrol Dial Transplant. 2000;15(7):1080–2.

Case 2.9

Kim YG, Kim B, Kim MK, Chung SJ, Han HJ, Ryu JA, … Oh HY. Medullary nephrocalcinosis associated with long-term furosemide abuse in adults. Nephrol Dial Transplant. 2001;16(12):2303–9.
Dyer RB, Chen MY, Zagoria RJ. Classic signs in uroradiology 1. Radiographics. 2004c;24 suppl 1:S247–80.

Case 2.10

Hidas G, Eliahou R, Duvdevani M, et al. Determination of renal stone composition with dual-energy CT: In Vivo analysis and comparison with X-ray diffraction. Radiology. 2010;257(2):394–401.

Case 2.11

Craig WD, Wagner BJ, Mark D, et al. Pyelonephritis: radiologic-pathologic review. Radiographics. 2008a;28:255–76.

Case 2.12

Craig WD, Wagner BJ, Travis MD. From the Archives of the AFIP: pyelonephritis: radiologic-pathologic review. Radiographics. 2008;28:255–76.
Huang JJ, Tseng CC. Emphysematous pyelonephritis: clinicoradiological classification, management, prognosis, and pathogenesis. Arch Intern Med [Internet]. 2000 Mar 27 [cited 2014 Apr 29];160(6):797–805. Available from: http://www.ncbi.nlm.nih.gov/pubmed/10737279.
Tasleem AM, Murray P, Anjum F, Sriprasad S. CT imaging is invaluable in diagnosing emphysematous pyelonephritis (EPN): a rare urological emergency. BMJ Case Rep [Internet]. 2014 Jan 4 [cited 2014 Apr 28];2014(apr03_2):bcr2014204040–. Available from: http://casereports.bmj.com/content/2014/bcr-2014-204040.long.

Case 2.13

Craig WD, Wagner B, Travis M. Pyelonephritis: radiologic-pathologic review. Radiographics. 2008c;28(1):255–76.
Hayes WS, Hartman DS, Sesterbenn IA. Xanthogranulomatous pyelonephritis. Radiographics. 1991;11:485–98.
Loffroy R, Guiu B, Watfa J, et al. Xanthogranulomatous pyelonephritis in adults: clinical and radiological findings in diffuse and focal forms. Clin Radiol. 2007;62:884–90.
Verswijvel G, Oyen R, Van Poppel H, Roskams T. Xanthogranulomatous pyelonephritis: MRI findings in the diffuse and the focal type. Eur Radiol. 2000;10:586–9.

Case 2.14

Di Fiori JL, Rodrigue D, Kapstein EM, et al. Diagnostic sonography of HIV-associated nephropathy: new observations and clinical correlation. AJR Am J Roentgenol. 1998;171:713–6.
Kay C. Renal diseases in patients with AIDS: sonographic findings. AJR Am J Roentgenol. 1992;159:551–4.
Symeonidou C, Standish R, Sahdev A, et al. Imaging and histopathologic features of HIV-related renal disease. Radiographics. 2008;28(5):1339–54.

Case 2.15

Kawashima A, Sandler CM, Goldman SM, Raval BK, Fishman EK. CT of renal inflammatory disease. Radiographics. 1997;17:851–66.

Case 2.16

Jung Y, Kim JK, Cho K-S. Genitourinary tuberculosis: comprehensive cross-sectional imaging. Am J Radiol. 2005;184:143–50.
Merchant S, Bharati A, Merchant N. Tuberculosis of the genitourinary system-Urinary tract tuberculosis: Renal tuberculosis-Part I. Indian J Radiol Imaging. 2013a;23(1):64–77.
Merchant S, Bharati A, Merchant N. Tuberculosis of the genitourinary system-Urinary tract tuberculosis: Renal tuberculosis-Part II. Indian J Radiol Imaging. 2013b;23(1):64–77.

Case 2.17

Kawashima A, Sandler CM, Corl FM, West OC, Tamm EP, Fishman EK, Goldman SM. Imaging of renal trauma: a comprehensive review. Radiographics. 2001;21(3):557–74.
Rezai P, Tochetto S, Galizia M, Yaghmai V. Perinephric hematoma: semi-automated quantification of volume on MDCT: a feasibility study. Abdom Imaging. 2011;36(2):222–7.

Case 2.18

Dopson S, Jayakumar S, Velez J. Page kidney as a rare cause of hypertension: case report and review of the literature. Am J Kidney Dis. 2009;54:334–9.
Smyth A, Collins S, Thorsteinsdottir B, Madsen B, et al. Page kidney: etiology, renal function outcomes and risk for future hypertension. J Clin Hypertens. 2012;14:216–21.

Case 2.19

Ross L, Titton RL, Debra A, et al. Urine leaks and urinomas: diagnosis and imaging-guided intervention. Radiographics. 2003;23(5):1133–47.

Case 2.20

Kamel IR, Berkowitz JF. Assessment of the cortical rim sign in posttraumatic renal infarction. J Comput Assist Tomogr. 1996;20:803–6.
Kawashima A, Sandler CM, Ernst RD, et al. CT evaluation of renovascular disease. Radiographics. 2000a;20(5):1321–40.
Siablis D, Liatsikos EN, Goumenos D, et al. Percutaneous rheolytic thrombectomy for treatment of acute renal-artery thrombosis. J Endourol. 2005;19:68–71.

Case 2.21

Harris SL, Smith MP, Laurie A, Darlow BA. Neonatal renal vein thrombosis and prothrombotic risk. Acta Paediatr. 2010;99(7):1104–7.
Kawashima A, Sandler CM, Ernst RD, et al. CT evaluation of renovascular disease. Radiographics. 2000b;20(5):1321–40.
Kim HS, Fine DM, Atta MG. Catheter-directed thrombectomy and thrombolysis for acute renal vein thrombosis. J Vasc Interv Radiol. 2006;17(5):815–22.

Case 2.22

Davenport MS, Neville AM, Ellis JH, Cohan RH, Chaudhry HS, Leder RA. Diagnosis of renal angiomyolipoma with hounsfield unit thresholds: effect of size of region of interest and nephrographic phase imaging. Radiology. 2011;260(1):158–65.
Logue LG, Acker RE, Sienko AE. Best cases from the AFIP: angiomyolipomas in tuberous sclerosis. Radiographics. 2003;23(1):241–6.
Pedrosa I, Sun MR, Spencer M, Genega EM, Olumi AF, Dewolf WC, et al. MR imaging of renal masses: correlation with findings at surgery and pathologic analysis. Radiographics. 2008;28(4):985–1003.

Case 2.23

Freire M, Remer EM. Clinical and radiologic features of cystic renal masses. Am J Roentgenol. 2009;192(5):1367–72.
Silver IMF, Boag AH, Soboleski DA. Multilocular cystic renal tumor: cystic nephroma. Radiographics. 2008;28(4):1221–5.
Zhou M, et al. Adult cystic nephroma and mixed epithelial and stromal tumor of the kidney are the same disease entity: molecular and histologic evidence. Am J Surg Pathol. 2009;33(1):72–80.

Case 2.24

Adamy A, Lowrance WT, Yee DS, Chong KT, Bernstein M, Tickoo SK, Coleman JA, Russo P. Renal oncocytosis: management and clinical outcomes. J Urol. 2011;185:795–801.
Bai X, Wu C-L. Renal cell carcinoma and mimics: pathologic primer for radiologists. AJR Am J Roentgenol. 2012;198:1289–93.

Gakis G, Kramer U, Schilling D, Kruck S, Stenzl A, Schlemmer H-P. Small renal oncocytomas: differentiation with multiphase CT. Eur J Radiol. 2011;80:274–8.

Harmon WJ, King BF, Lieber MM. Renal oncocytoma: magnetic resonance imaging characteristics. J Urol. 1996;155:863–7.

Kuroda N, Tanaka A, Ohe C, et al. Review of renal oncocytosis (multiple oncocytic lesions) with focus on clinical and pathobiological aspects. Histol Histopathol. 2012;27:1407–12.

Rosenkrantz AB, Hindman N, Fitzgerald EF, Niver BE, Melamed J, Babb JS. MRI features of renal oncocytoma and chromophobe renal cell carcinoma. AJR Am J Roentgenol. 2010;195:W421–7.

Schieda N, McInnes MDF, Cao L. Diagnostic accuracy of segmental enhancement inversion for diagnosis of renal oncocytoma at biphasic contrast enhanced CT: systematic review. Eur Radiol. 2014. doi:10.1007/s00330-014-3147-4.

Case 2.25

Ng CS, Wood CG, Silverman PM, et al. Renal cell carcinoma: diagnosis, staging, and surveillance". AJR Am J Roentgenol. 2008;191:1220–32.

Prasad SR, Humphrey PA, Catena JR, et al. Common and uncommon histologic subtypes of renal cell carcinoma: imaging spectrum with pathologic correlation. Radiographics. 2006; 26:1795–810.

Case 2.26

Browne RFJ, Meehan CP, Colville J, et al. Transitional cell carcinoma of the upper urinary tract: spectrum of imaging findings. Radiographics. 2005;25:1609–27.

Raza SA, Sohaib SA, Sahdev A, et al. Centrally infiltrating renal masses on CT: differentiating intrarenal transitional cell carcinoma from centrally located renal cell carcinoma. AJR Am J Roentgenol. 2012;198(4):846–53.

Case 2.27

Ganeshan D, Iyer R, Devine C, Bhosale P, Paulson E. Imaging of primary and secondary renal lymphoma. AJR Am J Roentgenol. 2013;201:W712–9.

Sheth S, Ali S, Fishman E. Imaging of renal lymphoma: patterns of disease with pathologic correlation. Radiographics. 2013;26:1151–68.

Zhang J, Lefkowitz RA, Bach A. Imaging of kidney cancer. Radiol Clin North Am. 2007; 45:119–47.

Chapter 3
Ureters

Case 3.1

Brief Case Summary: 35 year old male with abdominal pain

Imaging Findings CT urogram (excretory phase) of the abdomen demonstrates the right ureter lying posterior to the inferior vena cava (Fig. 3.1). Coronal reconstructed image demonstrates the presence of an abrupt narrowing of the ureter at this level (arrow, Fig. 3.2).

Differential Diagnosis Retrocaval ureter, medial deviation of the ureter related to retroperitoneal fibrosis.

Diagnosis and Discussion Retrocaval ureter.

A retrocaval ureter is an uncommon congenital anomaly with an incidence of 1:1,000. The etiology is related to abnormal development of the inferior vena cava (IVC), and not the ureter itself, resulting in a portion of the ureter passing behind the IVC. It is seen slightly more commonly in males (two to three fold increase) and typically occurs on the right side. Symptoms include intermittent pain related to ureteral obstruction as well as hematuria.

While imaging findings were first described with conventional urography and intravenous pyelography (IVP), both CT and MRI are used currently to diagnose this entity. Two subtypes have been described. Type 1 (or "low loop" form) manifests with the ureter passing behind the IVC at the level of the third or fourth vertebral body resulting a "reverse J" (also described as an "S" shape or "fish hook" deformity) configuration of the ureter at the point of transition. In the type 2 (or "high loop" form) subtype, the ureter passes behind the IVC at the level of or just above the ureteropelvic junction, resulting in a sickle shape at the point of transition. Type 1 is more common and is associated with higher degrees of ureteral obstruction.

Symptomatic patients or those with moderate to severe hydronephrosis are evaluated for surgical correction which involves ureteral transection with placement

M.G. Harisinghani, A. Rajesh, *Genitourinary Imaging: A Case Based Approach*, DOI 10.1007/978-1-4471-4772-5_3

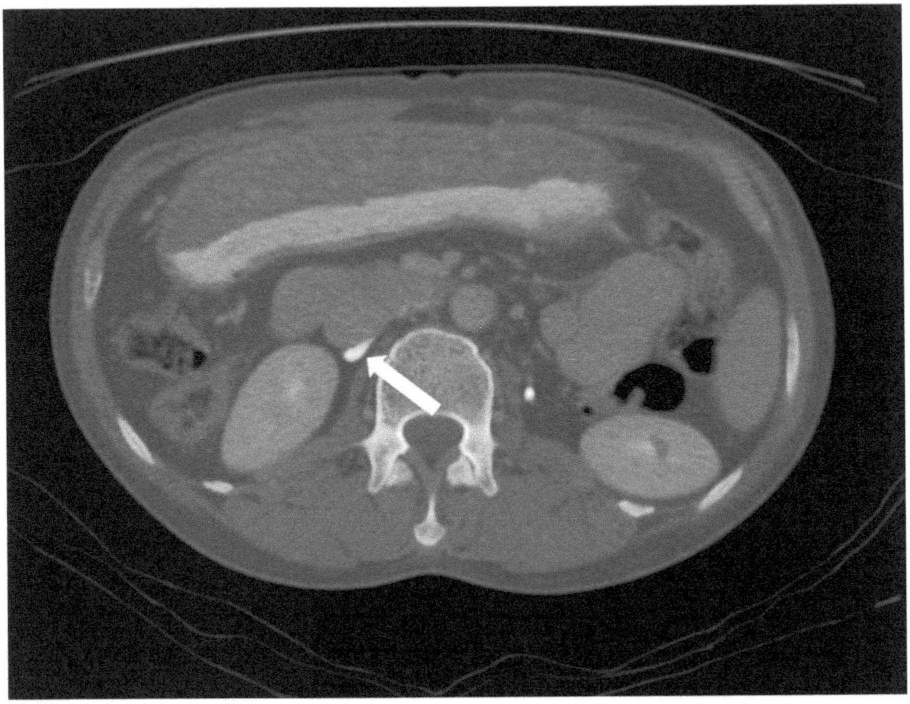

Fig. 3.1 CT urogram (excretory phase) of the abdomen demonstrates the right ureter (*arrow*) lying posterior to the inferior vena cava

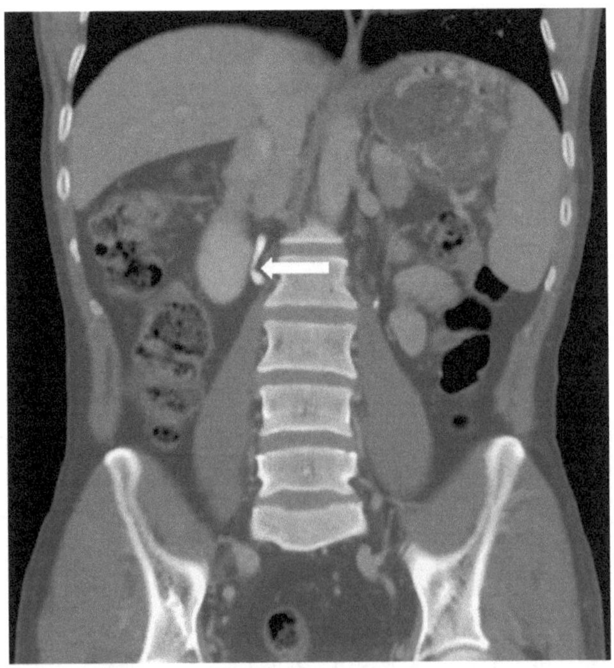

Fig. 3.2 Coronal reconstructed image demonstrates the presence of an abrupt narrowing of the ureter at this level (*arrow*)

of the affected ureteral segment anterior to the IVC. Treatment has traditionally been via an open surgical technique, though laparoscopic reconstructive techniques are being increasingly used with favorable outcomes.

Pitfalls The differential diagnosis for medial deviation of the ureter on IVP includes retroperitoneal fibrosis, a retroperitoneal mass or prior surgery. Definitive findings can be established using either a CT or MRI urogram protocol.

Teaching Points

1. Retrocaval ureter is a congenital abnormality which results in the ureter passing posterior to the IVC. The embryological anomaly is related to development of the IVC and not the ureter.
2. Two types exist. Type 1 is more common and results in worsening degrees of ureteral obstruction. Both types result in the ureter passing posterior to the IVC. In type 1, this transition occurs at the level of mid lumbar spine giving rise to a "reverse J", "S" shape or "fish hook" deformity. In type 2, the transition occurs at or above the level of the ureteropelvic junction resulting in a sickle shape appearance of the ureter.
3. Surgery is reserved for symptomatic patients or those with moderate to severe hydronephrosis

Case 3.2

Brief Case Summary: 45 year old male with hematuria.

Imaging Findings Conventional radiographs of the abdomen obtained as part of a retrograde urogram demonstrate the presence of multiple small filling defects in the left proximal ureter (arrows in Figs. 3.3, 3.4, and 3.5). The bladder is filled with contrast and a small amount of contrast is noted in the right mid to distal ureter.

Differential Diagnosis Transitional cell carcinoma, blood clots, ureteral stones, ureteritis cystica.

Diagnosis and Discussion Ureteritis cystica.

Ureteritis cystica is an uncommon benign process characterized by the formation of multiple epithelial lined submucosal cysts which protrude into the ureteral lumen. Histologically, the cysts are thought to represent cystic degeneration of invaginated epithelial cell nests. It is more commonly seen in older age groups and there is no gender predilection. Clinically, patients with ureteritis cystica usually have evidence of chronic urinary tract inflammation (such as a history of recurrent urinary tract infections) and may present with hematuria.

Conventional or CT urographic examinations are the imaging studies of choice. Ureteritis cystica typically presents as multiple small (often less than 5 mm), smooth filling defects which can, on occasion, given the ureter a scalloped appearance. The filling defects can be seen throughout any portion of the excretory system. Within the ureter, they can be unilateral or bilateral, though there is a predilection for the upper third. Urinary tract dilatation without hydronephrosis may be observed.

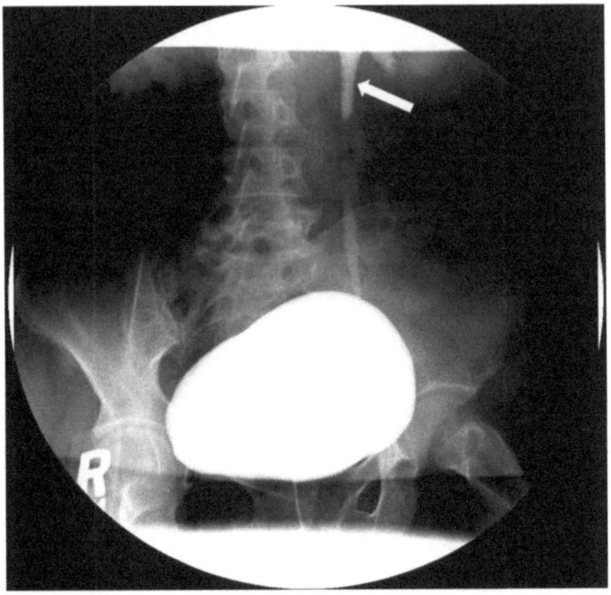

Fig. 3.3 Conventional radiograph of the abdomen obtained as part of a retrograde urogram demonstrating the presence of multiple small filling defects in the left proximal ureter (*arrow*)

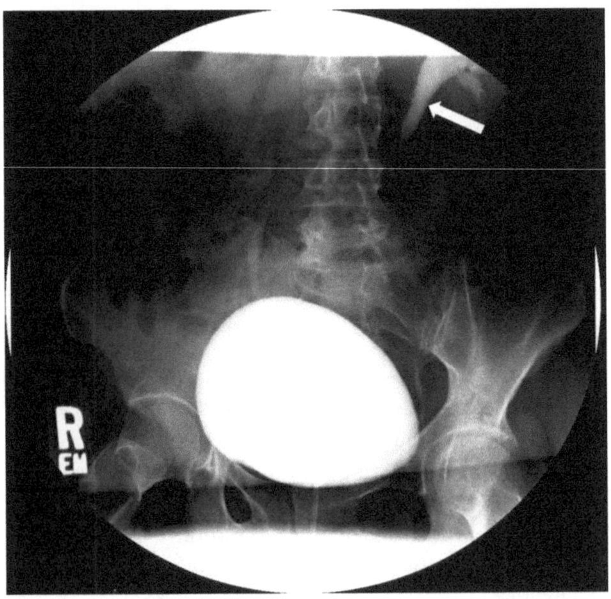

Fig. 3.4 Conventional radiograph of the abdomen obtained as part of a retrograde urogram demonstrating the presence of multiple small filling defects in the left proximal ureter (*arrow*)

The imaging findings are often non-specific, with uroepithelial malignancy being the most important mimicker. Urological evaluation with consideration of ureteroscopy is usually warranted when the imaging features are inconclusive. Treatment is conservative and is directed at treating the cause of inflammation. The imaging

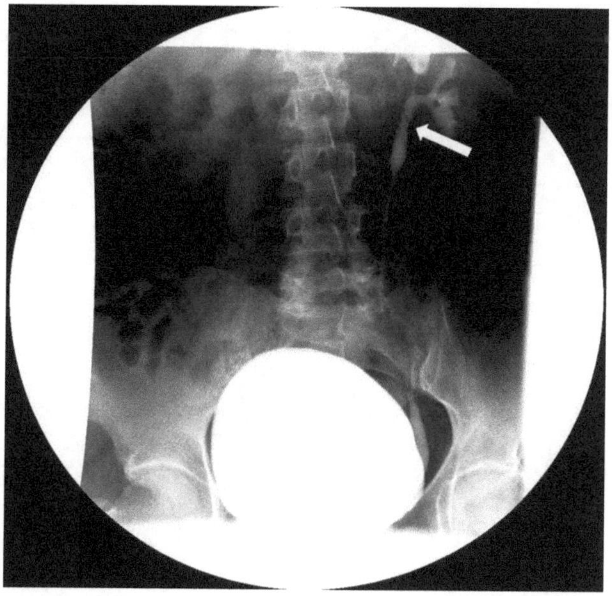

Fig. 3.5 Conventional radiograph of the abdomen obtained as part of a retrograde urogram demonstrating the presence of multiple small filling defects in the left proximal ureter (*arrow*)

appearance may regress or remain stable after the cessation of treatment. There is no definite increased risk for developing an uroepithelial malignancy.

Pitfalls Ureteritis cystica is included in the differential diagnosis of ureteral filling defects, along with transitional cell carcinoma, blood clots, and stones. Some of these mimickers can be excluded using a combination of the clinical information and the use of CT urographic imaging. The non-contrast portion of the exam allows evaluation for stones and blood clots, while the nephrographic and excretory phase images allows for the evaluation of enhancing soft tissue tumors. If imaging findings remain inconclusive, ureteroscopy should be considered.

Teaching Points

1. Ureteritis cystica is a benign condition characterized the presence of submucosal ureteral cysts which protrude into the lumen, manifesting radiographically as multiple filling defects. It is associated with conditions that promote chronic inflammation.
2. The most important differential diagnosis for ureteral filling defects is transitional cell carcinoma. A combination of clinical and CT urography findings can help make this distinction. A ureteroscopy should be considered to evaluate the entire urothelial system including the bladder and ureters for transitional cell carcinoma.
3. Treatment is aimed at managing the underlying cause of inflammation. Imaging findings may remain stable or improve following treatment. There is no definite increased risk for developing an uroepithelial malignancy.

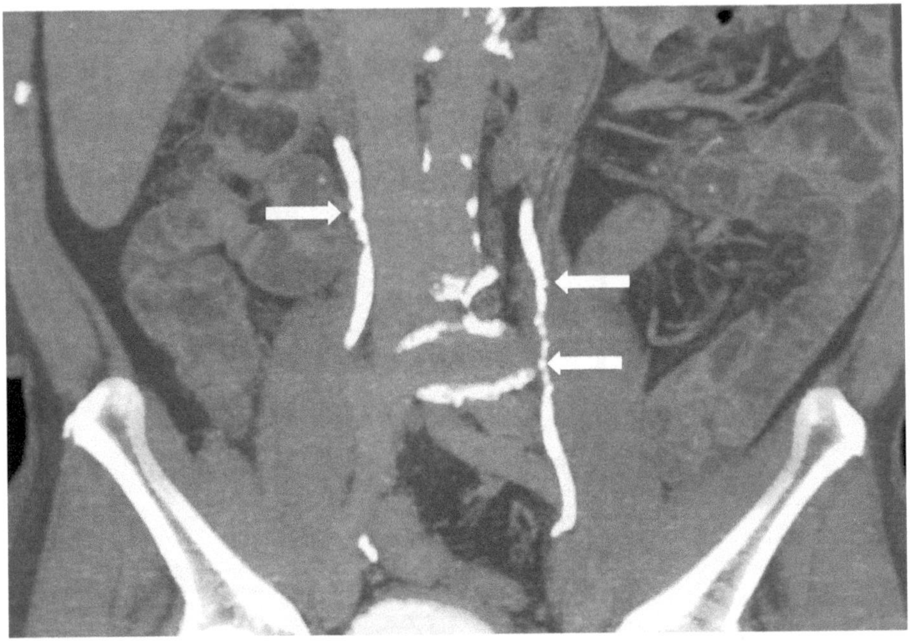

Fig. 3.6 Reconstructed coronal image from an excretory phase of a CT urogram demonstrates the presence of multiple outpouchings involving the mid portions of both ureters (*arrows*)

Case 3.3

Brief Case Summary: 47 year old male with hematuria

Imaging Findings Reconstructed coronal image from an excretory phase of a CT urogram demonstrates the presence of multiple outpouchings involving the mid portions of both ureters (arrows, Fig. 3.6). 3D reconstructed images shows the same findings (Fig. 3.7).

Differential Diagnosis Ureteral pseudodiverticulosis, ureteritis cystica, tuberculosis ureteritis, ureteral diverticula

Diagnosis and Discussion: Ureteral pseudodiverticulosis

Ureteral pseudodiverticulosis (UP) is typically an incidental finding seen in the workup for urinary symptoms. Histologically, UP represents a protrusion of hyperplastic transitional epithelium into the subepithelial connective tissue, typically in the background of underlying inflammation. The incidence is approximately 11 %.

Traditionally, UP has been diagnosed on conventional anterograde or retrograde urography studies where it is defined by multiple small ureteral outpouchings, measuring less than 4 mm. The lesions are often bilateral and commonly involve the mid to upper one-third of the ureter. If unilateral, UP is more commonly seen in the left ureter. There may be some mild narrowing of the associated ureteral segment. CT

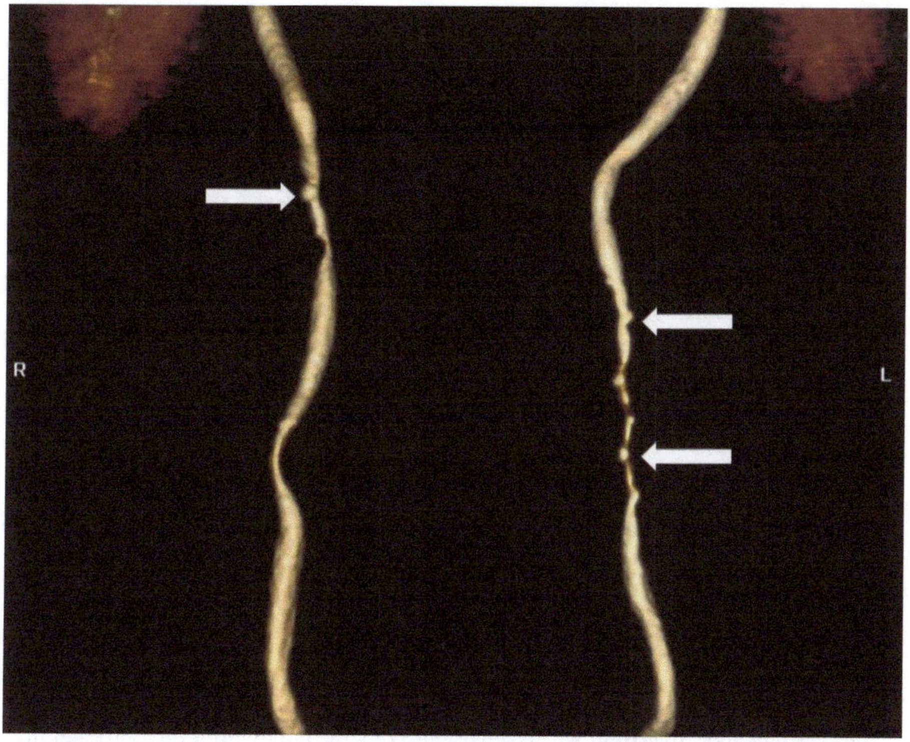

Fig. 3.7 3D reconstructed images demonstrates multiple outpouchings of the mid ureters (*arrows*)

urography, which has largely replaced conventional anterograde urography for the evaluation of the upper urinary tracts, demonstrates similar findings, best appreciated on coronal reconstructed images.

While UP is a benign lesion, it is associated with an increased risk for uroepithelial malignancy. While this risk has been traditionally quoted as 25 %, further studies by Wasserman et al. suggest a higher association reaching up to 71 % if UP is seen with radiolucent filling defects or strictures. The most common associated malignancy is transitional cell carcinoma, though squamous cell carcinoma has been reported. There is no known association between the number of outpouchings and the risk of malignancy and all cases should be closely monitored.

Pitfalls The appearance of UP is fairly pathognomonic on imaging studies. True diverticula of the ureter are exceedingly rare and usually present as a single large lesion. Histologically true diverticula of the ureter involve all the layers of the ureteral wall. Ureteritis cystica manifests as filling defects rather than focal small outpouchings. Tuberculosis ureteritis has a variety of imaging appearances but is usually associated with papillary necrosis, strictures, and calcifications.

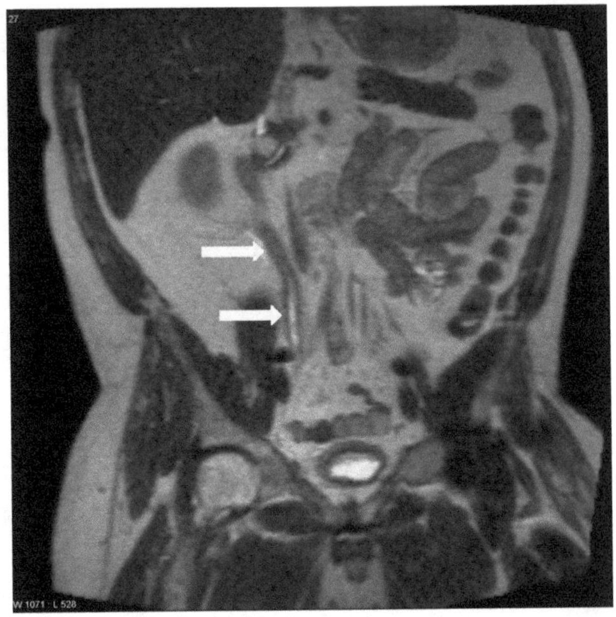

Fig. 3.8 Coronal T2 image shows circumferential right ureteral wall thickening (*arrows*)

Teaching Points

1. Ureteral pseudodiverticulosis is characterized by small ureteral outpouchings often less than 4 mm in size. Lesions are often bilateral and best appreciated on excretory phase images in the coronal plane.
2. There is an increased risk for developing uroepithelial malignancies, most often transitional cell carcinoma, warranting close monitoring in patients with UP.

Case 3.4

Brief Case Summary Elderly patient complaining of right sided abdominal pain.

Imaging Findings Coronal T2 image shows circumferential right ureteral wall thickening (Fig. 3.8) with associated diffuse enhancement of the urothelium on the postgadolinium images (Fig. 3.9).

Differential Diagnosis Transitional cell carcinoma

Diagnosis and Discussion Amyloidosis is a group of disorders characterized by extracellular deposition of insoluble proteins leading to impaired tissue function and significant patient morbidity and mortality. The incidence is eight out of one million people and is increasing. The diagnosis is made by demonstrating apple-green birefringence on tissue samples when Congo red staining is examined under polarized light.

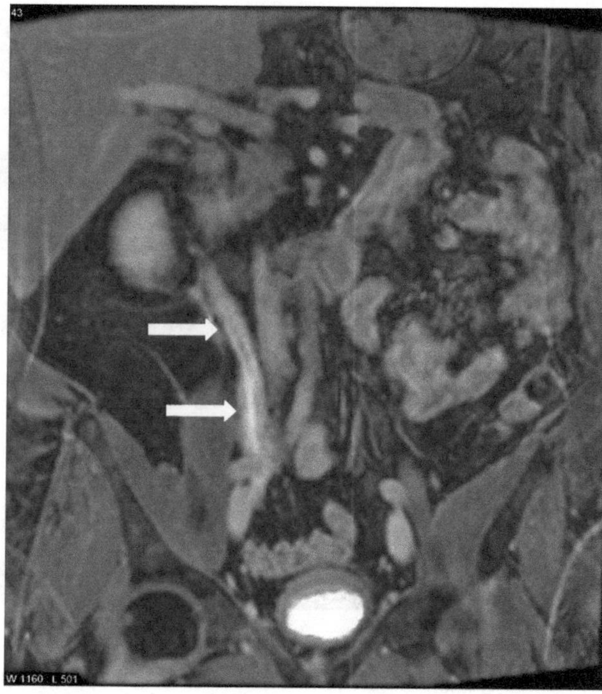

Fig. 3.9 Coronal T1 weighted gadolinium enhanced image shows circumferential right ureteral wall thickening, with associated diffuse enhancement of the urothelium (*arrows*) on the postgadolinium images

Amyloidosis can be categorized as primary or secondary forms based on the types of deposited proteins. Primary amyloidosis is defined as amyloid immunoglobulin light chain (AL) disease while secondary amyloidosis is associated with chronic inflammatory processes such as rheumatoid arthritis and inflammatory bowel disease.

Amyloidosis distribution can be classified as localized or diffuse. Amyloidosis is usually a systemic disease accounting for 80–90 % of cases whereby protein deposition occurs in multiple organ systems including the cardiovascular, gastrointestinal, musculoskeletal, and adipose tissue. The morbidity and mortality of systemic amyloidosis is high and usually results in renal and/or cardiac failure. Systemic amyloidosis often requires systemic treatment in contradistinction to localized amyloidosis where supportive and local treatment is sufficient as the disease is confined to one organ.

Localized amyloidosis affects one organ, typically the respiratory tract, urinary tract, or skin. The bladder is most commonly involved and the renal pelvis and ureter are less commonly affected. In the upper urinary tract, amyloid deposition is often unifocal and usually involves the lower ureter.

On imaging, amyloidosis of the ureter appears as focal or diffuse areas of urothelial thickening, filling defects, and urethral stricture and narrowing. Linear submucosal or intramural calcifications are characteristic of amyloidosis in the ureter and renal pelvis. CT and MR are the best imaging modalities to detect urethral wall thickening, intraluminal filling defects, and areas of narrowing.

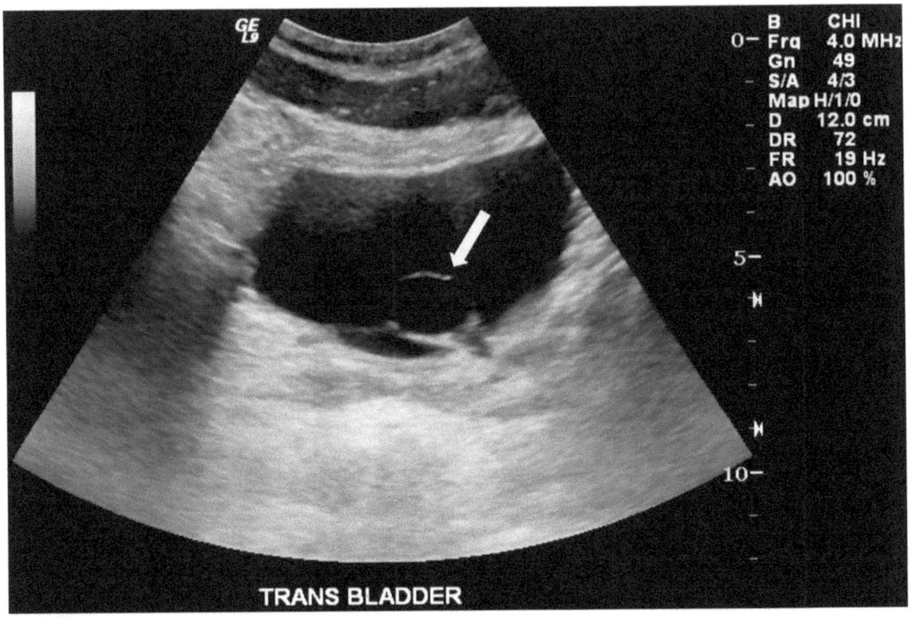

Fig. 3.10 Transverse gray scale US image demonstrates the presence of an anechoic intraluminal bladder mass with a thin echogenic wall (*arrow*), which appears to be attached to the bladder wall at the expected region of the left ureteovesicular junction

Pitfalls Urethral amyloidosis is indistinguishable from transitional cell carcinoma of the urethra by imaging. Cytologic analysis is crucial for accurate diagnosis and differentiation.

Teaching Point

1. Localized amyloidosis of the renal pelvis and urethra is rare but the imaging appearance is indistinguishable from transitional cell carcinoma.
2. On imaging, focal or diffuse areas of urothelial thickening, filling defects, and urethral stricture and narrowing.

Case 3.5

Brief Case Summary: 35 year old male with flank pain.

Imaging Findings Transverse gray scale US image demonstrates the presence of an anechoic intraluminal bladder mass with a thin echogenic wall (Fig. 3.10) which appears to be attached to the bladder wall at the expected region of the left ureteovesicular junction. Axial image from a CT at the level of the pelvis performed in the excretory phase demonstrates dense contrast within the corresponding mass seen on US (Fig. 3.11).

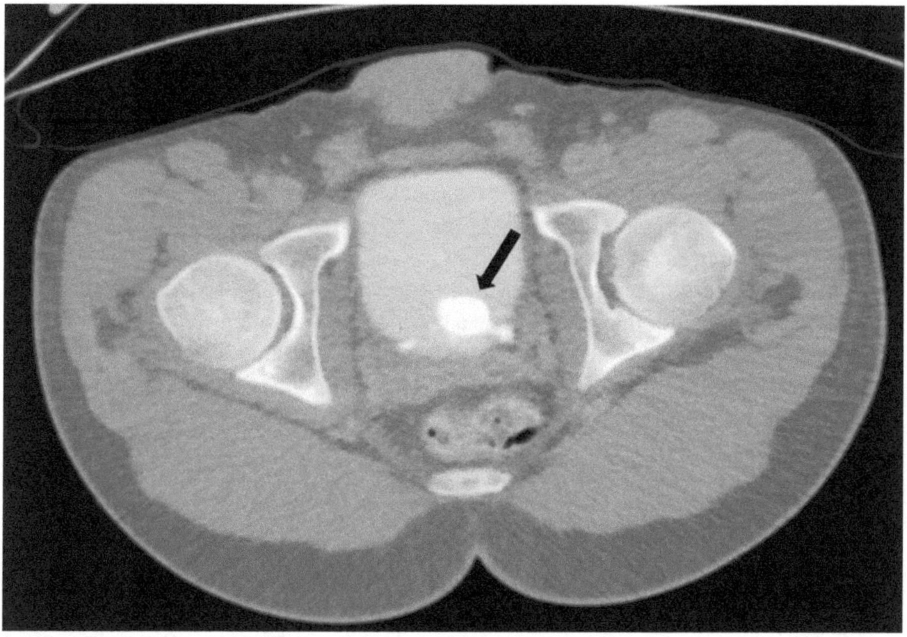

Fig. 3.11 Axial image from a CT at the level of the pelvis performed in the excretory phase demonstrates dense contrast within the corresponding mass (*arrow*) seen on US

Differential Diagnosis Ureterocele, bladder neoplasm (transitional cell carcinoma, pheochromocytoma), bladder stone.

Diagnosis and Discussion: Orthotopic ureterocele

A ureterocele is a saccular cystic outpouching of the intramural portion of the ureter. It is thought to occur secondary to failure of canalization of a congenital membrane (Chwalla's membrane) at the level of the ureteral orifice during intrauterine development. Ureteroceles can be categorized as orthotopic (20 % of cases) or ectopic (80 % of cases). Orthotopic cases are associated with single collecting system and appropriate positioning of the ureteral orifice. Ectopic ureterocele are associated with complete ureteral duplications, specifically the upper pole moiety, with the insertion site located more medial and caudal than the normally inserted lower pole collecting system. Symptoms are more commonly seen in infants with duplicated systems and include reflux, upper tract obstruction, and infection. Occasionally, ureteroceles may prolapse into the urethera resulting in bladder outlet obstruction.

Ureteroceles are often detected on voiding cystourethrography (VCUG), performed as part of a workup for infants with urinary tract infections. Early retrograde filling of the bladder demonstrates the presence of an oval or round lucency in the region of the bladder trigone. On US, the outpouching manifests as a cystic mass protruding into the bladder lumen from the region of the ureterovesicular junction (in orthotropic cases). Excretory urography images (conventional or CT) demonstrates the presence of a contrast filled mass (representing the lumen of the dilated intramural portion of the ureter) protruding into the bladder. A thin, smooth radiolucent halo, representing a double layer of ureteral and bladder wall mucosa, may be evident and is known as the "cobra head" sign.

Asymptomatic or incidentally detected ureteroceles require no treatment. A variety of surgical options are available for symptomatic cases.

Pitfalls The imaging appearance of ureteroceles on ultrasound allows differentiation from stones (echogenic foci with posterior shadowing) or a soft tissue mass. An incomplete distal ureteral obstruction from a stone or a mass may mimic an ureterocele on conventional urographic examination. Evaluation of the radiolucent halo is important as a thin smooth halo suggests a benign intravesicular ureterocele whereas a thick and irregular halo suggests the presence of a "pseudoureterocele" (with a stone or tumor being the underlying cause). This differentiation can easily be made on CT urogaphic examinations.

Teaching Point

1. Ureteroceles represent a congenital cystic dilation of the intramural portion of the distal ureter.
2. There are two types of ureteroceles: orthotopic and ectopic. Ectopic ureteroceles are more common accounting for 80 % of cases, are typically associated with the upper pole moiety of duplicated collecting system, and are usually symptomatic. Clinical presentations include reflux, obstruction and infection. Orthotopic ureteroceles account for 20 % of ureteroceles and there is anatomic insertion of the ureter.

Case 3.6

Brief Case Summary: A 65 year old man with dull flank pain and gross hematuria.

Imaging Findings On the coronal CT image (Fig. 3.12a), there is a soft tissue lesion in the left renal pelvis extending into the proximal ureter, which causes mild hydronephrosis. On MR, the T2 hypointense (arrow in Fig. 3.12b) enhancing lesion (Fig. 3.12c) expands the renal pelvis and has restricted diffusion with increased intensity on the DWI (Fig. 3.12d) and low signal on the ADC map (Fig. 3.12e).

Differential Diagnosis: Ureteral calculus, blood clot, tuberculosis.

Diagnosis and Discussion: Transitional cell carcinoma

Transitional cell carcinoma (TCC) is the most common primary malignancy involving the ureter. TCC involves the bladder most commonly due to the greatest number of transitional cells. The ureter is far less commonly involved than the renal pelvis which only in 1 % of TCCs of the urinary tract. The incidence is greater in males, mainly due to the risk factors including smoking and industrial exposure. It is a tumor of the elderly with the average age at diagnosis being 65. TCC is notorious for being multifocal with a high incidence of recurrence requiring rigorous urothelial

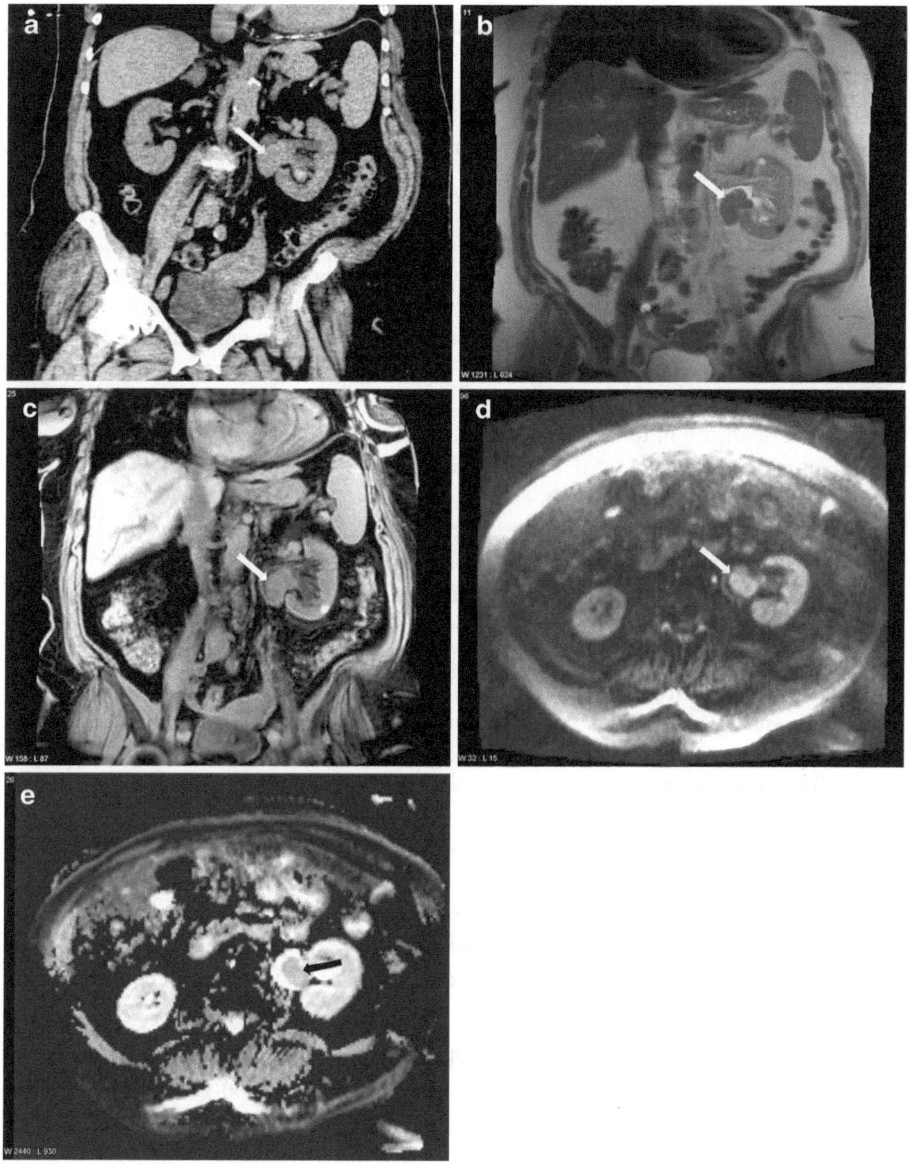

Fig. 3.12 (**a**–**e**) On the coronal CT image (**a**), there is a soft tissue lesion in the left renal pelvis extending into the proximal ureter, which causes mild hydronephrosis. (**b**) Coronal T2 weighted image shows lesion to be T2 hypointense filling the left renal pelvis (*arrow*). (**c**) Coronal T1 weighted post gadolinium enhanced image shows lesion enhancing in left renal pelvis. (**d**) On DWI, lesion appears hyperintense in left renal pelvis and shows restricted diffusion and appears low in signal on the ADC map (**e**)

surveillance. The distal ureter is more frequently affected which is thought to be due to more urinary stasis. Bilateral involvement is noted in 2–5 % of patients.

The diagnosis requires a high degree of clinical suspicion and most cases are diagnosed by imaging. Clinical presentation is relatively non-specific but hematuria and flank pain (due to obstructive hydronephrosis) are the most common symptoms.

Ultrasound is less useful in diagnosing ureteral tumors, however, it is most often the first imaging modality to in the evaluation of hydronephrosis. Intravenous pyelography can be performed and demonstrates the presence and site of obstruction. Obstruction may lead to hydronephrosis with or without hydroureter and may also result in a non-functioning kidney or a delayed nephrogram. If the collecting system is opacified, polypoid tumors may be seen as filling defects. The goblet sign, best seen on retrograde ureterography, is seen if there is partial long-standing obstruction resulting in focal dilatation of the ureter below the site of the tumor. The lesion may be eccentric or it may encircle the ureter, producing an apple-core appearance.

CT urography has largely replaced intravenous pyelography and is the mainstay for diagnosis and staging with high diagnostic accuracy. It allows for direct visualization of the obstructing soft tissue density filling defect in the ureter. Intramural lesions may infiltrate the ureteral wall; the lesion will demonstrate an irregular narrowing of the ureteral lumen with abrupt margins. Staging markers like infiltration of the periureteral tissues, multifocality and lymph node metastasis are also demonstrated.

MRI is equally efficacious in the diagnosis and staging of TCC of the ureter. MR urography can be useful in patients with bilateral obstructing tumors or in patients with unilateral functioning kidneys, where renal dysfunction may preclude intravenous CT contrast.

Treatment is a nephroureterectomy given the high risk for synchronous and metachronous tumors. In addition to the nephrectomy, the ureter and a cuff of bladder at the vesicoureteric junction are surgically excised.

Continued surveillance with cross sectional imaging is imperative for followup after a nephroureterectomy given the chance of local recurrence and distant metastases.

Pitfalls A radiolucent calculus or a blood clot may be difficult to differentiate from a polypoid tumor on intravenous pyelography, unless a typical goblet sign is demonstrated. CT may differentiate a calculus, blood clot, and tumor based on the Hounsfield units.

Teaching Points

1. The ureter is the least common site of TCC involvement in the urinary tract.
2. There is high incidence of multifocality and tumor recurrence of TCC requiring routine surveillance after surgical excision.
3. Goblet sign is typical of a polypoid tumour of the ureter on IVP; occasionally an apple core appearance can be demonstrated.
4. CT urography is better than conventional IVP for diagnosis and staging.

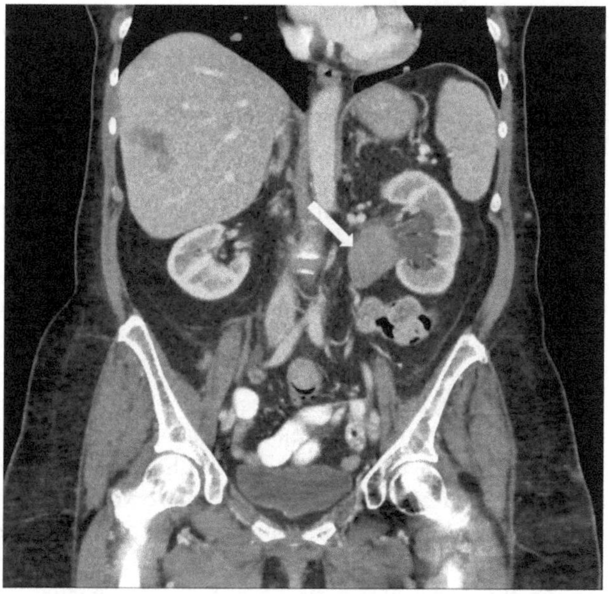

Fig. 3.13 A soft tissue lesion is seen in the left renal pelvis (*arrow*) on the contrast-enhanced CT coronal image in this patient with a history of melanoma. There is associated mild left hydronephrosis

Case 3.7

Brief Case Summary A 43 year old patient with history of melanoma complains of progressively increasing left sided flank pain. Ultrasound evaluation showed left sided hydronephrosis with a mass lesion filling the renal pelvis and proximal ureter.

Imaging Findings A soft tissue lesion is seen in the left renal pelvis (Fig. 3.13, arrow) on the contrast-enhanced CT coronal image in this patient with a history of melanoma. There is associated mild left hydronephrosis.

Differential Diagnosis Primary urothelial tumour

Diagnosis and Discussion Ureteral metastasis.

Ureteral metastasis is a very rare entity and an uncommon cause of ureteric obstruction. Breast and colorectal malignancies are the most common primary source followed by prostate, cervix, stomach and lung. There have been few reports of metastasis from pancreatic carcinoma as well.

Any part of the ureter may be affected with bilateral pathology seen in up to 25–70 % of cases. Although usually asymptomatic, ureteral metastases may present with urinary obstructive symptoms like pain, backache, UTI, dysuria, and hematuria.

The metastatic spread to the ureters occurs in one of the following ways:

Type I Infiltration of periadventitial layer by tumor cells. This is the commonest route of spread as the region as these are extensively vascularized by longitudinal vessels, which facilitates deposition of metastatic foci and promotes growth along the length of the ureter. Radiographically, there is stricture and compression of ureteral wall.

Type II Transmural involvement with tumor cells seen in muscular layer, perilymphatic and/or vascular layers. Transmural metastasis spread circumferentially, resulting in a focal stricture or ureteric obstruction similar to type I spread.

Type III mucosal and submucosal involvement with or without involvement of the muscularis. This route is less common due to lack of continuous network of blood vessels and lymphatics within the ureteral walls. Also, the lymphatic flow within the lower ureter and pelvic organs flow in opposite direction compared to urinary flow thereby creating a barrier against deposition in ureteral wall. Radiographically it presents as nodular filling defects within the lumen.

Diagnosis is made by cross sectional imaging including CT or MR urography or retrograde/conventional methods. Characteristic radiographic finding is isolated focal or diffuse narrowing of ureter with hydroureter and proximal hydronephrosis and the ureteral mucosa is generally preserved. There may be displacement of the ureter by adjacent lymphadenopathy as seen in lymphoma. CT is useful to characterize and measure the primary tumor, detect extraluminal extension, assess for lymphadenopathy, and evaluate for other metastasis. Features like encasement of ureter by metastatic deposits, periureteral fibrosis causing stenosis, or any external pressure on the ureter with secondary hydroureter/hydronephrosis are well seen on CT.

Ninety percent of patients presenting with ureteral metastasis have evidence of metastatic disease elsewhere and therefore carries a poor prognosis. Once detected, prompt management is necessary to preserve renal function which may otherwise lead to further morbidity.

Pitfalls Primary ureteric urothelial tumor simulates metastases as both may present as ureteric wall thickening. A key distinguishing point is mucosal irregularity which is common in urothelial tumors. Also the presence extraluminal extension of the ureteral wall thickening secondary to soft tissue infiltration can be seen in cases of ureteral metastases.

Teaching Point Although a rare entity, ureteric metastasis may be considered when a patient with a known primary presents with features of ureteral obstruction

Suggested Readings by Case

Case 3.1

Lautin E, Haramati N, Frager D, et al. CT diagnosis of circumcaval ureter. AJR Am J Roentgenol. 1988;150(3):591–4.

Li HZ, Ma X, Qi QL, Shi TP, et al. Retroperitoneal laparoscopic ureteroureterostomy for retrocaval ureter: report of 10 cases and literature review. Urology. 2010;76(4):873–6.

Uthappa MC, Anthony D, Allen C. Retrocaval ureter: MR appearances. Br J Radiol. 2002;75(890):177–9.

Case 3.2

Menendez V, Sala X, Alvarez-Vijande R, et al. Cystic pyeloureteritis: Review of 34 cases. Radiologic aspects and differential diagnosis. Urology. 1997;50(1):31–7.
Wasnik AP, Elsayes KM, Kaza RK, et al. Multimodality imaging in ureteric and periureteric pathologic abnormalities. AJR Am J Roentgenol. 2011;197(6):W1083–92.

Case 3.3

Spalluto LB, Woodfield CA. Ureteral pseudodiverticulosis: a unique case diagnosed by multidetector computed tomography. J Comput Assist Tomogr. 2009;33(2):286–7.
Wasserman NF, Zhang G, Posalaky IP, et al. Ureteral pseudodiverticula: frequent association with uroepithelial malignancy. AJR Am J Roentgenol. 1991;157(1):69–72.
Wasserman NF, La Pointe S, Posalaky IP. Ureteral pseudodiverticulosis. Radiology. 1985; 155(3):561–6.

Case 3.4

Kawashima A, Alleman WG, Takahashi N, et al. Imaging evaluation of amyloidosis of the urinary tract and retroperitoneum. Radiographics. 2011;31:1569–82.
Kim SH, Han JK, Lee KH, et al. Abdominal amyloidosis: spectrum of radiologic findings. Clin Radiol. 2003;58(8):610–20.
Sasatomi Y, Kiyoshi Y, Uesugi N, et al. Prognosis of renal amyloidosis: a clinicopathological study using cluster analysis. Nephron. 2001;87:42–9.

Case 3.5

Chavhan GB. The cobra head sign. Radiology. 2002;225(3):781–2.
Rowell AC, Sangster GP, Caraway JD, et al. Genitourinary imaging: part 1, congenital urinary anomalies and their management. AJR Am J Roentgenol. 2012;199(5):W545–53.

Chapter 4
Bladder and Urethra

Case 4.1

Brief Case Summary:

Case 1: 16 year old male with umbilical discharge
Case 2: Newborn male with midline mass
Case 3: 63 year old male with hematuria
Case 4: 44 year female with pelvic pain

Imaging Findings

Case 1: Sagittal transabdominal ultrasound image of the abdomen demonstrates a bilobed hypoechoic mass extending through the anterior abdominal wall, without detectable vascularity (Fig. 4.1a). Sagittal (Fig. 4.1b) and axial (Fig. 4.1c) images from a CT scan of the abdomen performed with intravenous and oral contrast demonstrate a sinus tract extending through the anterior abdominal wall at the level of the umbilicus (arrows, Fig. 4.1b, c).

Case 2: Transverse gray scale (Fig. 4.2a) and color Doppler (Fig. 4.2b) images at the level of the palpable abnormality demonstrate the presence of a hypoechoic midline mass in the region of the umbilicus without internal vascularity.

Case 3: Axial image from a CT scan of the pelvis (Fig. 4.3) performed in the excretory phase demonstrates the presence of a focal contained collection of contrast connected to the anterior bladder wall via a thin stalk.

Case 4: Sagittal image from a CT scan of the abdomen and pelvis performed with intravenous and oral contrast demonstrates the presence of an inflammatory tubular mass which is contiguous with the anterior and superior aspects of the bladder (arrow, Fig. 4.4a). Sagittal image from a CT scan of the abdomen and pelvis performed 3 years earlier demonstrates a tubular hypoattenuating mass in the same location (arrow, Fig. 4.4b).

M.G. Harisinghani, A. Rajesh, *Genitourinary Imaging: A Case Based Approach*, DOI 10.1007/978-1-4471-4772-5_4

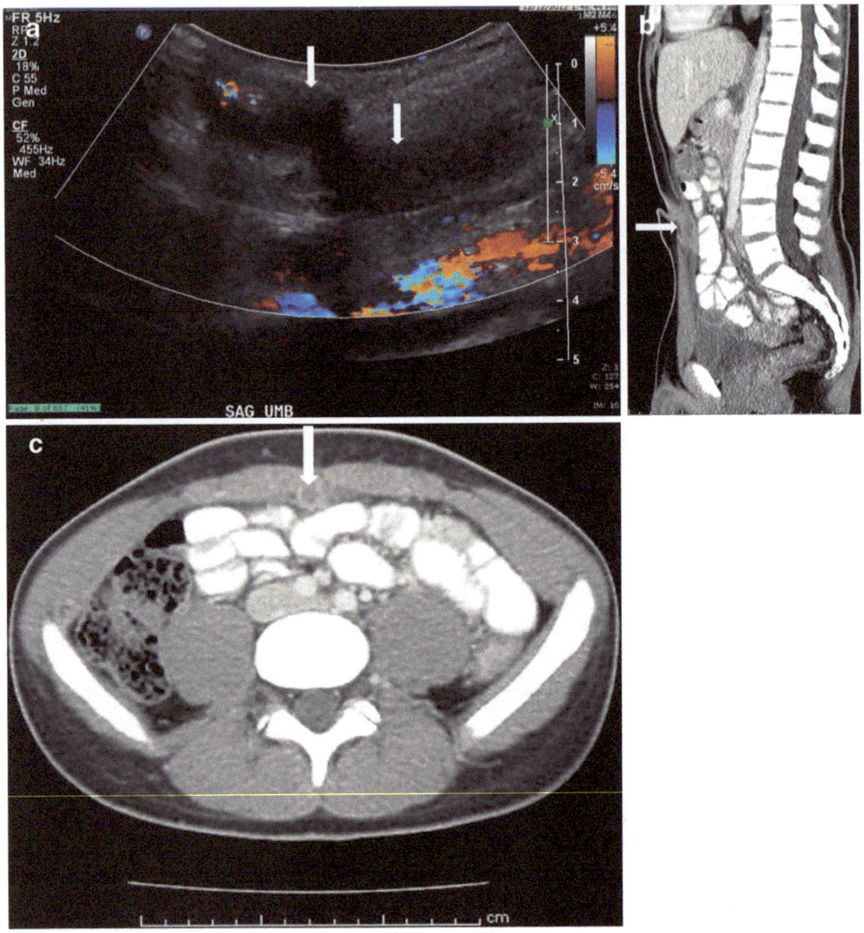

Fig. 4.1 Case 1. (**a**) Sagittal transabdominal ultrasound image of the abdomen demonstrates a bilobed hypoechoic mass extending through the anterior abdominal wall, without detectable vascularity. (**b**) Sagittal and (**c**) axial images from a CT scan of the abdomen performed with intravenous and oral contrast demonstrate a sinus tract extending through the anterior abdominal wall at the level of the umbilicus (*arrows*, **b**, **c**)

Differential Diagnosis Congenital urachal abnormalities (urachal sinus, urachal cyst, urachal diverticulum, patent urachus).

Diagnosis and Discussion:

Case 1: Umbilical-urachal sinus
Case 2: **Urachal cyst**
Case 3: **Urachal diverticulum**
Case 4: **Urachal diverticulitis**

The urachus is a midline tubular structure which connects the bladder apex to the umbilicus. It is derived in part from the allantois (an outpouching near the base of the yolk sac) as well as the ventral aspect of the cloaca. During fetal development,

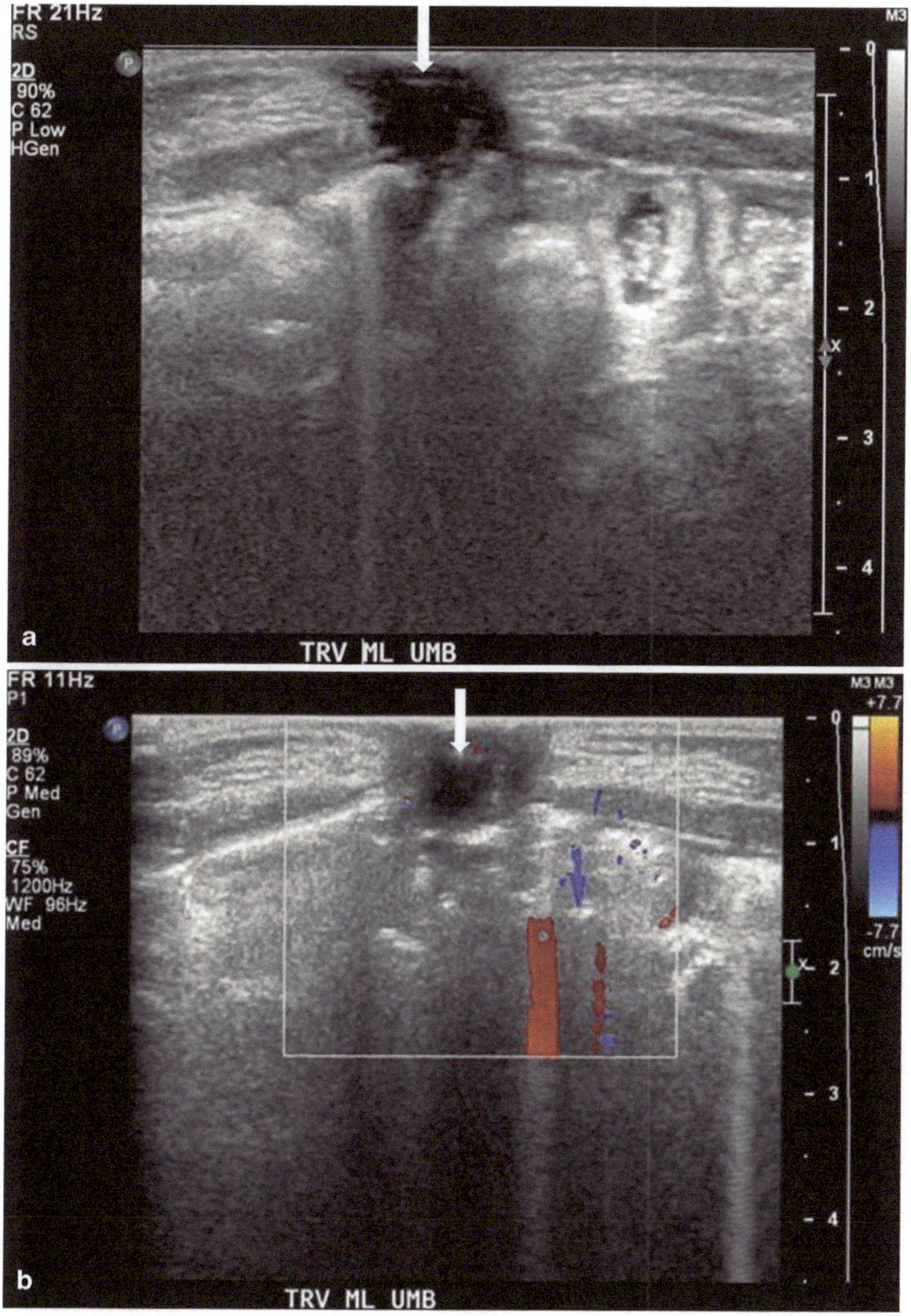

Fig. 4.2 Case 2. (**a**) Transverse gray scale and (**b**) color Doppler images at the level of the palpable abnormality demonstrate the presence of a hypoechoic midline mass (*arrow*) in the region of the umbilicus without internal vascularity

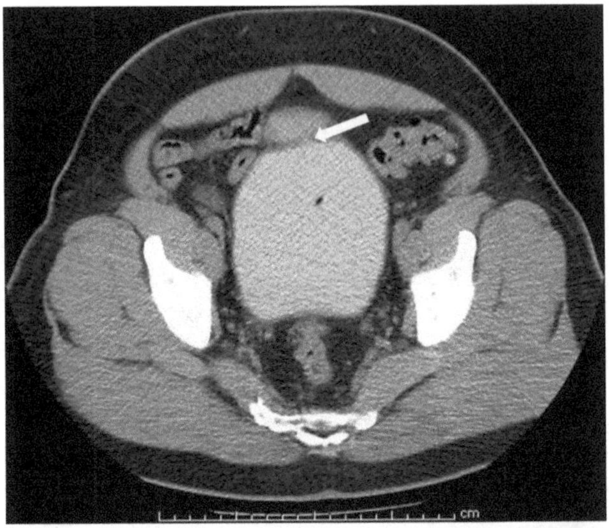

Fig. 4.3 Case 3. Axial image from a CT scan of the pelvis performed in the excretory phase demonstrates the presence of a focal contained collection of contrast connected to the anterior bladder wall via a thin stalk (*arrow*)

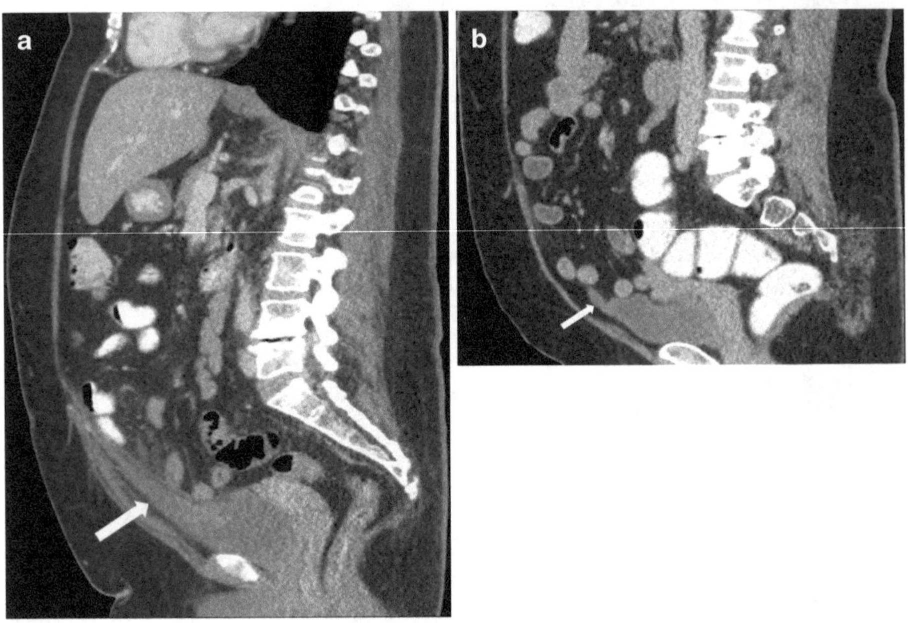

Fig. 4.4 Case 4. (**a**) Sagittal image from a CT scan of the abdomen and pelvis performed with intravenous and oral contrast demonstrates the presence of an inflammatory tubular lesion which is contiguous with the anterior and superior aspects of the bladder (*arrow*). (**b**) Sagittal image from a CT scan of the abdomen and pelvis performed 3 years earlier demonstrates a tubular hypoattenuating lesion in the same location (*arrow*)

the urachus undergoes progressive obliteration, such that it exists as a non-functioning fibrous band at the time of birth (also known as the median umbilical ligament). It is located in an extraperitoneal location, posterior to the transversalis fascia and anterior to the parietal peritoneum.

Congenital abnormalities of the urachus arise from failure of appropriate obliteration. Four discrete categories are recognized, and are as follows:

1. Patent urachus (50 %): the tract remains patent from the bladder apex to the umbilicus.
2. Umbilical-urachal sinus (approximately 15 %): the tract remains open at the umbilical end.
3. Urachal diverticulum (approximately 3–5 %): the tract remains open at the bladder apex.
4. Urachal cyst (approximately 30 %): The tract closes at the umbilical end and at the bladder apex, leaving a midline cystic structure.

The patent urachal variant is most symptomatic, often presenting as persistent urine discharge from the umbilicus after birth. Furthermore, patients with a patent urachus often have other genitourinary tract abnormalities, with posterior urethral valves or urethral atresia found in up to one third of cases. The remaining variants are often asymptomatic unless complicated by infection.

Findings can be seen on ultrasonography, particularly in the pediatric population, or may be incidental seen on CT or MRI. The presence of a midline hypoechoic mass, either isolated as in a urachal cyst, associated with the umbilicus as seen in a urachal sinus, or associated with the bladder as seen in a urachal diverticulum, is often seen. Superimposed infection may be suspected with the presence of thick, irregular walls and multiple low level internal echoes. Cross-sectional imaging demonstrates the presence of a midline fluid-attenuating mass, although the presence of hemorrhage or infection may give density values higher than simple fluid alone. The presence of a thick, irregularly enhancing rim with adjacent fat stranding suggests the presence of infection.

Incidentally discovered congenital urachal lesions in adults usually require no further treatment. Surgical excision should be considered for incidentally discovered lesions in the pediatric population given the potential risk of malignant transformation. Infected congenital urachal remnants require antibiotics with or without drainage, followed by consideration of resection, particularly in the pediatric population.

Pitfalls Patent urachus, umbilical-urachal sinus and urachal diverticula usually pose no diagnostic dilemma as a combination of ultrasound and CT or MR is sufficient for a definitive diagnosis. Urachal cysts can look similar to other benign entities such as a mesenteric cyst. An isolated cystic peritoneal metastasis from a mucinous primary may potentially have a similar appearance, although the presence of additional lesions and ascites is almost always present.

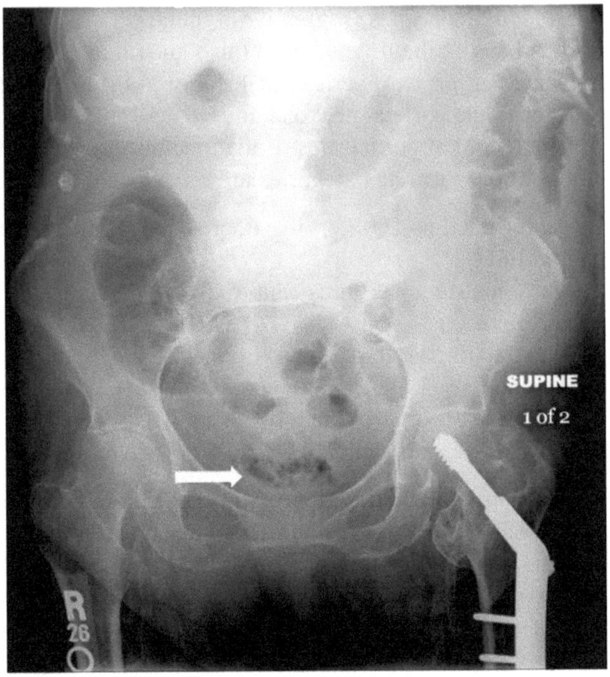

Fig. 4.5 Plain radiograph of the abdomen demonstrates multiple lucencies in the mid pelvis (*arrow*)

Teaching Points

1. The urachus connect the bladder apex to the umbilicus. It normally obliterates at the time of the birth and remains as an extra peritoneal fibrous structure called the median umbilical ligament.
2. Congenital urachal abnormalities result from a failure of this involution. Four categories exist: patent urachus, umbilical-urachal sinus, urachal diverticulum, and urachal cyst. These are most commonly asymptomatic with the exception of a patent urachus which may present with umbilical discharge.
3. Infected lesions require antibiotic with possible drainage. Incidental lesions in adults require no treatment, while most lesions regardless of symptoms in the pediatric population are excised due to the risk of potential malignant transformation.

Case 4.2

Brief Case Summary 76 year old female with abdominal pain and fever

Imaging Findings Plain radiograph of the abdomen demonstrates multiple lucencies in the mid pelvis (Fig. 4.5). A transverse gray scale US image demonstrates the presence of an abnormal curvilinear region of increased echogenicity over the

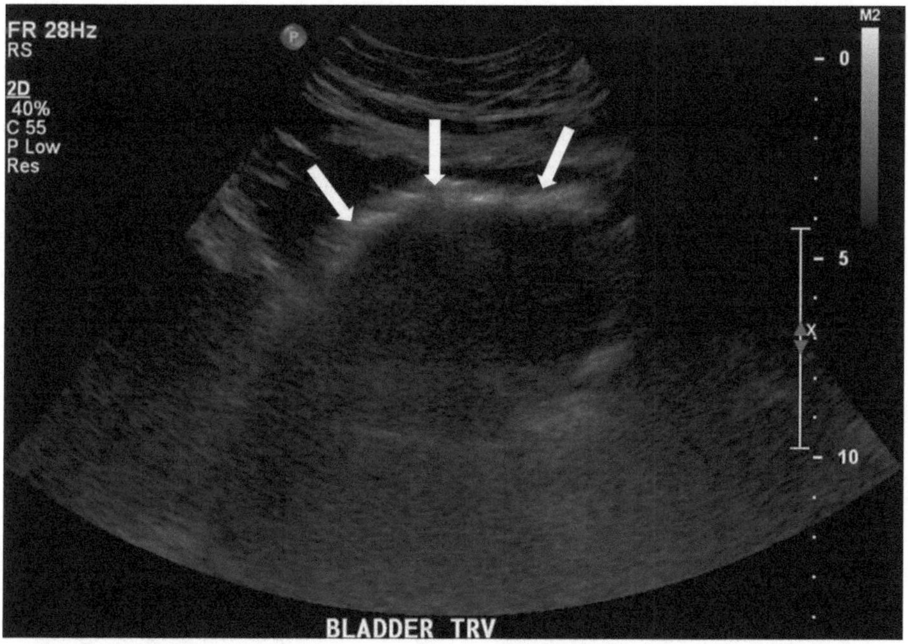

Fig. 4.6 A transverse gray scale US image demonstrates the presence of an abnormal curvilinear region of increased echogenicity (*arrows*) over the anterior aspect of the bladder with the presence of posterior "dirty" shadowing

anterior aspect of the bladder with the presence of posterior "dirty" shadowing (Fig. 4.6). Axial CT image (Fig. 4.7) at the level of the pelvis on lung windows demonstrates the presence of abnormal lucency's in the bladder wall (Fig. 4.7).

Differential Diagnosis: Emphysematous cystitis, recent Foley catheterization/cystoscopy, colovesicular or enterovesicular fistula.

Diagnosis and Discussion: Emphysematous cystitis.

Emphysematous cystitis (EC) is a rare complicated form of cystitis, characterized by the presence of air within the bladder wall and lumen. Risk factors for developing EC include the presence of diabetes, history of recurrent urinary tract infection (UTI) and conditions that promote urinary stasis such as neurogenic bladder or bladder outlet obstruction. Elderly diabetic females are the most commonly afflicted patient demographic. A variety of both bacterial and fungal organisms have been implicated, with *Escherichia coli, Enterobacter aerogenes and Klebsiella pneumonia* among the most commonly cultured organisms. The exact pathogenesis is debated but is likely related to fermentation of urinary glucose or albumin by organisms leading to the production of carbon dioxide bubbles that subsequently accumulate in the bladder lumen or wall. Clinical symptoms are typically indistinguishable from an uncomplicated UTI with patients complaining of dysuria or increased urinary frequency. Occasionally patients may be asymptomatic or present with pneumaturia.

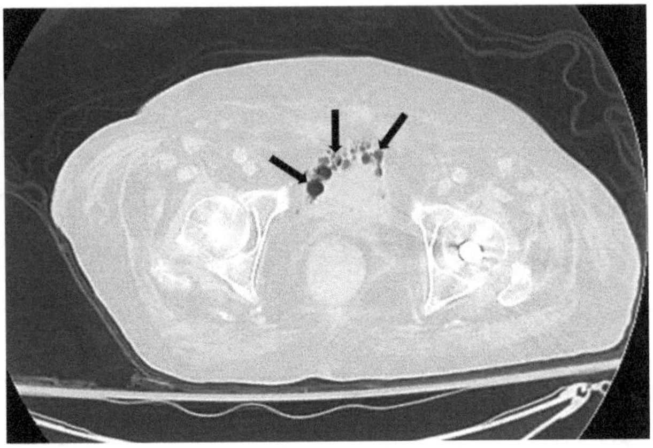

Fig. 4.7 Axial CT image at the level of the pelvis on lung windows demonstrates the presence of abnormal lucency's (*arrows*) in the bladder wall

Imaging can readily diagnosis EC and EC is often diagnosed on imaging. Conventional radiography demonstrates the presence of curvilinear lucency's in the lower midline pelvis, corresponding to the bladder wall. Bubbles of gas may also be seen within the bladder lumen itself. These findings can be confirmed sonographically where collections of intramural air are seen as curvilinear regions of increased echogenicity associated with posterior "dirty" shadowing. Further imaging with a CT examination is useful to confirm the diagnosis, as well as look for any signs of upper tract involvement, which typically require more aggressive treatment. Furthermore, CT can typically exclude other causes/mimickers of air in this location such as a colovesicular fistula or an underlying abscess.

Treatment is conservative and includes a combination of bladder drainage and antibiotics with appropriate control of comorbid conditions. Surgical options are reserved for patients who fail conservative therapy. Overall mortality rates are approximately 7 % in contrast to emphysematous pyelonephritis, where mortality rates have been reported up to 50 %.

Pitfalls Colovesicular or enterovesicular fistulas can mimic emphysematous cystitis though this distinction is usually apparent on cross-sectional imaging. A history of Crohn's disease, diverticulitis, or radiation treatment is associated with the formation of colovesicular fistulas. Foley catherization and/or recent cystoscopy can result in residual amounts of air typically isolated to the bladder lumen

Teaching Points

1. Emphysematous cystitis is a form of complicated UTI characterized by air in the bladder wall and lumen, most often seen in elderly diabetic females.
2. Treatment requires bladder drainage and antibiotics. Surgical intervention is rare, and reserved for failure of conservative management or severe infections.
3. Cross-sectional imaging should be used to detect upper tract disease which requires more aggressive treatment and is associated with a higher morbidity and to look for mimickers of EC such as colovesicular fistula.

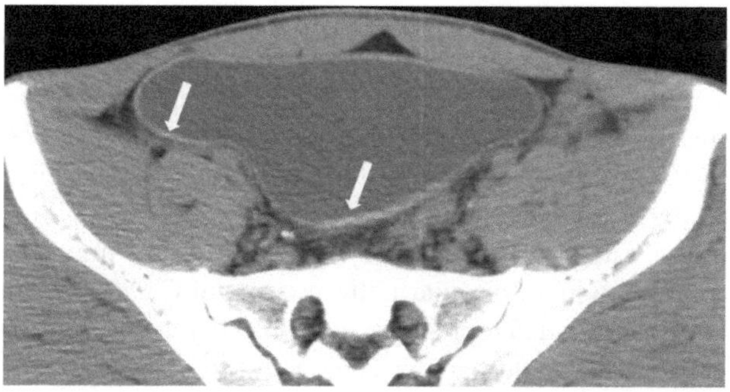

Fig. 4.8 Axial CT image through the bladder shows curvilinear calcifications (*arrows*) in the bladder wall

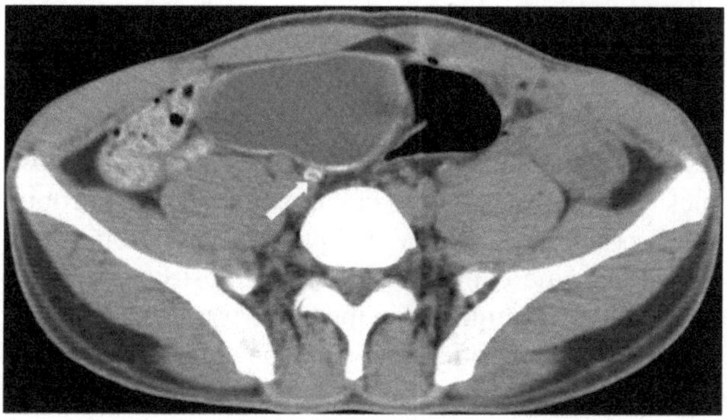

Fig. 4.9 On a more caudal axial CT image, calcifications are also seen involving the right ureter (*arrow*)

Case 4.3

Brief Case Summary: 40 year old man, an immigrant from sub-saharan country who presented with dysurea.

Imaging Findings: Axial CT image through the bladder (Fig. 4.8) shows curvilinear calcifications in the bladder wall. On a more caudal axial CT image (Fig. 4.9), calcifications are also seen involving the right ureter.

Differential Diagnosis Tuberculosis, primary carcinoma, radiation/cyclophospahamide cystitis, amyloidosis.

Diagnosis and Discussion: Bladder schistosomiasis

Genitourinary schistosomiasis is caused by Schistosoma hematobium, a parasitic fluke that is endemic in parts of Africa. Transmission is through contaminated water wherein the larvae penetrate human skin, pass through the lymphatic system, lungs, and liver at which time the larvae travel to the portal vein. After maturation, the worms travel to the pelvic veins and deposit eggs on the bladder wall inciting a granulomatous reaction causing cystitis. Calcification of these dead eggs causes the typical bladder and ureteral wall calcifications.

The clinical features depend on the stage of the disease ranging from dermatitis at the time of larvae penetration to urinary symptoms like dysuria, suprapubic pain, hematuria and local perineal lesions in later stages. Diagnosis is made by microscopic examination of urine.

Urinary bladder and lower ureters are the most commonly affected organs. Later stages of the disease may also show involvement of entire genitourinary system.

Earliest change is persistent ureteric filling on IVP followed by distal ureteric dilatation due to lack of peristalsis. Strictures with fibrosis and calcification are seen in later stages. The ureteric calcifications are fine initially followed by coalesced areas showing a circular pattern on axial CT and as linear parallel lines on X ray. Ureteritis cystica represents as bubble-like filling defects due to deposition of ova in ureteral walls and may be seen in children.

Bladder changes comprise of wall thickening, haziness initially followed by calcification, fibrosis and contraction with reduced capacity. The calcifications are more common in younger patients and can be varied in distribution. They may involve one side or both, the trigone or bladder base, and can be fine, granular, or thick and irregular. The imaging findings correlate to the pathologic course of disease with nodular wall thickening in the acute phase which progresses to a fibrotic, thick-walled bladder with calcifications in the chronic phase. Bladder decalcification is possible if there is resorption or excretion of the deposited eggs.

A syndrome called bladder neck obstruction can be seen where the eggs are deposited predominantly in the bladder trigone resulting in muscle hypertrophy followed by fibrosis and atrophy leaving elevated mucosa. This protrudes into the bladder lumen mimicking a mass like lesion causing obstruction of the bladder neck.

In children, mucosal inflammation may also cause formation of bud like masses in lamina propria which in turn may differentiate and result in cystitis cystica and cystitis glandularis.

Schistosomiasis is a strong predisposing factor for development of squamous cell carcinoma in endemic areas. It may present as a sessile focal mass or focal wall thickening arising from the trigone or lateral walls. Extravesical spread is common and carries a poor prognosis.

Pitfalls Tuberculosis affecting the urinary bladder results in a small capacity bladder with wall calcification, which can be easily differentiated from schistosomiasis where the bladder usually has a normal capacity until late chronic stages as the calcifications are submucosal. Tuberculosis generally affects the kidneys first unlike schistosomiasis which primarily affects the ureter and bladder.

Causes of bladder calcification other than schistosomiasis generally produce focal nodular calcific areas.

Teaching Points

1. Bladder and ureters are the main organs affected by the parasite schistosomiasis. The kidneys are affected only in late stage of the disease
2. Curvilinear bladder wall calcifications is the classic imaging feature of bladder schistosomiasis which is best delineated on noncontrast enhanced CT where ureteral involvement can also be assessed.
3. Chronic infection with schistosomiasis is a strong predisposing factor of squamous cell carcinoma.

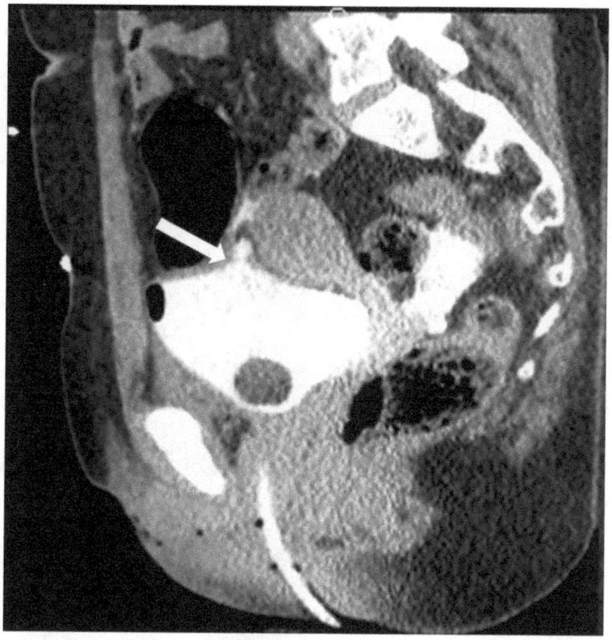

Fig. 4.10 Sagittal images from a CT cystogram demonstrates a focal bladder defect at the bladder dome with extravasation of contrast (*arrow*) between loops of bowel

Case 4.4

Brief Case Summary: Case 1 41 year old female pedestrian hit by car
Case 2 57 year old female with gross hematuria following instrumentation of urinary tract.

Imaging Findings: Sagittal (Fig. 4.10) and axial (Fig. 4.11) images from a CT cystogram demonstrates a focal bladder defect at the bladder dome with extravasation of contrast between loops of bowel. In another patient, axial (Fig. 4.12) and coronal (Fig. 4.13) images from a CT cystogram shows a focal defect in the right lateral bladder wall and extra vesicular contrast is visualized in the space of Retzius consistent with an extraperitoneal bladder rupture. Of note, both patients have a Foley catheter through which contrast was instilled for the CT cystogram.

Differential Diagnosis: Extraperitoneal bladder rupture, intraperitoneal bladder rupture, combined bladder rupture, bladder contusion, interstitial bladder injury.

Diagnosis and Discussion: Patient 1: Intraperitoneal bladder rupture
Patient 2: Extraperitoneal bladder rupture

Bladder rupture can be seen with either blunt or penetrating injuries, usually in the setting of significant polytrauma. Increased bladder distention at the time of

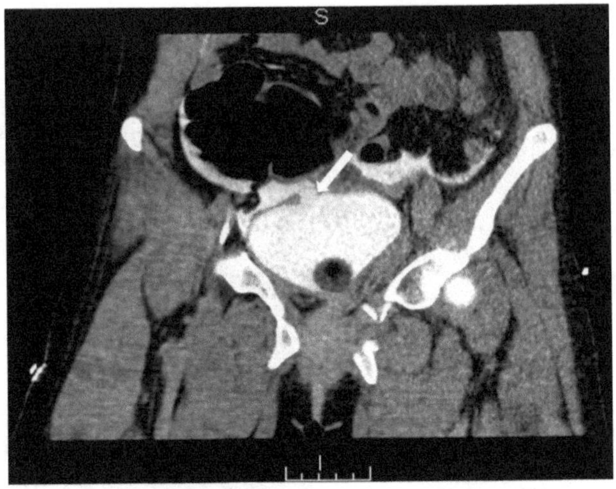

Fig. 4.11 Axial images from a CT cystogram demonstrates a focal bladder defect at the bladder dome (*arrow*) with extravasation of contrast between loops of bowel

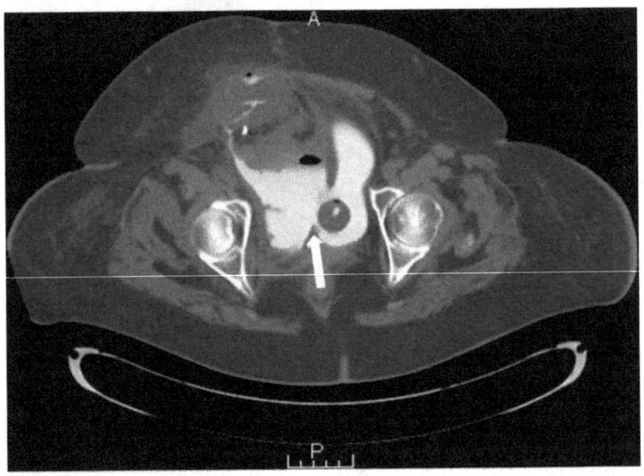

Fig. 4.12 In another patient, axial images from a CT cystogram shows a focal defect in the right lateral bladder wall (*arrow*) and extra vesicular contrast is visualized in the space of Retzius consistent with an extraperitoneal bladder rupture

injury is a predisposing factor to subsequent rupture. Bladder ruptures are classified into five different subtypes and are as follows:

- Type 1: Bladder contusion
- Type 2: Intraperitoneal rupture
- Type 3: Interstitial bladder injury
- Type 4: Extraperitoneal rupture (most common, approximately 80–90 % of cases)
- Type 5: Combined (intra and extraperitoneal rupture).

Accurate classification of the type of bladder injury is imperative for appropriate management. Intraperitoneal ruptures (type 2 and 5) require surgical management, while the remaining types may be managed conservatively with Foley catheterization.

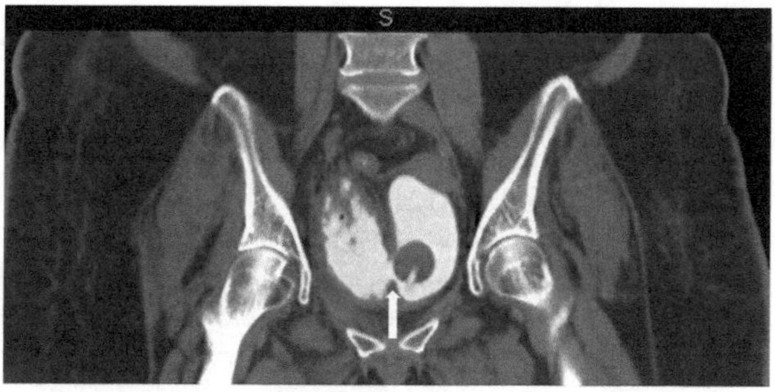

Fig. 4.13 In another patient, coronal images from a CT cystogram shows a focal defect in the right lateral bladder wall (*arrow*) and extra vesicular contrast is visualized in the space of Retzius consistent with an extraperitoneal bladder rupture

Conventional cystography has been the traditional imaging study of choice, though this has largely been replaced by CT cystography at many institutions. CT cystography requires retrograde instillation of contrast material into the bladder via a Foley catheter. Adequate bladder distention is imperative for detecting subtle leaks, with minimum volumes ranging from 250 to 300 ml. A non-contrast CT is obtained prior to the cystography in order to detect any regions of high attenuation, as can been seen with blood in the setting of trauma. A post drainage scan is usually not necessary, but can occasionally help detect small leaks.

Extraperitoneal bladder rupture can be seen in penetrating or blunt trauma, with pelvic fractures often causing direct injury to the bladder. The location of injury is typically at the bladder base. In simple extraperitoneal bladder rupture (type 4A), CT cystography demonstrates contrast extravasation into the perivesical space while complex injuries (type 4B) demonstrate extravasation beyond the perivesical space, often dissecting into various fascial planes. The appearance of contrast into the paravesical and perivesical spaces has been termed the "molar tooth" sign.

Intraperitoneal bladder rupture typically occurs at the bladder dome in the setting of a sudden increase in intravesical pressure upon a distended bladder. CT cystography demonstrates contrast extravasation into the mesentery, between loops of bowel, and extending into the paracolic gutters.

Imaging findings are normal in the setting of bladder contusion. Interstitial bladder injury (type 3) may demonstrate the presence of intramural hemorrhage and/or submuscosal dissection of contrast without extravasation beyond the serosa. Combined injuries (type 5) demonstrate features of both intra and extraperitoneal bladder ruptures.

Pitfalls Attention to technique is imperative in the accurate diagnosis of bladder ruptures which has therapeutic implications A non-contrast CT scan should always be obtained prior to the retrograde instillation of at least 300 ml to allow for adequate bladder distention. Complex extraperitoneal ruptures (type 4B) may be mistaken for intraperitoneal injuries: knowledge of the peritoneal anatomy is important to make this important distinction.

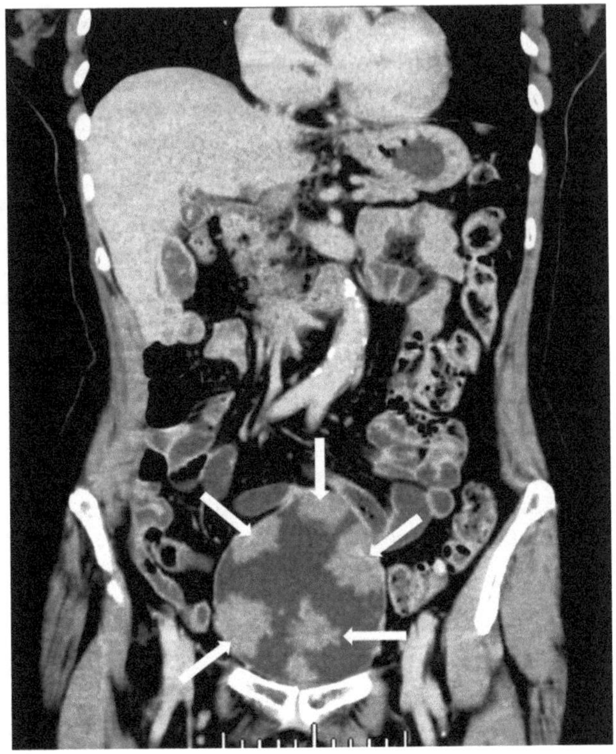

Fig. 4.14 Coronal contrast enhanced reformatted image shows multiple enhancing polypoid masses (*arrows*) projecting into the bladder lumen arising from the bladder wall

Teaching Points

1. Bladder injuries are classified into five types. For practical purposes, detection of an intraperitoneal component to the injury is the most important finding as this requires surgical treatment.
2. CT cystography has replaced conventional cystography as the imaging study of choice. A non-contrast exam and adequate distention of the bladder with at least 300 ml of contrast is necessary for an accurate exam.
3. Knowledge of the peritoneal anatomy is important to differentiate a complex extraperitoneal rupture, which is treated conservatively, from an intraperitoneal bladder rupture.

Case 4.5

Brief Case Summary Forty-nine year old male with hematuria.

Imaging Findings Coronal contrast enhanced reformatted image shows multiple enhancing polypoid masses projecting into the bladder lumen arising from the bladder wall (Fig. 4.14).

Differential Diagnosis Squamous cell carcinoma, adenocarcinoma.

Diagnosis and Discussion: Transitional Cell Carcinoma bladder.

TCC most commonly occurs in the bladder and of all bladder tumors, TCC is the most common. It mostly occurs in older patients and is three times more common in males. Smoking has the strongest correlation with smokers being five times more likely to develop TCC than non smokers.

The hallmark of TCC is synchronous and metachronous lesions. Tumors can be within the bladder, renal pelvis, or ureter, and given the high incidence of synchronous and metachronous lesions, complete imaging of the entire urinary tract is essential. Cystoscopy with biopsy is the gold standard for the diagnosis of bladder TCC and imaging is used to diagnose upper tract disease, assess local disease and distant metastases.

CT is usually the first imaging modality in a case of hematuria where TCC manifests as multiple enhancing masses within the bladder. Delayed urography images are the best imaging modality to evaluate for upper urinary tract lesions that are seen as irregular filling defects with possible tumor infiltration into the renal parenchyma. On MRI, tumors are T1 iso- to hypointense and T2 iso to hyperintense relative to renal parenchyma.

Tumors arising within bladder diverticula have a poorer prognosis due their propensity to spread early as diverticula lack a muscular wall which acts as a barrier to tumor spread.

Treatment of TCC is total nephroureterectomy and bladder cuff excision given the high incidence of multifocality.

Pitfalls Imaging of the upper urinary tract is crucial given the propensity of TCC to have synchronous and metachronous lesions. TCC cannot be differentiated from squamous cell carcinoma (SCC) or adenocarcinoma on imaging but patient history is helpful. SCC is less common and occurs in the setting of chronic irritation from bladder calculi, indwelling catheter, and schistosomiasis infection. Adenocarcinoma is the least common subtype and occurs either in bladder or within a urachal remnant.

Teaching Point

1. TCC is associated with synchronous and metachronous lesions and evaluation of the entire urinary tract is essential.
2. MRI provides better soft tissue contrast and is superior to CT in evaluation of muscle invasion however, cystoscopy with biopsy is still necessary to diagnose bladder TCC the gold standard to evaluate TCC
3. Tumors in diverticula have a poorer prognosis and might be inaccessible by cystoscopy. Imaging can be useful in this particular clinical setting.

Case 4.6

Brief Case Summary Thirty-five year old man with uncontrolled hypertension.

Imaging Findings On the axial contrast enhanced CT image (Fig. 4.15), there is nodular thickening of the anterior bladder wall (arrows). The I-123 MIBG whole

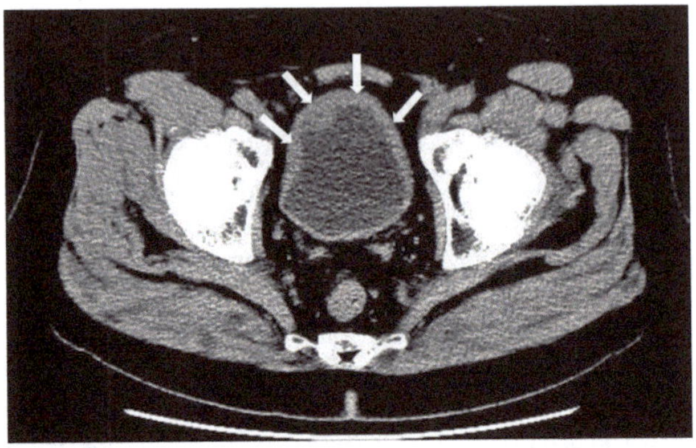

Fig. 4.15 On the axial contrast enhanced CT image, there is nodular thickening of the anterior bladder wall (*arrows*)

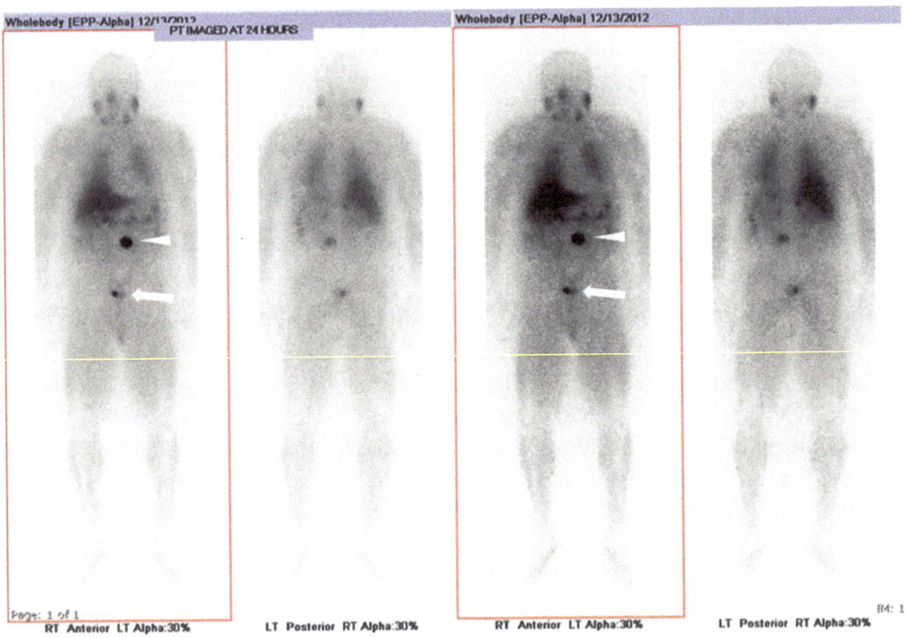

Fig. 4.16 The I-123 MIBG whole body scans demonstrates two foci of tracer uptake, one in the mid abdomen (*arrowhead*) and the second in the pelvis (*arrows*)

body scans (Fig. 4.16) demonstrates two foci of tracer uptake, one in the mid abdomen (arrowhead) and the second in the pelvis (arrow).

Differential Diagnosis Bladder transitional cell carcinoma, cystitis

Diagnosis and Discussion: Bladder pheochromocytoma

Bladder pheochromocytomas are rare tumors accounting for less than 1 % of paragangliomas and less than 0.05 % percent of bladder tumors. They arise from paraganglion chromaffin cells in sympathetic nervous system present in all layers of bladder wall. They are seen usually between third and fifth decades and affect men and women equally. They are seen in the submucosal or intramural layers, commonly in the bladder trigone or dome of bladder. The clinical features can be either due to release of catecholamines or the mass effect caused depending on the location of tumor. Characteristic symptoms are hypertension and hematuria accompanied by tremors, palpitations, sweating, and headache following micturition or bladder distension. Ten percent of the tumors may be malignant and present with metastasis to regional lymph nodes or distant organs. Tumors of the trigone can rarely present as urinary retention.

Imaging modalities include IVP, Ultrasound, CT, MRI and MIBG scans.

IVP may show nonspecific filling defects in the bladder. Ultrasound demonstrates bladder pheochromocytomas as sharply defined heterogeneously hypoechoic lesions. Due to their submucosal and intramural location, the overlying mucosa appears continuous and smooth. Internally there may be foci of hemorrhage and necrosis. Doppler US shows abundant internal vascularity. On CT, the lesions are seen as hypervascular enhancing mass owing to the rich capillary network, which may have heterogeneous enhancement due to hemorrhage and necrosis. Ten percent may show calcifications. Due to the improved tissue contrast, MR is better than CT for tumor characterization. Pheochromotyctomas appear enhancing hypo- to isointense on T1 and have a typical bright appearance on T2, however, approximately one-third of cases are not T2 hyperintense. MIBG scans are used for the detection of extraadrenal pheochromocytomas and to evaluate for metastases with a high degree of sensitivity (80–90 %) and specificity (90–100 %). The diagnosis of pheochromocytoma is made by detecting elevated urine levels of vanillylmandelic acid (VMA).

Preoperative diagnosis of pheochromocytoma is important so that adequate medical therapy is administered with α and β-adrenergic blockers before, during, and after surgery. Surgical excision is performed for both benign and malignant pheochromocytoma given the metastatic potential and long-term, continued surveillance imaging is necessary.

Pitfalls Transitional cell carcinoma can be differentiated from bladder pheochromocytoma on CT as TCC tend to be hypovascular whereas pheochromocytomas are hypervascular.

Teaching Points

1. Most (90 %) of pheochromocytomas arise from the adrenal medulla and 10 % are extraadrenal with most arising from the Organ of Zuckerkandl or near the urinary bladder.
2. CT and MR findings reflect the hypervascular nature of pheochromocytoma owing to their rich capillary network. Typical imaging characteristics are a very T2 hyperintense lesion with bright enhancement.
3. I-123 MIBG is the best imaging modality to detecte extraadrenal tumors and metastatic disease in a malignant pheochromocytoma.

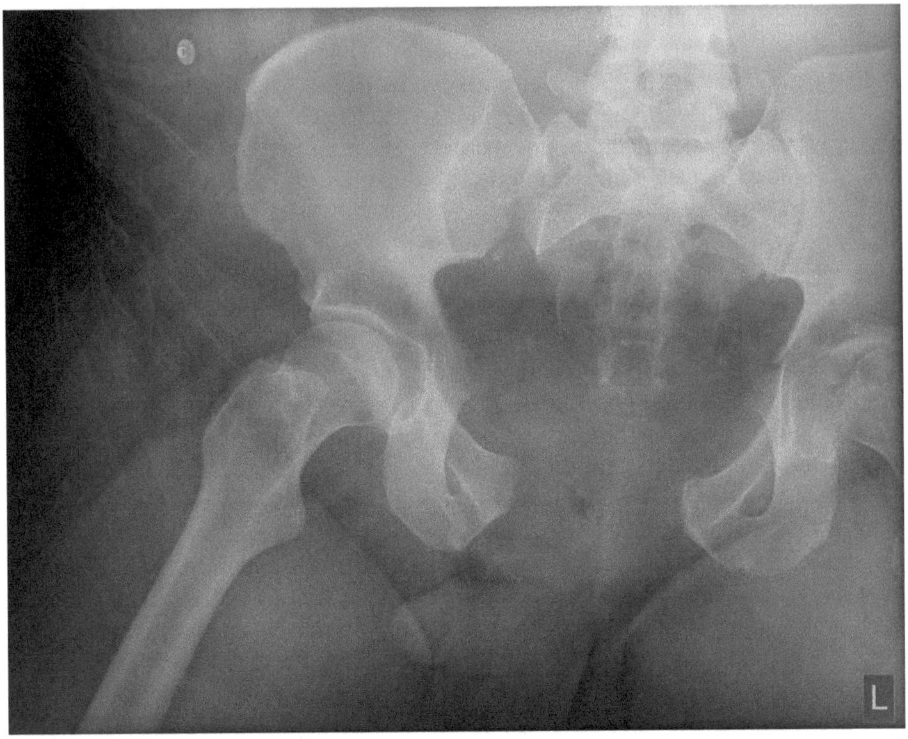

Fig. 4.17 An open-book pelvic fracture is seen on the radiograph with severe diastasis of the pubic symphysis and widening and separation of the right sacroiliac joint

Case 4.7

Brief Case Summary A 45 year old male with history of motor vehicle accident.

Imaging Findings An open-book pelvic fracture is seen on the radiograph (Fig. 4.17) with severe diastasis of the pubic symphysis and widening and separation of the right sacroiliac joint. Axial (Fig. 4.18a) and saggital (Fig. 4.18b) images from a CT cystogram demonstrate a linear focus of extraluminal contrast along the anterior prostatic urethral consistent with a urethral injury.

Differential Diagnosis Bladder injury

Diagnosis and Discussion: Urethral injury

Urethral injury is a common finding in pelvic trauma and carries significant morbidity due to possible complications like urethral stricture, incontinence and impotence. Accurate diagnosis and triage are crucial to minimize complications.

The male urethra can be divided into anterior and posterior parts. The posterior urethra is composed of the membranous and prostatic urethra while the anterior urethra is composed of the penile and bulbar urethra. Posterior urethral injuries

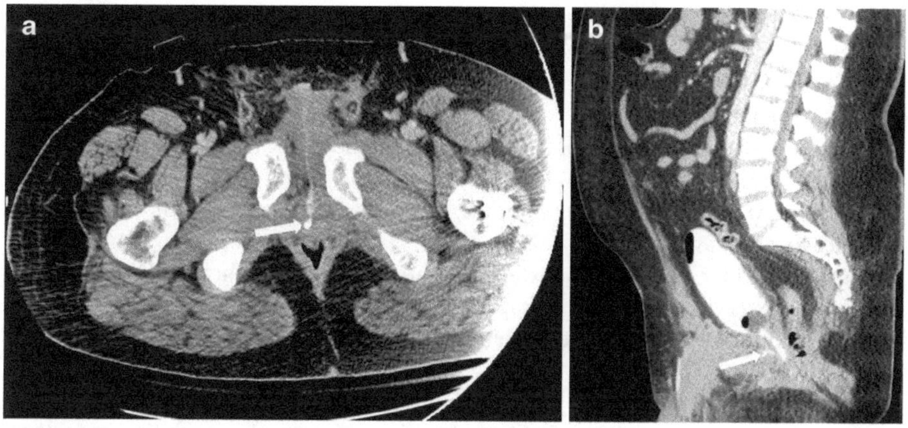

Fig. 4.18 Axial (**a**) and saggital (**b**) images from a CT cystogram demonstrate a linear focus of extraluminal contrast (*arrow*) along the anterior prostatic urethra consistent with a urethral injury

are common owing to its restricted mobility and are usually associated with pelvic fractures. Anterior urethral injuries are associated with straddling injuries wherein the urethra is pressed against the pubis. Pelvic fractures are rarely seen in anterior urethral injuries. Injury to the urethra must be suspected in a trauma patient presenting with pelvic fracture, hematuria, blood at the meatus, inability to void, and scrotal or perineal hematoma/edema. The female urethra anatomy is less complex and female urethral injury is more rare, accounting for less than 6 % of female pelvic fractures.

The imaging modality of choice is retrograde urethrogram. The correct technique requires patient to be placed in a 30–45° oblique position with the penis stretched away from the legs. In case of patients who sustain polytrauma, CT is the study used to assess for other traumatic injuries but a urethrogram should be performed if a urethral injury is clinically suspected. If a transurethral catheter had been previously placed, then the catheter should remain in place until the presence of a urethral injury has been evaluated. A pericatheter technique should be utilized where either a small gauge pediatric catheter is placed adjacent to the indwelling urethral catheter or a small bore feeding tube can be inserted along the urethral catheter.

Accurate classification of urethral injuries is imperative for effective treatment. The classification system by Goldman and colleagues takes into account the anatomical location to grade injuries, specifically whether the injury is near the urogenital diaphragm/external sphincter. Classification of urethral injury is as follows:

Grade I- rupture of puboprostatic ligament causing stretching or elongation of the posterior urethra with no tear. RUG shows stretched but intact urethra. No contrast extravasation is seen and continuity with the bladder is maintained. On CT a distance of 2 cm between the prostatic apex and urogenital diaphragm is specific for grade I injury

Grade II -disruption proximal to urogenital diaphragm with an intact membranous urethra. Contrast extravasation is seen in extraperitoneal pelvis above the urogenital diaphragm. The intact diaphragm restricts contrast extravasation into the perineum.

Grade III - disruption of membranous urethra extending beyond the urogenital diaphragm into anterior urethra. RUG shows contrast extravasation in the extraperitoneal pelvis and in the perineum, the extravasated amount depending upon the exact location and degree of tear.

Grade IV- bladder neck injury extending into posterior urethra. RUG may show contrast extravasation in the extraperitonal pelvis near the proximal urethra. This type of injury carries a risk of damage to internal sphincter thereby affecting continence.

Grade IVa- bladder base injury simulating a grade IV injury where there is periurethral contrast extravasation from bladder in periurethral, simulating a urethral tear. Differentiation between the two is important as the management of Type IV injury is surgical. Dynamic RUG under fluoroscopic guidance helps in differentiation.

Grade V- isolated injury to anterior urethra. RUG shows contrast extravasation below the level of urogenital diaphragm near anterior urethra and is confined to the anterior urethra.

Antegrade and retrograde urethrogaphy may be performed simultaneously to determine the length of the defect in case of complete urethral transaction. Additional findings seen on CT are obscuration of urogenital fat planes, hematoma in ischiocavernous and obturator internus muscles and obscuration/distortion of prostatic contour and bulbocavernous muscle.

Pitfalls Type IV and IVa injuries may be radiologically indistinguishable and differentiation requires careful evaluation with dynamic fluoroscopy. Reflux of contrast into Cowper's duct may mimic extravasation from anterior urethra. Evaluation of subsequent films may help in distinguishing Foley catheters in the urethra during a CT may prevent contrast extravasation in the presence of a urethral injury thus leading to false negative result.

Teaching Point

1. Anatomical localization of the urogenital diaphragm is essential to determine whether the anterior or posterior urethra is injured, which has a great impact on the management.
2. In order to minimize the morbidity associated with traumatic urethral injuries, accurate and prompt detection and appropriate treatment is essential.
3. Retrograde urethrogram is the imaging study of choice to diagnose and classify ureteral injuries. RUG are essential for accurate diagnosis and require familiarity with urethral anatomy and the classification system along with the surgical implications.

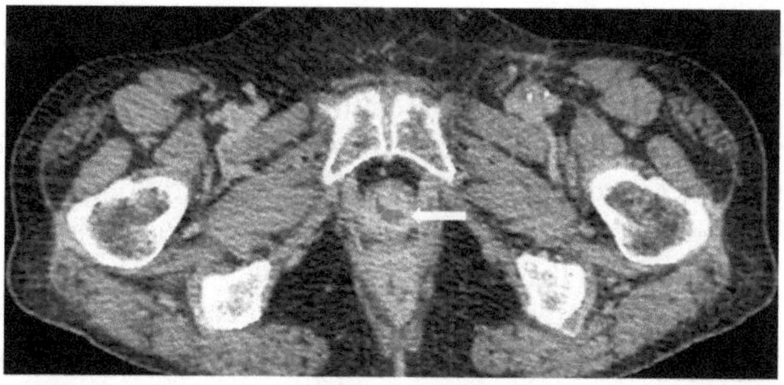

Fig. 4.19 Axial noncontrast CT through the pelvis shows a low density lesion located posterior to the urethra (*arrow*)

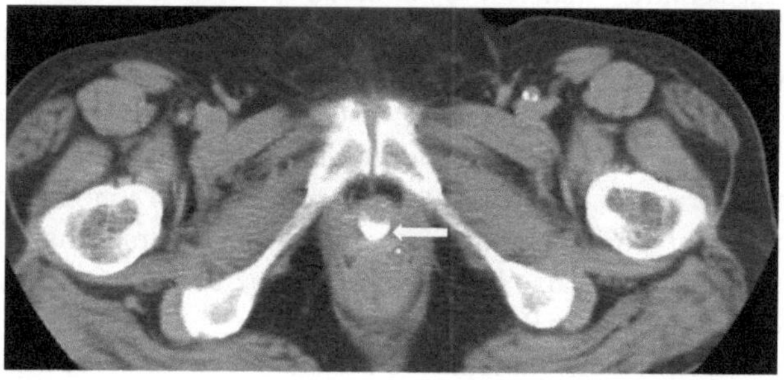

Fig. 4.20 On the axial delayed CT, there is contrast opacification of the collection (*arrow*) confirming continuity to the urethra

Case 4.8

Brief Case Summary A 60 year old female with history of dribbling

Imaging Findings Axial noncontrast CT (Fig. 4.19) through the pelvis shows a low density lesion located posterior to the urethra (arrow). On the axial delayed CT (Fig. 4.20) there is contrast opacification of the collection (arrow) confirming continuity to the urethra.

Differential Diagnosis vaginal wall cyst, Skene gland abscess, Skene duct cyst, Bartholin gland cyst/ abscess.

Diagnosis and Discussion Urethral diverticulum (UD) is a focal outpouching extending from and is contiguous with the true urethral lumen. The diagnosis is made far more commonly in females. It occurs in up to 6 % of females, especially those with stress urinary incontinence. The pathophysiology leading to the formation of a UD is still hypothetical, with the most accepted theory being rupture of dilated and infected periurethral glands, which results in pseudodiverticulum formation. In males, the causative factors include urethral stricture, chronic indwelling urethral catheters and post surgery for complex anorectal anomalies. UD can be narrow or wide necked, uni or multiloculated. The location is posterolateral to the urethra and anterior to the vagina.

The classical symptomatology includes the "three Ds" (dysuria, postvoid dribbling, and dyspareunia). On examination, an anterior vaginal wall mass may be palpated and compression of this mass may result in purulent discharge from the urethra. Urethral diverticula may be complicated by infection, stone formation (up to 10 % of patients), and malignant degeneration.

The radiological report of a UD should mention the number, location, size, configuration, and the position of the neck of the diverticulum. The diagnostic finding is a cystic periurethral lesion communicating with the urethral lumen. VCUG has a sensitivity of 65 % and diagnoses most of the wide-necked diverticula. A Double balloon (positive pressure) urethrography is more sensitive than VCUG and facilitates contrast material to be forced into a diverticular ostium by creating a relatively closed urethral system. However, this technique is rarely used due to practical difficulties.

Cross-sectional imaging, both CT and MRI, are more useful in the diagnosis of UD and excluding other periurethral pathologies. MRI, in particular, has the added advantage of high spatial resolution with no ionizing radiation. At CT, a voiding urethographic technique is required for accurate diagnosis of a UD. Transvaginal ultrasound has also been reported to be useful in the diagnosis of UD with efficacy comparable to MRI.

Symptomatic patients are treated operatively, the most common procedure being transvaginal diverticulectomy. A VCUG is performed 2 weeks after surgery to evaluate for urethral healing and presence of postoperative complications.

Pitfalls Narrow-necked or noncommunicating diverticula are difficult to differentiate from other periurethral/ vaginal cysts like the Gartner cyst, Skene gland cyst or Bartholin cyst. A helpful finding is the location, which is classically posterolateral to the mid-urethra.

Teaching Points

1. Urethral diverticulum is far more common in females than males.
2. The diagnostic finding is a cystic periurethral lesion communicating with the urethral lumen.
3. Diagnostic modalities include VCUG, transvaginal sonography, CT voiding urethrography and MRI, the latter being the most specific and sensitive.
4. The radiological report should mention the number, location, size, configuration and the position of the neck of the diverticulum

Case 4.9

Brief Case Summary Fifty-five year old female with hematuria and pain on micturition.

Imaging Findings Axial (Fig. 4.21) and sagittal (Fig. 4.22) postgadolinium images demonstrate a well defined heterogeneously enhancing mass centered in the urethra which is heterogeneously hyperintense on the T2 images (Fig. 4.23).

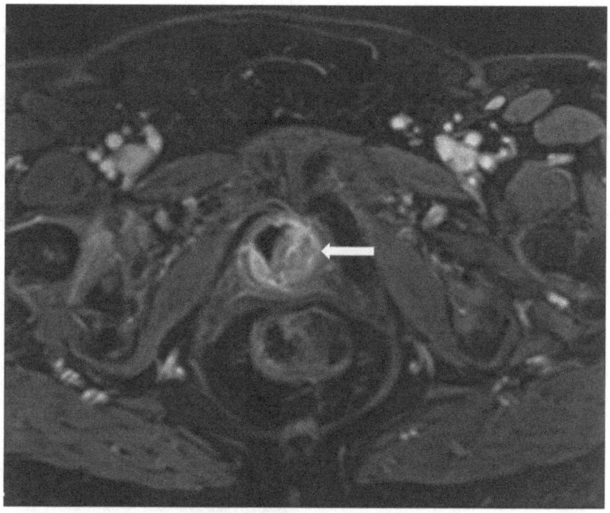

Fig. 4.21 Axial postgadolinium images demonstrate a well defined heterogeneously enhancing mass (*arrow*) centered in the urethra which is heterogeneously hyperintense on the T2 images (see Fig. 4.23)

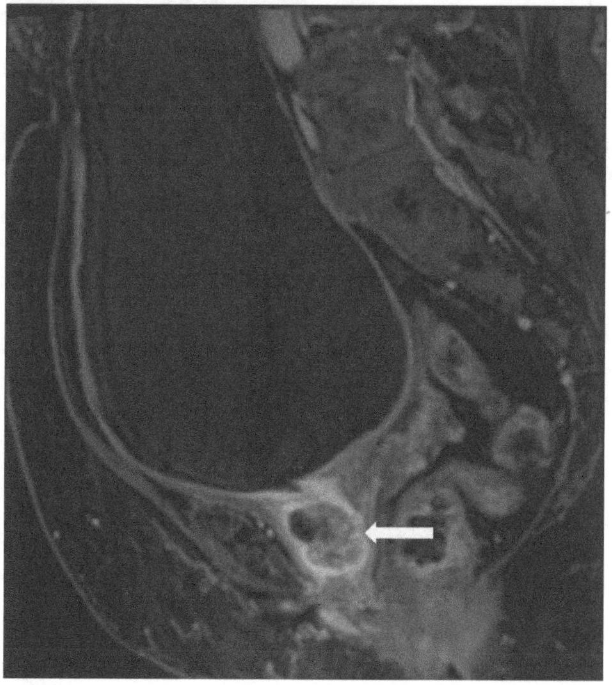

Fig. 4.22 Sagittal postgadolinium images demonstrate a well defined heterogeneously enhancing mass (*arrow*) centered in the urethra which is heterogeneously hyperintense on the T2 images (see Fig. 2.23)

Differential Diagnosis Secondary spread from prostate, rectum or bladder TCC, amyloidosis, urethral bulking agents.

Diagnosis and Discussion: Urethral carcinoma

Urethral carcinoma is a rare malignancy and has a male to female ratio of 1:4. Patients are usually over 50 years of age. Chronic HPV infection, presence of

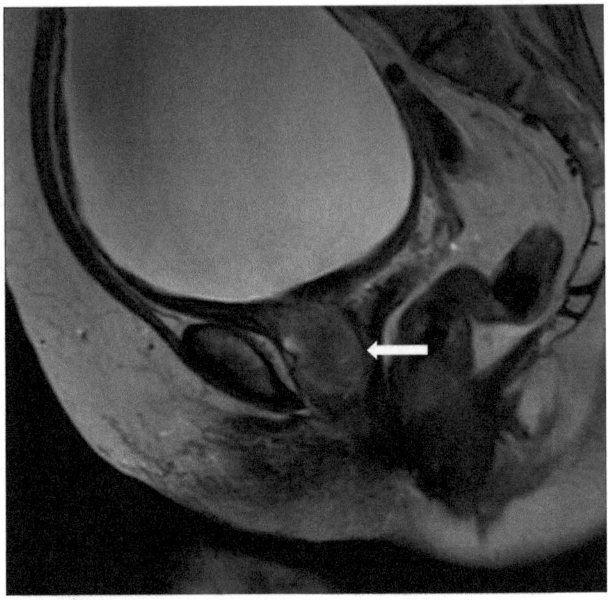

Fig. 4.23 T2 images

urethral diverticula, sexual activity, and child birth are risk factors, these risk factors differ from those of the male counterparts. A majority of urethral carcinomas (95 %) are epithelial carcinomas with squamous cell carcinoma accounting for 80 % of the subtypes followed by transitional cell carcinoma (15 %) and adenocarcinoma (5 %).

In males, the bulbomembranous urethra is most commonly affected (60 %) while the penile and prostatic urethra are involved in 30 and 10 % of cases, respectively. Approximately half of urethral carcinomas in females involve the anterior urethra (distal one-third) of the urethra while the other half involve the entire urethra which is defined as the proximal 2/3rd and/or the distal urethra

On imaging, a perineal mass with irregular narrowing of the urethra is seen. Retrograde urethrograms, voiding cystourethrograms, CT and MR can be used for evaluation of a perineal mass. Urethral narrowing that is irregular with filling defects is seen on RUG and VCUG. CT is limited in anatomic localization and soft tissue characterization given the limited spatial and contrast resolution compared to MR. On MRI, the perineal mass is low signal on T1 and T2 images and the normal "target appearance"(hypointense mucosa and outer muscular layer and hyperintense submucosa.) of urethra on T2 axial images is lost. MR is the most sensitive and specific modality for diagnosing urethral carcinoma, assessing involvement of surrounding organs and corpus cavernosa, and for staging.

Pitfalls Urethral metastases is usually secondary to contiguous spread from surrounding organs, specifically the prostate gland, rectum, and bladder. MR is very useful to assess surrounding organs and to accurately differentiate metastases from adjacent organs from primary urethral carcinoma. Urethral bulking agents can be confused for urethral carcinoma. These agents are injected for urinary incontinence and are composed of a collagen suspension which is hyperintense on T2 if recently injected and gradually becomes isointense with time. Coated microbeads are T2 hypointense- injected bulking agents do not enhance.

Teaching Points

1. Urethral carcinoma are rare malignancies and occur more frequently in women.
2. MRI is the imaging modality of choice for diagnosing urethral carcinoma, assessing involvement of surrounding organs and corpus cavernosa, and for staging

Suggested Readings by Case

Case 4.1

Rowell AC, Sangster GP, Caraway JD, et al. Genitourinary imaging: part 1, congenital urinary anomalies and their management. AJR Am J Roentgenol. 2012;199(5):W545–53.

Yu JS, Kim KW, Lee HJ, et al. Urachal remnant diseases: spectrum of CT and US findings. Radiographics. 2001;21(2):451–61.

Case 4.2

Levenson R, Mai-Lan HO. Imaging of genitourinary emergencies. Emergency radiology. New York: Springer; 2013. p. 85–98.

Thomas AA, Lane BR, Thomas AZ, et al. Emphysematous cystitis: a review of 135 cases. BJU Int. 2007;100(1):17–20.

Case 4.3

Shebel HM, Elsayes KM, Abou El Atta HM, et al. Genitourinary schistosomiasis: life cycle and radiologic-pathologic findings. Radiographics. 2012;32(4):1031–46.

Wong-you-cheong JJ, Woodward PJ, Manning MA, et al. From the archives of the AFIP: inflammatory and nonneoplastic bladder masses: radiologic-pathologic correlation. Radiographics. 2006;26(6):1847–68.

Case 4.4

Ishak C, Kanth N. Bladder trauma: multidetector computed tomography cstography. Emerg Radiol. 2011;18(4):321–7.

Matlock KA, Tyroch AH, Kronfol ZN, et al. Blunt traumatic bladder rupture: a 10-year prospective. Am Surg. 2013;79(6):589–93.

Vaccaro JP, Brody JM. CT cystography in the evaluation of major bladder trauma1. Radiographics. 2000;20(5):1373–81.

Case 4.5

Cheung G, Sahai A, Billia M, et al. Recent advances in the diagnosis and treatment of bladder cancer. BMC Med. 2013;11:13.

Hafeez S, Huddart R. Advances in bladder cancer imaging. BMC Med. 2013;11:104.

Lawrentschuk N, Lee ST, Scott AM. Current role of PET, CT, MR for invasive bladder cancer. Curr Urol Rep. 2013;14(2):84–9.

Vikram R, Sandler CM, Ng CS. Imaging and staging of transitional cell carcinoma: part 1, lower urinary tract. AJR Am J Roentgenol. 2009;192(6):1481–7.

Wong-You-Cheong JJ, Wagner BJ, Davis CJ. Transitional cell carcinoma of the urinary tract: radiologic-pathologic correlation. Radiographics. 1998;18(1):123–42.

Case 4.6

Baez JC, Jagannathan JP, Krajewski K, et al. Pheochromocytoma and paraganglioma: imaging characteristics. Cancer Imaging. 2012;12(1):153–62.

Mallat F, Hmida W, Slama A, et al. Unexpected small urinary bladder pheochromocytoma: a non-specific presentation. Case Rep Urol. 2013;2013:496547.

Vyas S, Kalra N, Singh SK, et al. Pheochromocytoma of urinary bladder. Indian J Nephrol. 2011;21(3):198–200.

Case 4.7

Ingram MD, Watson SG, Skippage PL, et al. Urethral injuries after pelvic trauma: evaluation with urethrography. Radiographics. 2008;28(6):1631–43.

Rosenstein DI, Alsikafi NF. Diagnosis and classification of urethral injuries. Urolo Clin North Am. 2006;33(1):3019.

Case 4.8

Chou CP, Levenson RB, Elsayes KM, et al. Imaging of female urethral diverticulum: an update. Radiographics. 2008;28(7):1917–30.

Hahn WY, Israel GM, Lee VS. MRI of female urethral and periurethral disorders. AJR Am J Roentgenol. 2004;182(3):677–82.

Kawashima A, Sandler CM, Wasserman NF, et al. Imaging of urethral disease: a pictorial review. Radiographics. 2004;24 Suppl 1:S195–216.

Prasad SR, Menias CO, Narra VR, et al. Cross-sectional imaging of the female urethra: technique and results. Radiographics. 2005;25(3):749–61.

Case 4.9

Del Gaizo A, Silva AC, Lam-Himlin DM, et al. Magnetic resonance imaging of solid urethral and peri-urethral lesions. Insights Imaging. 2013;4:461–9.

Hickey N, Murphy J, Herschorn S. Carcinoma in a urethral diverticulum: magnetic resonance imaging and sonographic appearance. Urology. 2000;55:588–9.

Surabhi VR, Menias CO, George V, et al. Magnetic resonance imaging of female urethral and periurethral disorders. Radiol Clin North Am. 2013;51:941–53.

Tunitsky E, Goldman HB, Ridgeway B. Periurethral mass: a rare and puzzling entity. Obstet Gynecol. 2013;120:1459–64.

Chapter 5
Retroperitoneum

Tumor

Case 5.1

Brief Case Summary: 64 year old female with abdominal pain

Imaging Findings Axial image from a contrast enhanced CT scan of the abdomen and pelvis demonstrates the presence of a heterogeneous, soft tissue mass expanding the inferior venae cava (IVC) (arrow, Fig. 5.1a). The cephalocaudal extent of the lesion is better demonstrated on the coronal reformatted image (Fig. 5.1b).

Axial images from a three phase (non-contrast, arterial and portal venous) CT scan in another patient demonstrate the presence of an enhancing soft tissue mass expanding the inferior vena cava (Fig. 5.2a–c). The mass contains a punctate calcification, best visualized on the non-contrast image (arrow, Fig. 5.2a). Coronal reformatted image from the same patient demonstrates the cephalocaudal extension of the lesion, with involvement of both the left renal vein (arrow, Fig. 5.2d) and the suprahepatic IVC (double arrow, Fig. 5.2d).

Differential Diagnosis Bland thrombus involving the IVC, Primary leiomyosarcoma of the IVC, Primary retroperitoneal sarcoma extending into the IVC, Exophytic mass arising from an adjacent organ (adrenal glands, kidney).

Diagnosis and Discussion: Primary leiomyosarcoma of the IVC.

Primary leiomyosarcoma of the IVC is a rare, slow growing neoplasm that arises from the smooth muscle layer of the tunica media. Clinical symptoms may relate to the specific segment of involved IVC where infra-renal IVC involvement may present with sign of venous obstruction, while tumor at or above the level of the renal veins may give rise to renal failure or Budd Chiari syndrome. The imaging

M.G. Harisinghani, A. Rajesh, *Genitourinary Imaging: A Case Based Approach*, DOI 10.1007/978-1-4471-4772-5_5

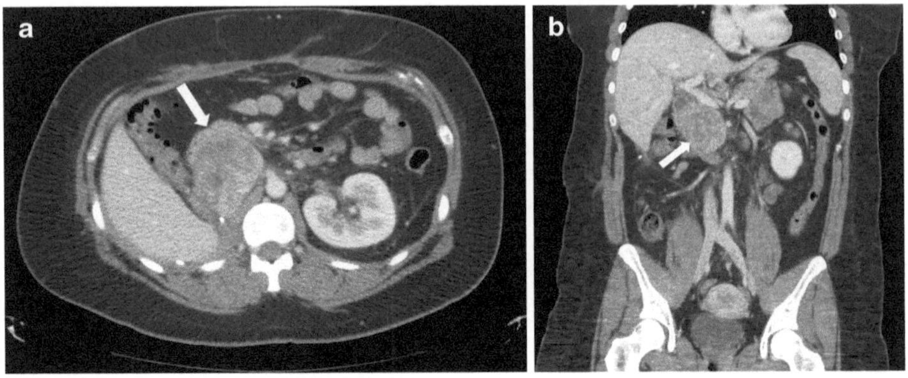

Fig. 5.1 (**a**) Axial image from a contrast enhanced CT scan of the abdomen and pelvis demonstrates the presence of a heterogeneous, soft tissue mass expanding the inferior venae cava (IVC) (*arrow*). (**b**) Cephalocaudal extent of the lesion is better demonstrated on the coronal reformatted image

appearance is non-specific, manifesting as a heterogeneous mass expanding the IVC with variable area of soft tissue enhancement and necrosis. Calcifications within the lesion are rare.

The tumor may be confined to the IVC lumen or may extend extrinsically to involve adjacent structures. Metastases to the liver, lung, lymph nodes, skeleton and brain usually occur late in the disease process. Aggressive surgical resection is the mainstay of therapy with no established consensus on the role for adjuvant/neoadjuvent therapy. Tumors confined to the level of hepatic veins are least amenable to surgical therapy.

Pitfalls Benign mimickers of IVC filling defects include bland thrombus and flow related phenomenon. Contiguous extension of a primary retroperitoneal leiomyosarcoma into the IVC may be difficult to distinguish from a primary IVC neoplasm. A heterogeneous mass in the IVC may also result from tumor extension from renal cell carcinoma, hepatocellular carcinoma and adrenocortical carcinoma.

Teaching Points

1. Unlike bland thrombus, IVC tumor thrombus/neoplasm expand the lumen and show variable degrees of enhancement and necrosis.
2. Differentiation of a primary IVC leiomyosarcoma from contiguous involvement of the IVC from a retroperitoneal soft tissue mass is challenging. Complete effacement of the IVC at the point of maximal contact with the neoplasm may be suggestive of a primary IVC neoplasm.
3. Overall prognosis is poor with aggressive surgical resection being the mainstay of treatment. Tumors confined above the level of hepatic veins are least amenable to surgical therapy.

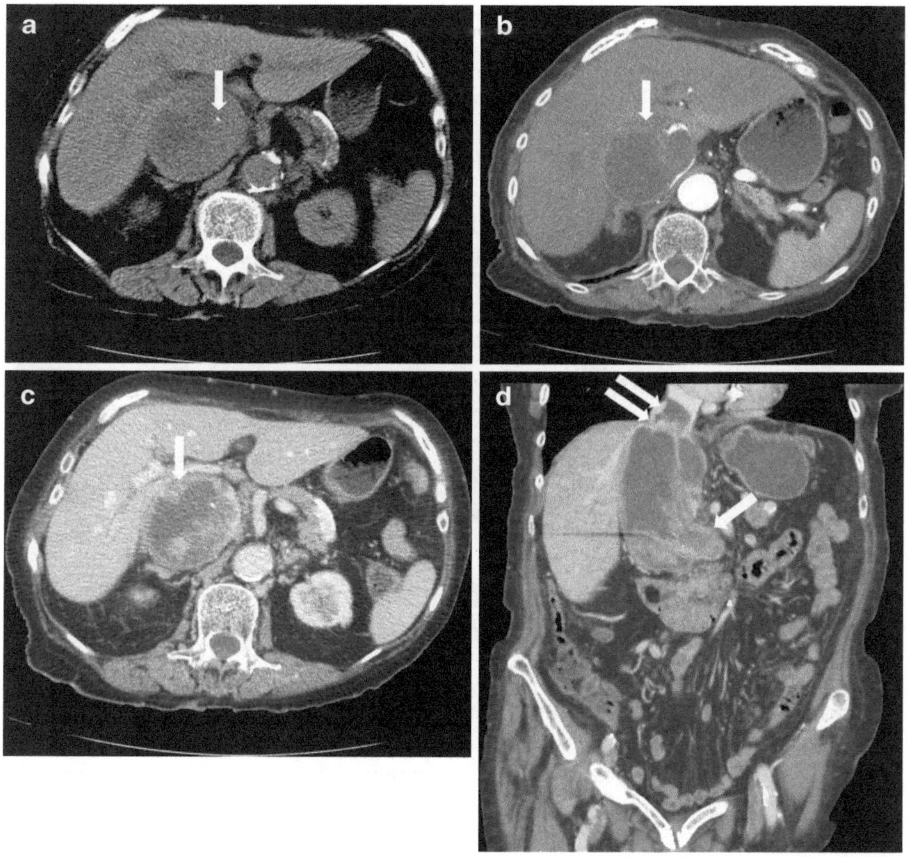

Fig. 5.2 Axial images from a three phase (non-contrast, arterial and portal venous) CT scan in another patient demonstrate the presence of an enhancing soft tissue mass expanding the inferior vena cava (**a–c**). The mass contains a punctate calcification, best visualized on the non-contrast image (*arrow*, **a**). Coronal reformatted image from the same patient demonstrates the cephalocaudal extension of the lesion, with involvement of both the left renal vein (*arrow*, **d**) and the suprahepatic IVC (*double arrow*, **d**)

Case 5.2

Brief Case Summary: 76 year old male with abdominal pain.

Imaging Findings CT scan of the abdomen and pelvis with intravenous and oral contrast demonstrates the presence of a large, complex, predominantly fat containing right sided retroperitoneal mass displacing both the right kidney and loops of bowel anteromedially (Fig. 5.3, arrow). Several septations are noted within the lesion and there are focal areas of higher attenuation (Fig. 5.3, curved arrow).

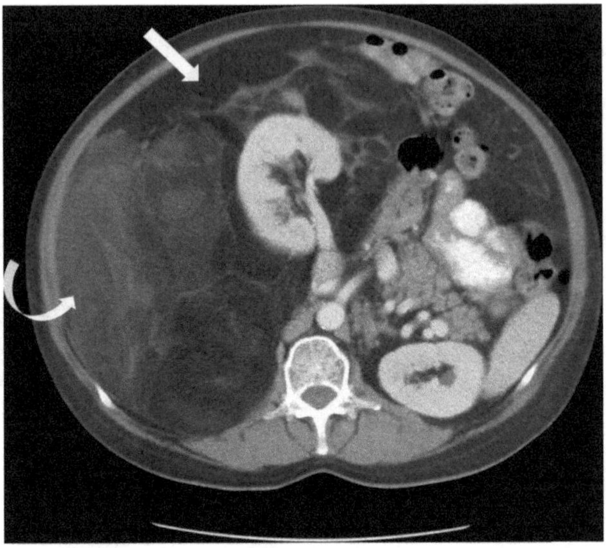

Fig. 5.3 CT scan of the abdomen and pelvis with intravenous and oral contrast demonstrates the presence of a large, complex, predominantly fat containing right sided retroperitoneal mass displacing both the right kidney and loops of bowel anteromedially (*arrow*). Several septations are noted within the lesion and there are focal areas of higher attenuation (*curved arrow*)

Differential Diagnosis Primary retroperitoneal Liposarcoma, Lipoma, Lipoblastoma, Exophytic renal angiomyolipoma (AML), extraadrenal myelolipoma, Hibernoma, Teratoma

Diagnosis and Discussion: Primary retroperitoneal Liposarcoma, well-differentiated.

Primary retroperitoneal liposarcoma is a rare neoplasm, but constitutes the most common malignant retroperitoneal soft tissue tumor in adults. The neoplasm is most often discovered during the fifth to seventh decades of life, either presenting incidentally, or related to mass effect on adjacent structures. The different histological subtypes have been grouped into three categories. Group 1 includes atypical lipomatous tumor (ALT), well differentiated and dedifferentiated liposarcomas, group 2 is composed of myxoid and round cell subtypes while group 3 consists of pleomorphic liposarcoma. Despite the variable aggressiveness of these subtypes, tumor recurrence is common.

Well differentiated and ALT subtype liposarcomas are the least aggressive neoplasms and do no metastasize. Both are indistinguishable by imaging and typically present as predominantly fat attenuation masses, with variable degrees of septal thickening and nodular soft tissue masses <1 cm. Dedifferentiation within these neoplasm may occur over time, manifesting by new and enlarging areas of focal soft tissue nodules >1 cm in size. Cystic components are rare, and calcifications within the lesion are a poor prognostic factor, usually suggesting the presence of dedifferentiation. Metastases from dedifferentiated liposarcoma may occur in the liver, lung and rarely, the peritoneum.

Myxoid and round cell subtypes are thought to be a continuum of the same histological entity and most often occur within the extremities. Imaging findings are somewhat distinct from group 1 and 2 lesions, manifesting as enhancing multilobulated low attenuation masses with a paucity of intralesional fat. Pleomorphic liposarcoma is an aggressive neoplasm which manifest as heterogeneous soft tissue masses, often with internal hemorrhage and necrosis, with lacy, linear or amorphous foci of fat.

Treatment involves wide surgical excision, with or without adjacent or neoadjuvent chemotherapy dependent on the size and histology of the neoplasm.

Pitfalls

1. Lipoma and well differentiated liposarcoma may be indistinguishable. However, primary retroperitoneal lipomas are exceedingly rare, and a fat containing primary retroperitoneal lesion should be assumed to be a well-liposarcoma as evaluated as such.
2. Lipoblastoma is a fat containing mass found in infants and young children
3. Large exophytic AML or myelolipoma may potentially mimic a liposarcoma, though careful evaluation usually reveals the origin from the kidney and adrenal gland respectively. Extraadrenal myelolipoma most often occurs in the presacral space.
4. Hibernomas are uncommon lesions composed of brown fat. They rarely occur in the retroperitoneum and demonstrate higher levels of FDG 18 fluorodeoxyglucose uptake on Positron emission tomography (PET) scans.
5. Retroperitoneal teratomas typically occur in a younger patient demographic, and demonstrate the presence of distinct calcifications (toothlike, well defined) and a fat-fluid level (due to sebum).

Teaching Point

1. Three groups of liposarcoma have been established. Group 1 is the most common, least aggressive, and is predominantly fat containing. Increase in size of the soft tissue component and the absence of calcifications suggests dedifferentiation with potential risk for metastatic disease.
2. Group 2 liposarcoma are multilobulated and may appear cystic, however enhancement will be demonstrated after administration of intravenous contrast.
3. Group 3 lesions are the most aggressive and appear as heterogenous soft tissue masses with a paucity of fat.

Case 5.3

Brief Case Summary: 53 year old male with abdominal pain.

Imaging Findings Coronal T1 precontrast (Fig. 5.4) and coronal T1 postcontrast (Fig. 5.5), coronal T2 (Fig. 5.6) and axial T2 (Fig. 5.7) weighted images of the abdomen and pelvis demonstrate the presence of a well-circumscribed multicystic right sided retroperitoneal mass with thickened septations and enhancing soft tissue, displacing the right kidney anteriorly.

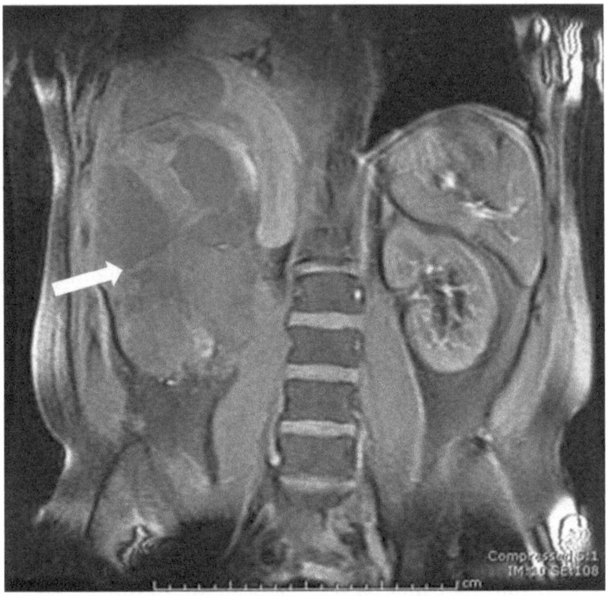

Fig. 5.4 Coronal T1 precontrast weighted image of the abdomen and pelvis demonstrating the presence of a well-circumscribed multicystic right sided retroperitoneal mass (*arrow*) with thickened septations and soft tissue, displacing the right kidney anteriorly

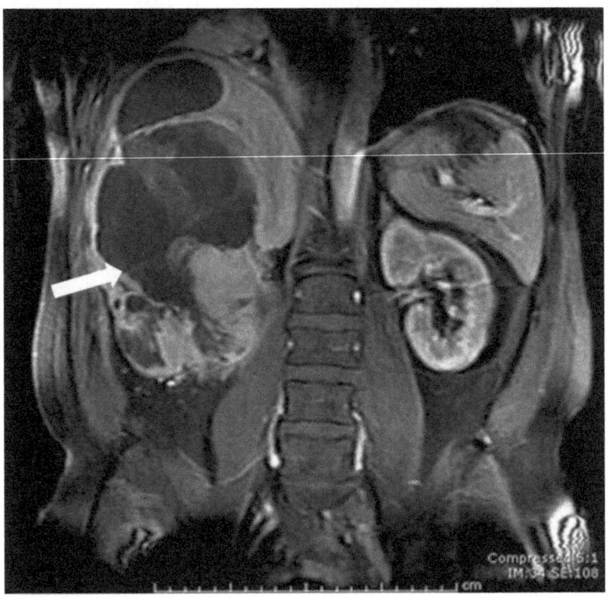

Fig. 5.5 Coronal T1 postcontrast weighted image of the abdomen and pelvis demonstrating the presence of a well-circumscribed multicystic right sided retroperitoneal mass (*arrow*) with thickened septations and enhancing soft tissue, displacing the right kidney anteriorly

Differential Diagnosis Malignant fibrous histiocytoma, leiomyosarcoma, liposarcoma, malignant peripheral nerve sheath tumor

Diagnosis /Discussion: Malignant fibrous histiocytoma

Malignant fibrous histiocytoma (MFH) is the third most common primary retroperitoneal sarcoma following liposarcoma and leiomyosarcoma. Patients with

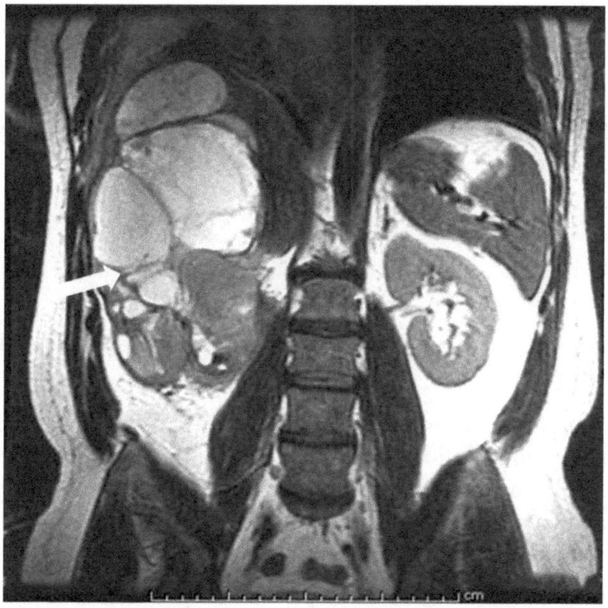

Fig. 5.6 Coronal T2 weighted image of the abdomen and pelvis demonstrating the presence of a well-circumscribed multicystic right sided retroperitoneal mass (*arrow*) with thickened septations and soft tissue, displacing the right kidney anteriorly

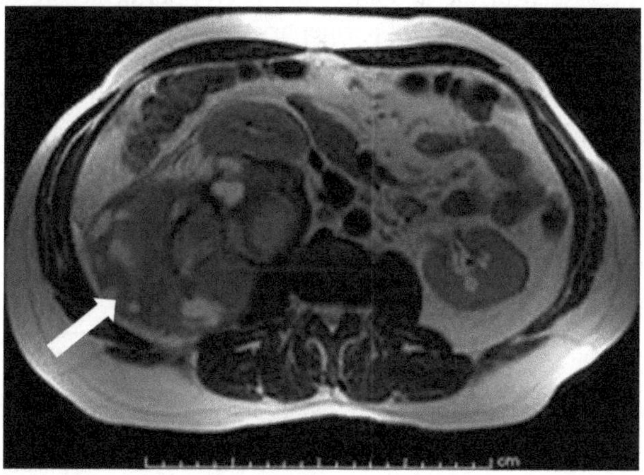

Fig. 5.7 Axial T2 weighted image of the abdomen and pelvis demonstrating the presence of a well-circumscribed multicystic right sided retroperitoneal mass (*arrow*) with thickened septations and soft tissue, displacing the right kidney anteriorly

retroperitoneal MFH often manifest late with tumors growing greater than 10 cm in diameter on presentation. Imaging finding are non-specific with MFH typically demonstrating heterogeneous soft tissue enhancement with variable area of necrosis, hemorrhage and calcification. Surgical excision is the mainstay of therapy, with limited role of chemotherapy and radiation.

Pitfalls There are no specific features that allow confident differentiation of MFG from other primary retroperitoneal sarcomas. Leiomyosarcomas calcify less often than MFH and have a tendacy to invade vasculaure, while liposarcomas often contain fat.

Teaching Points

1. MFH is the third most common retroperitoneal sarcoma, often growing greater than 10 cm on presentation.
2. It is difficult to differentiate MFH from other primary retroperitoneal sarcomas.
3. Surgical excision is the mainstay of therapy.

Case 5.4

Brief Case Summary: 27 year old male with abdominal pain after doing situps.

Imaging Findings Axial image from a CT scan of the abdomen and pelvis after the administration of intravenous and oral contrast demonstrates the presence of a low attenuating, partially septated midline retroperitoneal mass. The IVC is flattened and compressed posteriorly by the mass (arrow, Fig. 5.8).

Plain radiograph in another patient done for abdominal pain demonstrates the presence of a mass overlying the expected region of the right kidney (Fig. 5.9a). Coronal noncontrast (Fig. 5.9b) and axial contrast enhanced (Fig. 5.9c) images from a CT scan of the abdomen and pelvis performed re demonstrates the lesion and localizes it to the right perinephric space. Left para-aortic lymphadenopathy is also noted (double arrow, Fig. 5.9c).

Axial and coronal image from a CT scan of the abdomen and pelvis after the administration of intravenous and oral contrast in another patient demonstrates the presence of confluent retroperitoneal lymphadenopathy with a homogenous soft tissue attenuation (Fig. 5.10a, b). Notice the anterior elevation of the aorta off the upper lumbar spine (arrow, Fig. 5.10a).

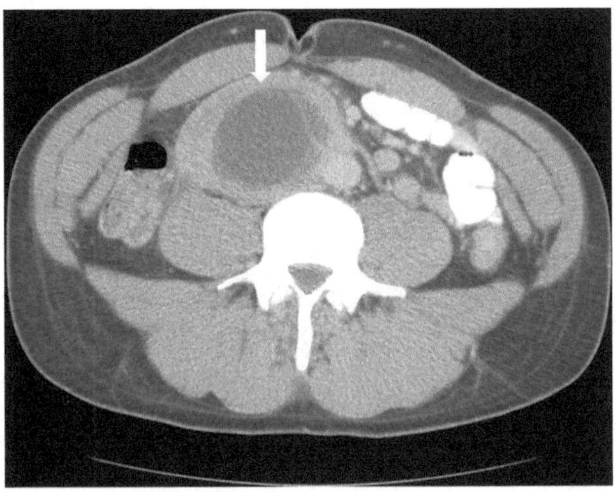

Fig. 5.8 Axial image from a CT scan of the abdomen and pelvis after the administration of intravenous and oral contrast demonstrates the presence of a low attenuating, partially septated midline retroperitoneal mass. The IVC is flattened and compressed posteriorly by the mass (*arrow*)

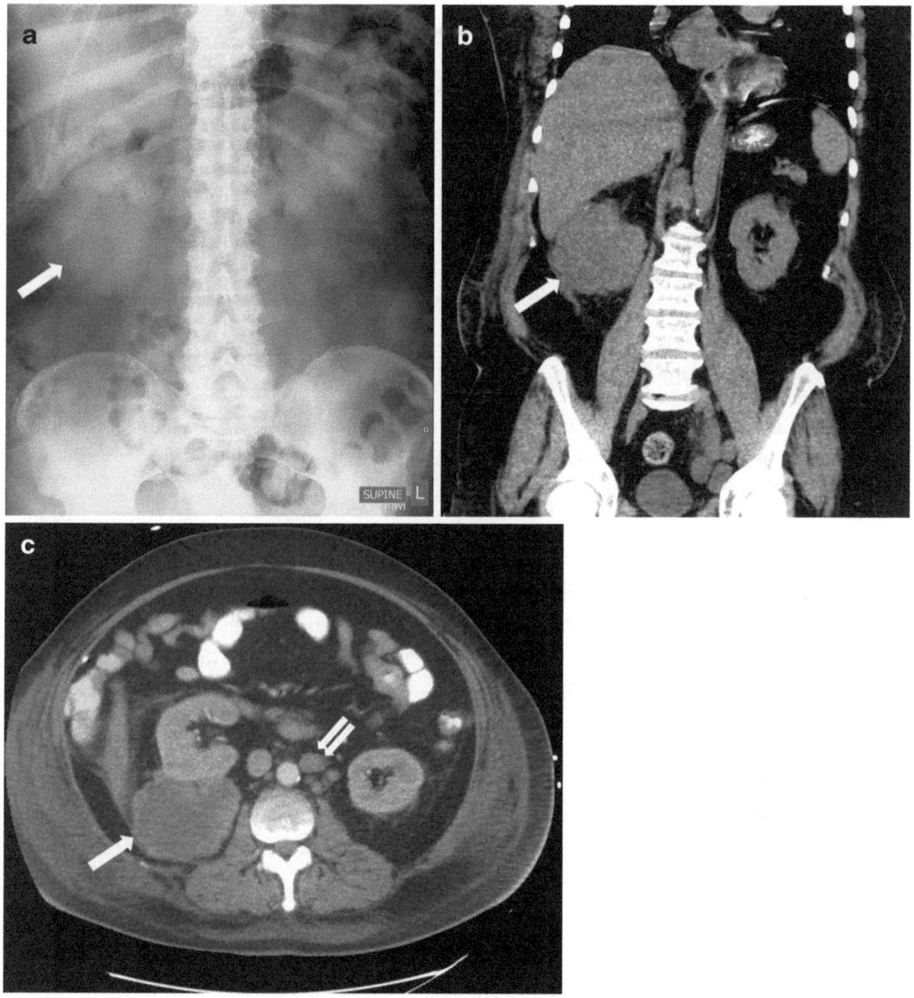

Fig. 5.9 Plain radiograph in another patient done for abdominal pain demonstrates the presence of a mass overlying the expected region of the right kidney (**a**). Coronal noncontrast (**b**) and axial contrast enhanced (**c**) images from a CT scan of the abdomen and pelvis performed re demonstrates the lesion and localizes it to the right perinephric space. Left para-aortic lymphadenopathy is also noted (*double arrow*, **c**)

Differential Diagnosis Metastatic disease, primary retroperitoneal sarcoma, lymphoma, lymphadenopathy due to infection

Diagnosis and Discussion: Metastatic disease (germ cell tumor in Fig. 5.8, **melanoma in** Fig. 5.9, **non-Hodgkin lymphoma in** Fig. 5.10).

Retroperitoneal lymph nodes are a common pathway for regional spread of intratesticular neoplasms. Metastatic nodes are typically larger than 10 mm in short axis dimension and may manifest as homogenous or heterogeneous density,

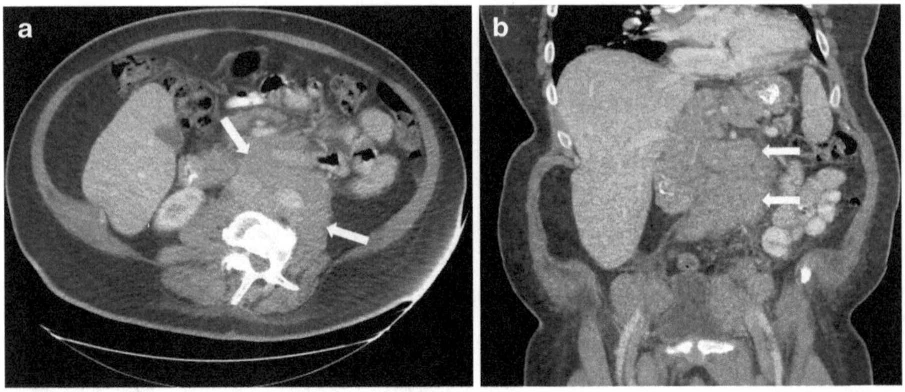

Fig. 5.10 Axial and coronal image from a CT scan of the abdomen and pelvis after the administration of intravenous and oral contrast in another patient demonstrates the presence of confluent retroperitoneal lymphadenopathy with a homogenous soft tissue attenuation (**a**, **b**). Notice the anterior elevation of the aorta off the upper lumbar spine (*arrows*, **a**)

particularly with nonseminomatous primary testicular neoplasms. Other notable neoplasms to give rise to retroperitoneal metastatic disease include ovarian, prostate, and colorectal cancer, as well as lung and breast. Metastases to the perirenal space are uncommon, but have been described for melanoma, lung, breast and prostate cancer.

Lymphoma represents the most common malignant retroperitoneal tumor. The two broad categories are Hodgkin and non-Hodgkin lymphoma. The latter typically presents at an advanced age with extranodal disease involving the liver, spleen and bowel, and often has mesenteric and retroperitoneal lymphadenopathy at presentation. Hodgkin lymphoma has a bimodal age of distribution of disease and typically presents with isolated disease, often involving the mediastinum. On imaging, retroperitoneal lymphadenopathy related to lymphoma is mildly enhancing, confluent and homogenous, typically insinuating between normal viscera and vessels without compression or obstruction. The aorta may be lifted off the spine resulting in the "floating aorta" sign.

Chemotherapy and radiation are the cornerstones of treatment, and patient are typically followed using positron emission tomography (PET) imaging with viable tumors demonstrating 18 fluorodeoxyglucose (FDG) uptake. Focal areas of calcification and necrosis may be seen after therapy.

Pitfalls Retroperitoneal soft tissue masses may potentially mimic primary retroperitoneal sarcomas, however the multiplicity, proximity to vessels and the often homogenous attenuation of the lesions typically favors lymphadenopathy

Teaching Point

1. Retroperitoneal lymphadenopathy in an otherwise healthy young male adult should warrant a search for an underlying testicular neoplasm (ultrasound).

2. Lymphoma is the most common malignant retroperitoneal tumor. Distinction from primary retroperitoneal sarcoma is critical as the former is treated medically and the latter is treated with surgery.
3. Confluent, mildly enhancing lymphadenopathy, insinuating between viscera and vessels without compression or obstruction is characteristic of lymphoma. Heterogeneity with calcifications and necrosis may be seen post chemotherapy and radiation.

Case 5.5

Brief Case Summary: 43 year old male with abdominal pain

Imaging Findings Axial (Fig. 5.11a) and coronal (Fig. 5.11b) CT images of the abdomen and pelvis performed with intravenous and oral contrast demonstrate an enhancing, heterogenous soft tissue aortocaval mass (arrows).

Axial image from a CT scan of the abdomen and pelvis performed with intravenous and oral contrast in another patient with the same diagnosis demonstrates a homogenously enhancing mass anterior to the left adrenal gland (arrow, Fig. 5.12).

Axial (Fig. 5.13a) and coronal (Fig. 5.13b) image from a CT scan of the abdomen and pelvis performed with intravenous and oral contrast in a third patient with the same diagnosis demonstrates the presence of a heterogeneously enhancing mass just inferior to the bifurcation of the abdominal aorta (arrows).

Differential Diagnosis Paraganglioma, Ganglioneuroma, Peripheral nerve sheath tumor, Metastases.

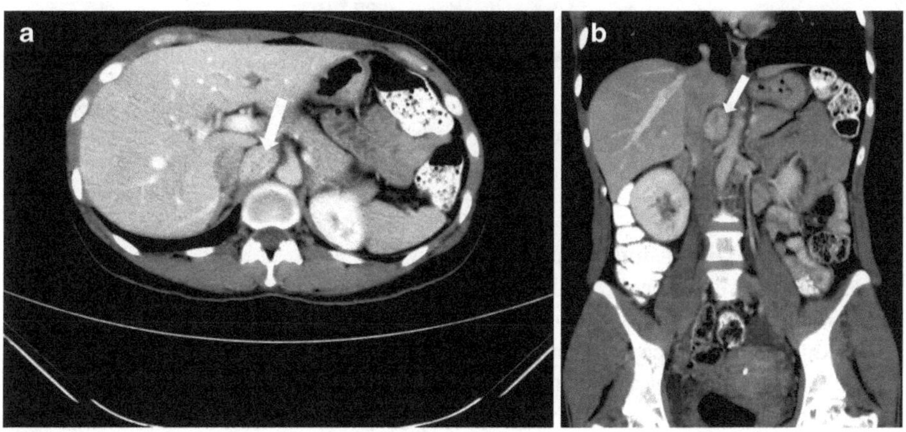

Fig. 5.11 Axial (**a**) and coronal (**b**) CT images of the abdomen and pelvis performed with intravenous and oral contrast demonstrate an enhancing, heterogenous soft tissue aortocaval mass (*arrows*)

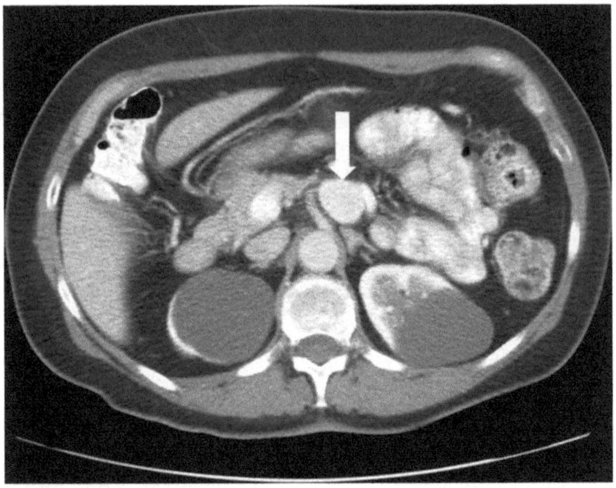

Fig. 5.12 Axial image from a CT scan of the abdomen and pelvis performed with intravenous and oral contrast in another patient with the same diagnosis demonstrates a homogenously enhancing mass anterior to the left adrenal gland (*arrow*)

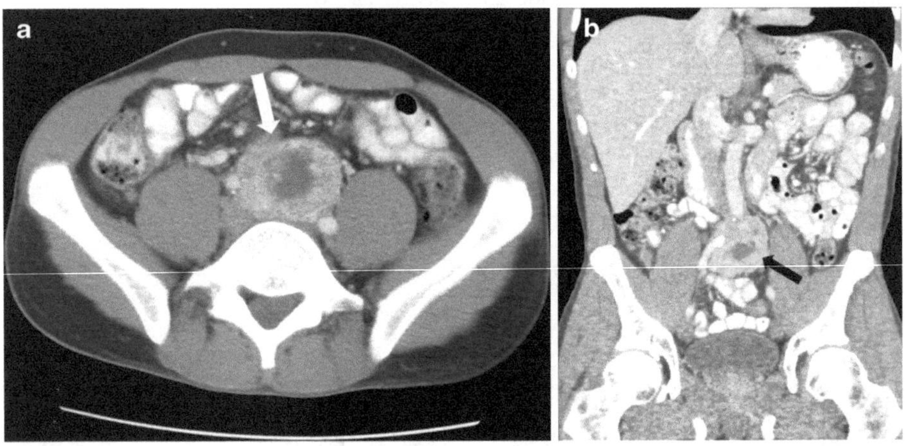

Fig. 5.13 Axial (**a**) and coronal (**b**) image from a CT scan of the abdomen and pelvis performed with intravenous and oral contrast in a third patient with the same diagnosis demonstrates the presence of a heterogeneously enhancing mass just inferior to the bifurcation of the abdominal aorta (*arrows*)

Diagnosis and Discussion: Paraganglioma.

Paragangliomas are neuroendocrine tumors that originate from neural crest cells found in the paraganglionic system. The paraganglionic system consists of the adrenal medulla, chemoreceptors, and clusters of cells associated with ganglia in the thoracic cavity and retroperitoneum. The most common location is the adrenal medulla (where these tumors are referred to as pheochromocytoma) and approximately 10 % arise in extra adrenal sites, most commonly at the abdominal aortic bifurcation, also referred to as the organ of Zukerkandl. The tumors may be sporadic or hereditary; hereditary cases are more often multicentric and are associated with multiple endocrine neoplasia (MEN) type 2, NF-1, von-Hippel Lindau disease, familial paranganglioma and Carney triad.

While the majority of tumors are non-functional, a small percentage will present with symptoms of excess catecholamine secretion (palpitations, headache, sweating, hypertension) for which a biochemical workup is mandated prior to imaging. Rarely, these tumors may rupture and present with retroperitoneal hemorrhage. If the biochemical workup is positive, cross-sectional imaging is performed where a paraganglioma typically manifests as a hypervascular mass with a variable degree of hemorrhage or necrosis. Approximately 80 % of lesions demonstrate very hyperintense T2 signal ("light bulb" bright) on MR imaging. Occasionally, hemorrhagic necrosis can occur, resulting in fluid-fluid levels. Whole body radionuclide imaging utilizing 131-iodine metaiodobenzylguanidine may be used to identify an anatomically occult lesion in a patient with a positive biochemical workup and to evaluate for metastatic disease.

Imaging cannot reliably differentiate benign from malignant paragangliomas, however, contiguous or metastatic spread is diagnostic of malignancy. Overall, paragangliomas are more aggressive than pheochromocytomas with increased risk for metastatic disease. Common sites of metastases include the regional lymph nodes, liver, bone and lung. Surgical resection preceded by medical management (adrenergic blockade) to decrease the potential risk of intra-operative hypertension crisis is the mainstay of treatment.

Pitfalls

1. Neuroendocrine tumor of the pancreas or a pseudoaneurysm may mimic a paraganglioma.
2. Differentiation from other neurogenic tumors may be difficult, particularly without clinical evidence for hypercatecholamine secretion. Unlike other primary retroperitoneal sarcomas, paragangliomas do not contain fat and tend to be smaller in size with less mass effect.
3. Paragangliomas in patients with MEN syndrome may be small and more subtle than in sporadic cases.

Teaching Points

1. If there is suspicion for a paraganglioma, a biochemical workup should always be obtained prior to imaging. Similarly, a biochemical workup should be obtained before biopsy or surgical resection of any mass thought to represent a paraganglioma.
2. The most common location of an extra adrenal paraganglioma is the organ of Zukerkandl.
3. On imaging, paragangliomas are often hypervascular and the "lightbulb" bright hyperintense T2 signal is present in approximately 80 % of cases. Occasionally, hemorrhagic necrosis can occur, resulting in fluid-fluid levels

Case 5.6

Brief Case Summary: 65 year old female with nausea, vomiting and abdominal pain

Imaging Findings Supine radiograph of the abdomen demonstrates the presence of a space-occupying lesion in the left abdomen with superior and medial displacement of the adjacent bowel loops (arrow, Fig. 5.14a). Coronal reformatted image from a non-contrast CT scan of the abdomen and pelvis demonstrates a low attenuation mass in the abdomen (Fig. 5.14b). A few subtle septations are noted within the medial aspect of the mass (arrows, Fig. 5.14b). Axial T2 fat saturated image of the abdomen demonstrates a multiseptated cystic mass in the left retroperitenum, just lateral to the abdominal aorta (Fig. 5.14c).

CT scan of the abdomen and pelvis with intravenous and oral contrast in a 26 year old female with the same diagnosis demonstrates a heterogeneous retroperitoneal soft tissue mass with internal low attenuation components (Fig. 5.15). The mass compresses the IVC and is intimately associated with the anterior aspect of the right psoas muscle.

Differential Diagnosis Malignant fibrous histiocytoma, leiomyosarcoma, liposarcoma, metastases, peripheral nerve sheath tumor

Diagnosis and Discussion: Malignant peripheral nerve sheath tumor.

Malignant peripheral nerve sheath tumors (MPNST's) are rare soft tissue sarcomas which arise from peripheral nerve branches or the nerve sheath. Peak age of incidence is in the seventh decade of life, although the lesions can occur in the third or fourth decades in patients with neurofibromatosis type 1 (NF-1). Malignant peripheral nerve sheath tumors can also develop after radiation therapy for other neoplasms, with a latency period of greater than 10 years.

A rapid increase in size of a palpable mass or new onset/rapidly progressing neurological symptoms in a patient with a known history of NF-1 should raise suspicion for an underlying MPNST. Imaging cannot reliably differentiate a MPNST from a benign lesion such as a neurofibroma or schwannoma. On MR, both benign and malignant lesions may demonstrate hypointense T1 signal and variable T2 signal (high in the setting of myxoid tissue, low if cellular tissue) and soft tissue enhancement. Malignant lesions tend to be larger (>5 cm) with more infiltrative, ill-defined margins and demonstrate rapid growth on serial imaging studies. Necrosis and calcifications are more often seen in malignant lesions, though internal degeneration of otherwise benign lesions may give a similar appearance.

Surgical resection is the cornerstone of therapy. Chemotherapy and radiation are often given, though the effect of these therapies on overall survival benefit is limited. Prognosis of MPNST is poor, with high rate of local tumor recurrence and distant metastatic disease.

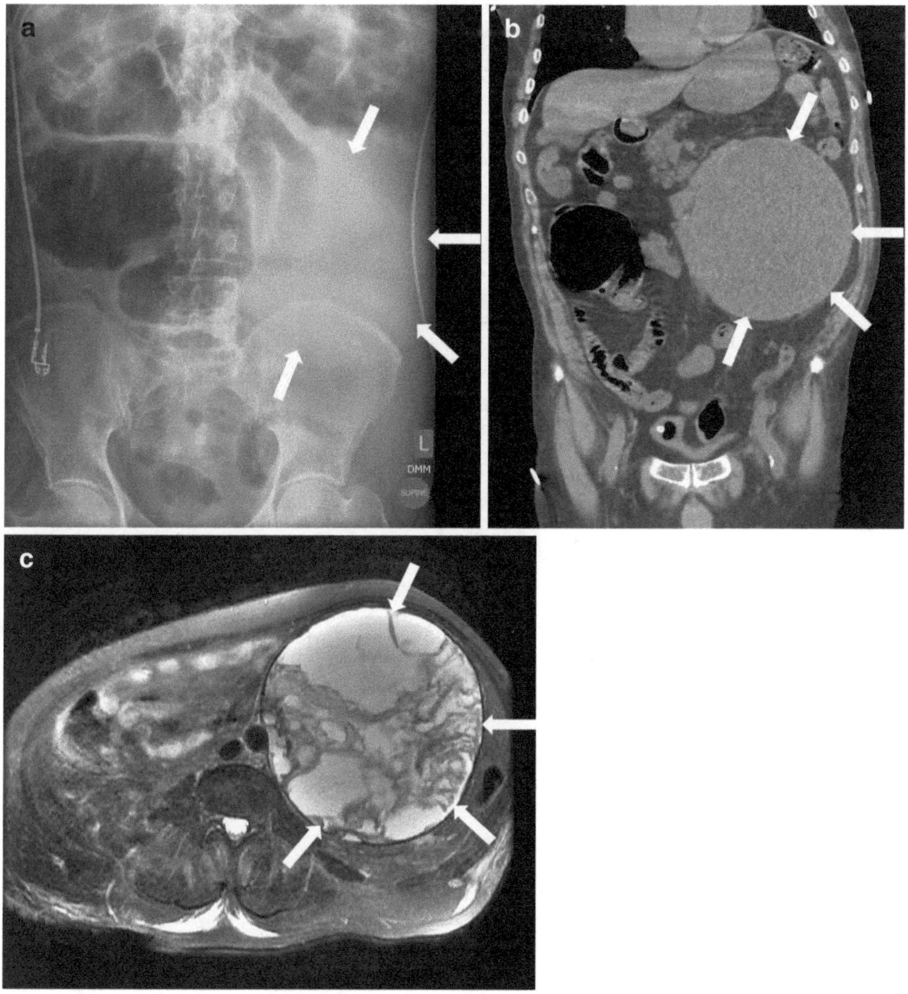

Fig. 5.14 Supine radiograph of the abdomen demonstrates the presence of a space-occupying lesion in the left abdomen with superior and medial displacement of the adjacent bowel loops (*arrows*, **a**). Coronal reformatted image from a non-contrast CT scan of the abdomen and pelvis demonstrates a low attenuation mass in the abdomen (**b**). A few subtle septations are noted within the medial aspect of the mass (*arrows*, **b**). Axial T2 fat saturated image of the abdomen demonstrates a multiseptated cystic mass in the left retroperitoneum, just lateral to the abdominal aorta (**c**)

Pitfalls

1. It may be impossible to differentiate a MPNST from a primary retroperitoneal soft tissue sarcoma. Group 1 liposarcomas have a predominant fatty component while a leiomyosarcoma does not typically demonstrate the high T2 signal of myxoid stroma. Metastases should be considered if there a history of a primary neoplasm.
2. A clinical syndrome of excess catecholamine release associated with a briskly enhancing mass is suggestive of a retroperitoneal paraganglioma

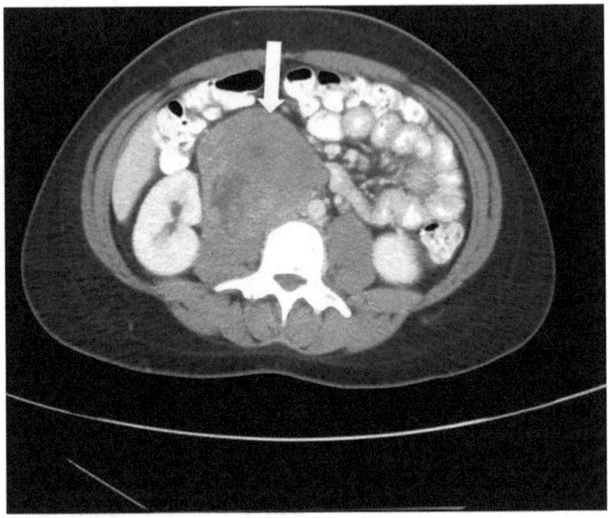

Fig. 5.15 CT scan of the abdomen and pelvis with intravenous and oral contrast in a 26 year old female with the same diagnosis demonstrates a heterogeneous retroperitoneal soft tissue mass (*arrow*) with internal low attenuation components. The mass compresses the IVC and is intimately associated with the anterior aspect of the right psoas muscle

Teaching Point

1. A tumor of neurogenic origin should be considered in the differential of a retroperitoneal mass, particularly if there is a history of radiation or NF-1
2. Imaging cannot reliable differentiate a benign from a malignant nerve sheath tumor.
3. Rapid increase in size, new or progressive neurological symptoms, large mass (>5 cm) with infiltrative, ill –defined margins is suggestive of a MPNST.

Case 5.7

Brief Case Summary: 69 year old man with incidentally detected mass on physical examination.

Imaging Findings Axial (Fig. 5.16a) and coronal (Fig. 5.16b) images from a contrast-enhanced CT examination demonstrates a large, heterogeneous, well-circumscribed mass in the retroperitoneum. The mass has central hypodensity, correlating to necrosis, and multiple surrounding large blood vessels are visualized. Note that the right kidney is displaced superiorly. Slightly more caudal (Fig. 5.16c), engorgement of the right spermatic vein is seen secondary to compression of the infrarenal IVC by the large retroperitoneal mass.

Differential Diagnosis: Desmoid, high-grade sarcoma, angiosarcoma, leiomyosarcoma, solitary vascular metastatic lesion.

Diagnosis and Discussion Solitary fibrous tumors (SFTs) is a rare mesenchymal neoplasm of fibroblastic or myofibroblastic origin and account for less than 2 % of soft tissue tumors. These tumors can involve any body part and extrapleural SFTs

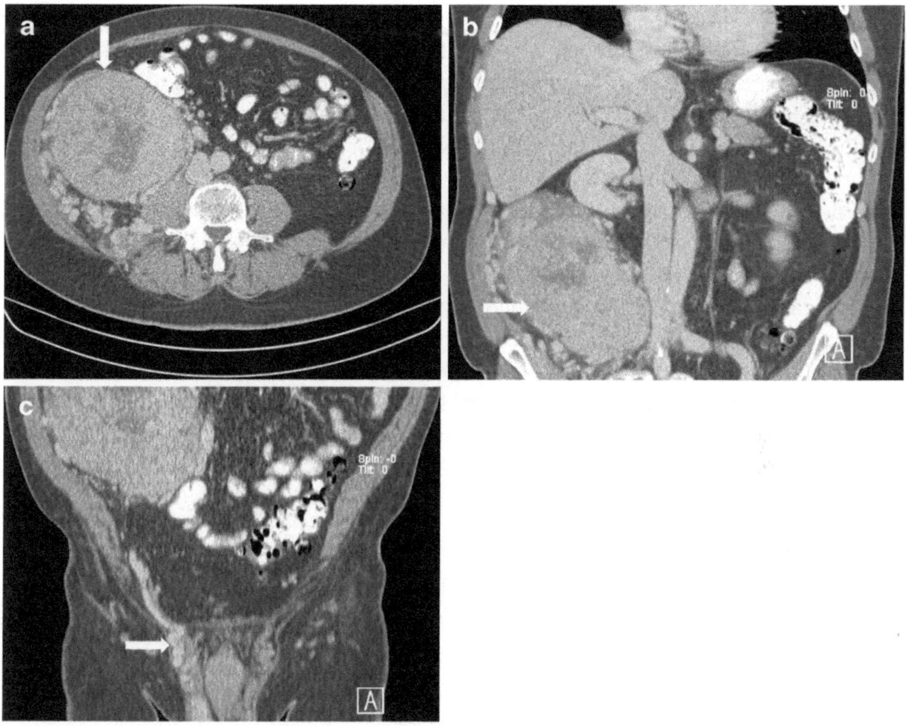

Fig. 5.16 Axial (**a**) and coronal (**b**) images from a contrast-enhanced CT examination demonstrates a large, heterogeneous, well-circumscribed mass (*arrow*) in the retroperitoneum. The mass has central hypodensity, correlating to necrosis, and multiple surrounding large blood vessels are visualized. Note that the right kidney is displaced superiorly. Slightly more caudal (**c**) engorgement of the right spermatic vein is seen secondary to compression of the infrarenal IVC by the large retroperitoneal mass

are more common than pleural SFTs. Extrapleural SFTs manifest clinically as slow-growing masses in middle-aged adults with equal frequency in women and men and are typically asymptomatic, however, symptoms may develop secondary to compression of adjacent parenchyma or viscera. Approximately 5 % of SFTs are associated with hypoglycemia due to excess production of insulinlike growth factors and hypoglycemia is more commonly seen with large SFTs.

Any body part can be affected with SFTs in the abdomen and pelvis including the liver, pancreas, intestine and mesentery, kidneys, retroperitoneum, pelvis and prostate gland. Somatic tissues can also be involved including the extremities, anterior abdominal wall, and the head and neck.

On imaging, CT is the initial imaging modality of choice and manifest as well-circumscribed, discrete, lobulated hypervascular masses that usually exert mass effect on adjacent organs. Central necrosis or cystic change may be present and is seen as a hypoenhancing central area within the tumor. Calcifications are rare but tend to be seen in larger tumors. In addition to detection of SFTs, CT assesses local extent as well as distant metastases.

On MR, SFTs are T1 isointense and T2 heterogeneously hypointense with flow voids. Avid enhancement is seen after gadolinium and areas of heterogeneous enhancement can be seen depending on the tissue composition. Areas of hypervascularity intensely enhance whereas necrotic or cystic areas do not enhance. Hypercellular areas exhibit persistent or prolonged enhancement in the venous and delayed phases of contrast and fibrous and collagenous stroma have mild arterial enhancement with increasing enhancement in the delayed phase. On angiography, SFTs are seen as a vascular mass with collateral feeding vessels.

Surgical resection is the treatment and is usually curative in benign cases. Surgical excision can be difficult secondary to the hypervascularity and presence of collateral vessels. Preoperative embolization may be considered. SFTs with malignant components and lesions larger than 10 cm carry a higher risk of local recurrence and metastatic disease. Some cases previously classified as benign were found to have metastases which necessitate long-term follow-up despite benign histopathologic features.

Pitfalls SFTs are rare and frequently confused with other tumors such as leiomyosarcoma, high-grade sarcomas, and even solitary hypervascular metastases. Although these tumors are rare and are often confused with other tumors, familiarity with the imaging features is important.

Teaching Point

1. Solitary fibrous tumors are rare neoplasms of mesenchymal origin composed of fibroblasts or myofibroblasts.
2. SFTs are slow growing and are typically asymptomatic masses but may have symptoms secondary to mass effect on adjacent organs.
3. SFTs present as large, well-defined, heterogeneous and hypervascular masses with areas of necrosis and cystic change and surgical excision is the treatment of choice.

Miscellaneous

Case 5.8

Brief Case Summary: 86 year old female with abdominal pain.

Imaging Findings Coronal reformatted image from a CT scan of the abdomen and pelvis performed with intravenous and oral contrast demonstrates an extensive amount of both intra and extra-abdominal air (Fig. 5.17). Within the abdomen and pelvis, the air is located mostly in the retroperitoneal space surrounding both kidneys, medial to the psoas musculature and surrounding portions of the rectum. Subcutaneous emphysema extending to the soft tissue of the breast as well

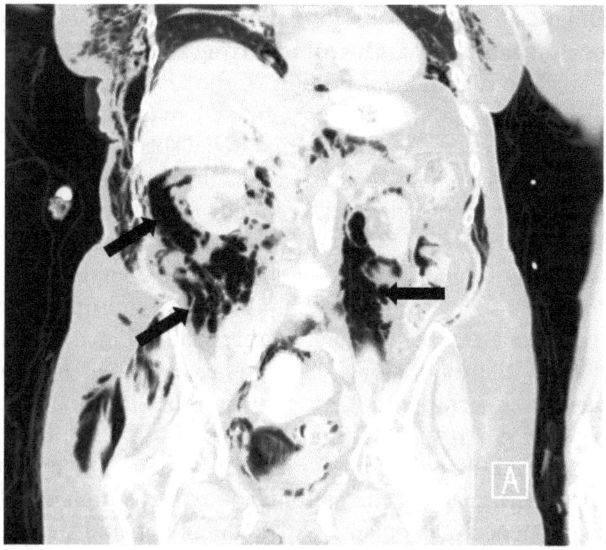

Fig. 5.17 Coronal reformatted image from a CT scan of the abdomen and pelvis performed with intravenous and oral contrast demonstrates an extensive amount of both intra and extra-abdominal air (*arrows*)

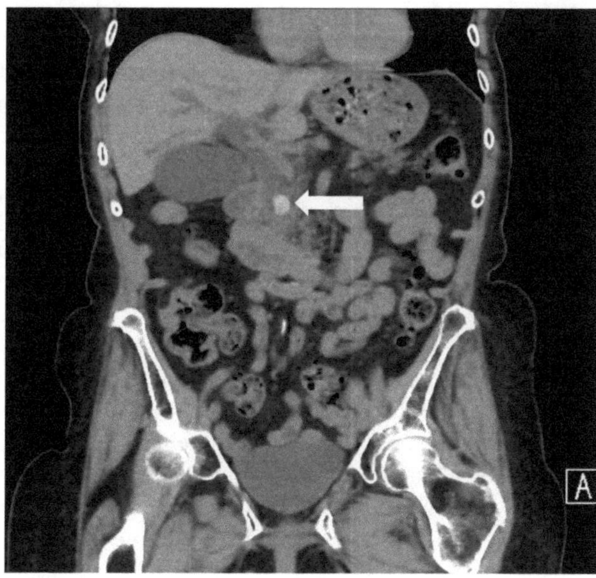

Fig. 5.18 On the coronal image in soft tissue windows, a large calcified gallstone (*arrow*) is visualized in the distal common bile duct

as pneumomediastinum is also noted. On the coronal image in soft tissue windows (Fig. 5.18), a large calcified gallstone is visualized in the distal common bile duct.

Differential Diagnosis Perforated retroperitoneal viscus (peptic ulcer, perforated neoplasm, diverticulitis, iatrogenic). Alternatively, the pneumoretroperitoneum may be the result of pneumomediastinum or subcutaneous emphysema secondarily dissecting into the abdomen.

Diagnosis and Discussion: Pneumoretroperitoneum secondary to duodenal perforation, post endoscopic retrograde cholangiopancreatography (ERCP).

The retroperitoneal portion of the abdominal cavity can be divided into three distinct spaces: the anterior pararenal space, the perirenal space, and the posterior pararenal space. The anterior pararenal space contains the retroperitoneal portion of the duodenum, pancreas as well as the ascending and descending colon, while the perirenal space contains the kidney and adrenal glands. The posterior pararenal space is delineated by the posterior aspect of the perirenal fascia and the muscles of the posterior abdominal wall and as such, contains fat.

Injury to the organs contained by the retroperitoneal compartments can lead to pneumoretroperitoneum. Rarely, pneumomediastinum and pneumothorax may dissect inferiorly along fascial planes leading to retroperitoneal air. Iatrogenic causes, as seen post colonoscopy and ERCP, are another source for retroperitoneal air. The risk of ERCP related perforation is less than 1 % in patients with normal anatomy, although the presence of asymptomatic pneumoretroperitoneum on post-ERCP CT scans of the abdomen may be as high as 29 %. The presence of pneumoperitoneum associated with abdominal pain and underlying retroperitoneal fluid collections post-ERCP portends a worse prognosis, requiring more urgent surgical intervention. Rarely, pneumoperitoneum can lead to subcutaneous emphysemsa, pneumomediastinum and pneumothorax.

The patient in this case had undergone an ERCP for choledocholiathiasis (Fig. 5.18) earlier that day and developed severe abdominal pain, prompting cross sectional evaluation of the abdomen and pelvis.

Pitfalls It may difficult to differentiate intra and extraperitoneal free air on plain abdominal radiographs. In addition, subcutaneous emphysema may project over the abdomen, thus mimicking findings of intra-abdominal free air. An intra-abdominal abscess may present as a localized collection of air on an abdominal radiograph.

Teaching Points

1. Plain abdominal radiographs are useful to detect the presence of intra-abdominal air, although the etiology is often non-specific. If the patient is stable, a CT scan of the abdomen and pelvis should be the next step.
2. Closely evaluate the retroperitoneal organs to look for evidence of perforation.
3. Rarely, pneumoretroperitoneum may secondarily result from air leaks outside the abdomen/pelvis (pneumomediastinum, pneumothorax).

Case 5.9

Brief Case Summary 39 year old male with left lower quadrant pain

Imaging Findings Sagittal grayscale ultrasound image shows a solid lesion along the anterior aspect of the abdominal aorta (Fig. 5.19). Axial contrast enhanced CT examination of the abdomen at the level of the kidneys (Fig. 5.20) demonstrates a

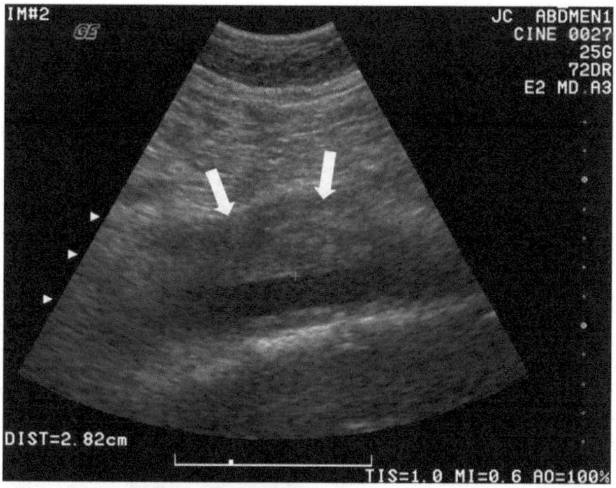

Fig. 5.19 Sagittal grayscale ultrasound image shows a solid lesion (*arrows*) along the anterior aspect of the abdominal aorta

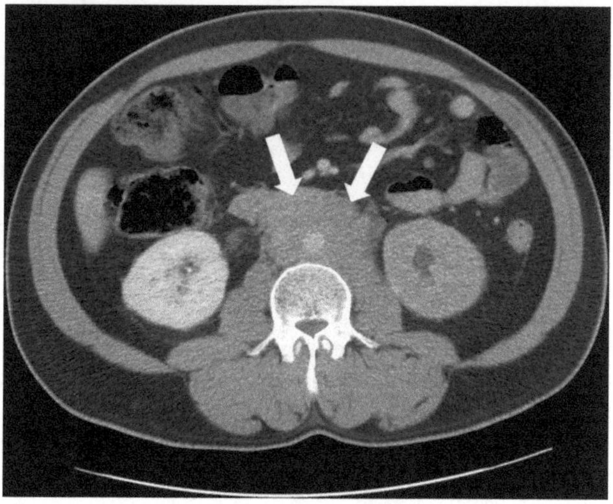

Fig. 5.20 Axial contrast enhanced CT examination of the abdomen at the level of the kidneys demonstrates a retroperitoneal soft tissue mass (*arrows*) surrounding the inferior vena cava and aorta

retroperitoneal soft tissue mass surrounding the inferior vena cava and aorta. The left kidney shows a delayed nephrogram with no excretion of contrast on the coronal reformatted delayed phase images (Fig. 5.21). Note the encasement of both ureters by the soft tissue mass with medial deviation of the right ureter (Fig. 5.21).

Differential Diagnosis: Lymphoma, metastatic disease, retroperitoneal fibrosis, periaortic hematoma

Diagnosis and Discussion: Retroperitoneal Fibrosis.

Retroperitoneal fibrosis (RPF) is an uncommon fibrotic process with an incidence of 1 in 200,000. Most cases are idiopathic (greater than 70 %), with the remainder associated with malignancy (most commonly lymphoma), retroperitoneal hemorrhage, urine extravasation, prior radiation or medications (methysergide

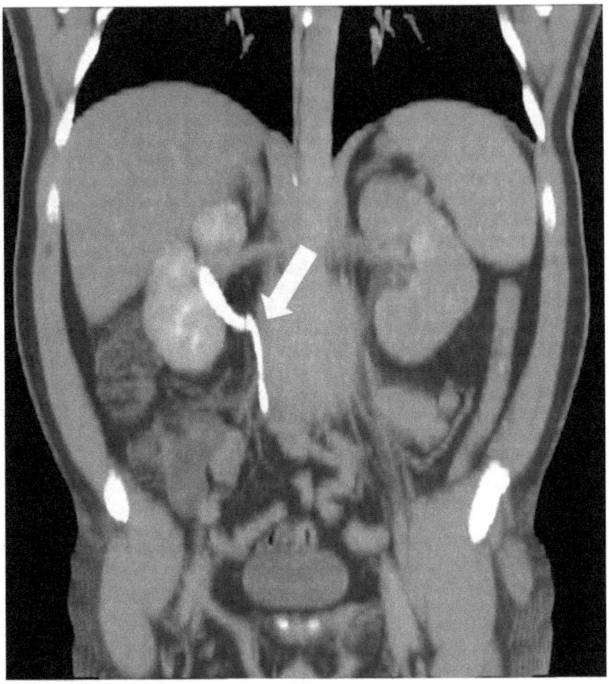

Fig. 5.21 The left kidney shows a delayed nephrogram with no excretion of contrast on the coronal reformatted delayed phase images. Note the encasement of both ureters by the soft tissue mass (*arrow*) with medial deviation of the right ureter

and bromocriptine). There is increasing literature suggesting that RPF may be a manifestation of an immune mediated systemic disease associated with other entities such as primary biliary cirrhosis and mediastinitis.

Sonographic findings are non-specific, with RPF manifesting as a well-defined hypo to anechoic retroperitoneal mass with irregular contours. On CT, RPF typically presents as a soft tissue attenuation mass extending cephalad from the proximal common iliac arteries to the renal hilum, without associated osseous destruction. The extent of soft tissue enhancement correlates with the chronicity of the fibrotic process. Malignant etiologies for RPF (such as lymphoma or metastasis) tend to present as bulky masses with lobulated contours, classically lifting the aorta and IVC off the spine. The fibrotic process often deviates the ureters medially resulting in obstructive uropathy. RPF presents as T1 hypointense mass on MR imaging, with the T2 signal and enhancement varying depending on the chronicity of the disease (acute disease has more enhancement and higher T2 signal compared to chronic RPF). Differentiating malignant from benign etiologies remains a challenge, with malignant RPF having a tendency to demonstrate more heterogeneous T2 signal and enhancement. Given the advent of CT and MR urography, there is limited role for conventional excretory urography in the workup of RPF.

Pitfalls Specific differentiation of benign from malignant causes of RPF remains elusive with current imaging modalities; a tissue biopsy is required for a definitive diagnosis.

Teaching Points

1. RPF may be idiopathic or may be associated with benign or malignant conditions.
2. A bulky retroperitoneal soft tissue mass with lobulated contours that causing lifting the vasculature (aorta and IVC) off the spine and lateral displacement of the ureters suggest a malignant cause such as lymphoma.
3. Imaging differentiation of benign from malignant causes is not specific; a tissue biopsy is ultimately required for a definitive evaluation.

Case 5.10

Brief Case Summary 55 year old male status post cardiac catherization with hematocrit drop.

Imaging Findings Axial and coronal images (Fig. 5.22a, b) from a CT scan of the abdomen and pelvis performed without the administration of contrast demonstrates the presence of a large left sided retroperitoneal collection. Note the presence of a fluid level within the collection (arrow, Fig. 5.22a).

Differential Diagnosis Retroperitoneal hematoma, other retroperitoneal collections (abscess, seroma, lymphocele, pancreatic pseudocyst), retroperitoneal sarcoma

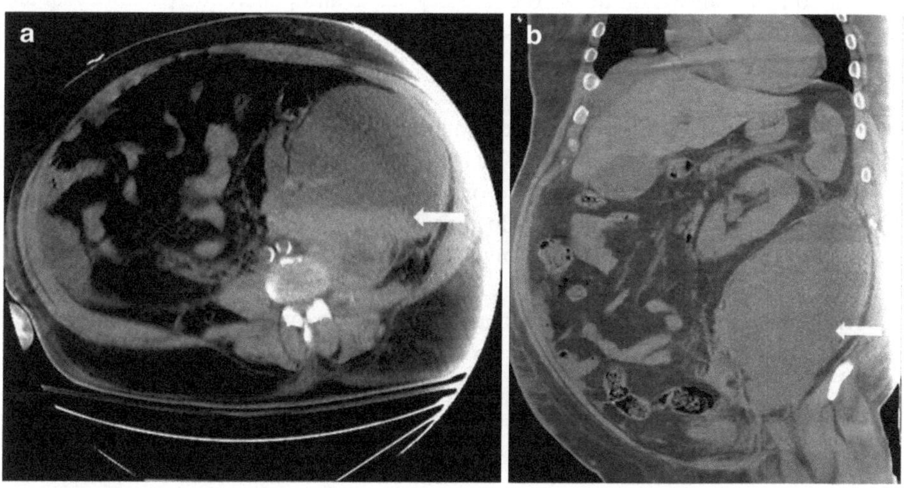

Fig. 5.22 Axial and coronal images (**a**, **b**) from a CT scan of the abdomen and pelvis performed without the administration of contrast demonstrates the presence of a large left sided retroperitoneal collection. Note the presence of a fluid level within the collection (*arrow*, **a**)

Diagnosis /Discussion: Retroperitoneal hematoma

Retroperitoneal hematoma (RPH) may be seen in the setting of trauma, ruptured abdominal aortic aneurysm, renal tumors, or can be spontaneous in the setting of anticoagulation medication, underlying blood dyscrasia, or vasculitis. In addition, RPH may be iatrogenic and can be seen in up to 1 % of percutaneous coronary interventions. Common presenting symptoms include hypotension and abdominal/back pain.

The imaging appearance varies with the acuity of the underlying event. Acute to subacute hematomas have a higher attenuation value due to the formation of blood clot, while chronic hematoma have a relatively lower attenuation on non-contrast CT scans due to the breakdown of blood products. Active bleeding is seen as extravasation of intraluminal contrast that is isodense to opacified blood vessels and should be linear in distribution and flame-shaped. The "sentinel clot" sign are areas of high attenuation corresponding to areas of acute clotted hemorrhage that are more likely to localize anatomic sites of hemorrhage. No enhancement is seen on post-contrast images. A fluid-hematocrit level may be occasionally seen (as in this case, arrow in Fig. 5.22b).

Pitfalls

1. The heterogeneous appearance of a RPH may be confused for a primary sarcoma, however, the lack of enhancement, well marginated borders, and change in appearance and decrease in size over time favors the presence of a hematoma.
2. Other non-neoplastic retroperitoneal collections may be differentiated by a combination of clinical history and imaging findings. Lymphoceles typically occur after lymph node dissection and may demonstrate areas of internal fat, urinomas will collect contrast on delayed excretory scans and pancreatic pseudocysts are seen with a history of pancreatitis.

Teaching Points

1. Hypotension, abdominal pain, and hematocrit drop should warrant a search for a retroperitoneal hematoma. A non-contrast CT scan is the next best imaging step.
2. Hematomas change in appearance over time: acute to subacute hematomas are relatively high in attenuation while chronic hematomas are of lower attenuation due to breakdown of blood products. A fluid hematocrit level is highly specific for a hematoma.
3. The lack of enhancement and change in appearance over time favors a hematoma over a primary retroperitoneal sarcoma.

Suggested Readings By Case

Case 5.1

Hartman DS, Hayes WS, Choyke PL, et al. From the archives of the AFIP. Leiomyosarcoma of the retroperitoneum and inferior vena cava: radiologic-pathologic correlation. Radiographics. 1992;12(6):1203–20.

Kandpal H, Sharma R, Gamangatti S, et al. Imaging the inferior vena cava: a road less traveled. Radiographics. 2008;28(3):669–89.

Webb EM, Wang ZJ, Westphalen AC, et al. Can CT features differentiate between inferior vena cava leiomyosarcomas and primary retroperitoneal masses? AJR Am J Roentgenol. 2013;200(1):205–9.

Case 5.2

Craig WD, Fanburg-Smith JC, Henry LR, et al. Fat-containing lesions of the retroperitoneum: radiologic-pathologic correlation. Radiographics. 2009;29(1):261–90.

O'Regan KN, Jagannathan J, Krajewski K, et al. Imaging of liposarcoma: classification, patterns of tumor recurrence, and response to treatment. AJR Am J Roentgenol. 2011; 197(1):W37–43.

Rajiah P, Sinha R, Cuevas C, et al. Imaging of uncommon retroperitoneal masses. Radiographics. 2011;31(4):949–76.

Case 5.3

Elsayes KM, Staveteig PT, Narra VR, et al. Retroperitoneal masses: magnetic resonance imaging findings with pathologic correlation. Curr Probl Diagn Radiol. 2007;36(3):97–106.

Rajiah P, Sinha R, Cuevas C, et al. Imaging of uncommon retroperitoneal masses. Radiographics. 2011;31(4):949–76.

Case 5.4

Dalal PU, Sohaib SA, Huddart R. Imaging of testicular germ cell tumours. Cancer Imaging. 2006;6(1):124–34.

Eberhardt SC, Johnson JA, Parsons RB. Oncology imaging in the abdomen and pelvis: where cancer hides. Abdom Imaging. 2013;38(4):641–71.

Rajiah P, Sinha R, Cuevas C, et al. Imaging of uncommon retroperitoneal masses. Radiographics. 2011;31(4):949–76.

Case 5.5

Fujita T, Kamiya K, Takahashi Y, et al. Mesenteric paraganglioma: report of a case. World J Gastrointest Surg. 2013;5(3):62–7.

Rha SE, Byun JY, Jung SE, et al. Neurogenic tumors in the abdomen: tumor types and imaging characteristics. Radiographics. 2003;23(1):29–43.

Case 5.6

Gupta G, Mammis A, Maniker A. Malignant peripheral nerve sheath tumors. Neurosurg Clin N Am. 2008;19(4):533–43.

Lin J, Martel W. Cross-sectional imaging of peripheral nerve sheath tumors: characteristic signs on CT, MR imaging, and sonography. AJR Am J Roentgenol. 2001;176(1):75–8.

Nishino M, Hayakawa K, Minami M, et al. Primary retroperitoneal neoplasms: CT and MR imaging findings with anatomic and pathologic diagnostic clues. Radiographics. 2003;23(1):45–57.

Case 5.7

Shanbhogue AK, Prasad SR, Takahashi N, et al. Somatic and visceral solitary fibrous tumors in the abdomen and pelvis: cross-sectional imaging spectrum. Radiographics. 2011;31(2):393–408.

Vallat-Decouvelaere AV, Sm D, Fletcher CD. Atypical and malignant solitary fibrous tumors in extrathoracic locations: evidence of their comparability to intra-thoracic tumors. Am J Surg Pathol. 1998;22:1501–11.

Wignall OJ, Moskovic EC, Thyway K, et al. Solitary fibrous tumors of the soft tissues: review of the imaging and clinical features with histopathologic correlation. AJR Am J Roentgenol. 2010;195(1):W55–62.

Case 5.8

Ozgonul A, Cece H, Sogut O, et al. Pneumoperitoneum, pneumoretroperitoneum and bilateral pneumothorax caused by ERCP. J Pak Med Assoc. 2010;60(1):60–1.

Silbergleit R, Silbergleit A, Silbergleit R, et al. Benign pneumoperitoneum associated with pneumomediastinum and pneumoretroperitoneum in ambulatory outpatients. J Emerg Med. 1999;17(1):81–5.

Tirkes T, Sandrasegaran K, Patel AA, et al. Peritoneal and retroperitoneal anatomy and its relevance for cross-sectional imaging. Radiographics. 2012;32(2):437–51.

Wu HM, Dixon E, May GR, et al. Management of perforation after endoscopic retrograde cholangiopancreatography (ERCP): a population-based review. HPB (Oxford). 2006;8(5):393–9.

Case 5.9

Cronin CG, Lohan DG, Blake MA, et al. Retroperitoneal fibrosis: a review of clinical features and imaging findings. AJR Am J Roentgenol. 2008;191(2):423–31.

Goenka AH, Shah SN, Remer EM. Imaging of the retroperitoneum. Radiol Clin North Am. 2012;50(2):333–55.

Case 5.10

Farouque HM, Tremmel JA, Raissi Shabari F, et al. Risk factors for the development of retroperitoneal hematoma after percutaneous coronary intervention in the era of glycoprotein IIb/IIIa inhibitors and vascular closure devices. J Am Coll Cardiol. 2005;45(3):363–8.

Rajiah P, Sinha R, Cuevas C, et al. Imaging of uncommon retroperitoneal masses. Radiographics. 2011;31(4):949–76.

Yang DM, Jung DH, Kim H, et al. Retroperitoneal cystic masses: CT, clinical, and pathologic findings and literature review. Radiographics. 2004;24(5):1353–65.

Chapter 6
Female Pelvis

Ovaries

Case 6.1

Brief Case Summary: 25 year old woman, annual check up

Imaging Findings Grey scale transvaginal ultrasound demonstrates several small follicles at cortex of the left ovary (Fig. 6.1).

Differential Diagnosis Polycystic ovaries

Diagnosis and Discussion: Ovarian Follicles

Ovarian follicles are the basic units of female reproductive biology, and contain a single oocyte (immature ovum or egg). These structures are periodically initiated to grow and develop, culminating in ovulation of usually a single competent oocyte in humans. These eggs/ova are developed once every menstrual cycle.

Approximately 10 ovarian follicles begin to mature in during a normal menstrual cycle and out of these usually one will turn into a dominant ovarian follicle. During ovulation, the primary follicle forms the secondary follicle, then becomes the mature vesicular follicle (also known as a Graafian follicle). After rupture, the follicle turns into a corpus luteum. Rupture of the follicle can result in abdominal pain (Mittelschmerz) and should be considered in the differential diagnosis in women of childbearing age who present with pain.

In the normal physiological state, one of the follicles typically becomes a dominant follicle which subsequently grows up to 2.9 cm. If the follicle is larger than 3.0 cm, then it is considered a follicular cyst.

On ultrasound following maturations under the development of gonadotropins, follicles can be seen as round, thin-walled, anechoic, less than 1 cm. in diameter around the ovary.

M.G. Harisinghani, A. Rajesh, *Genitourinary Imaging: A Case Based Approach*, DOI 10.1007/978-1-4471-4772-5_6

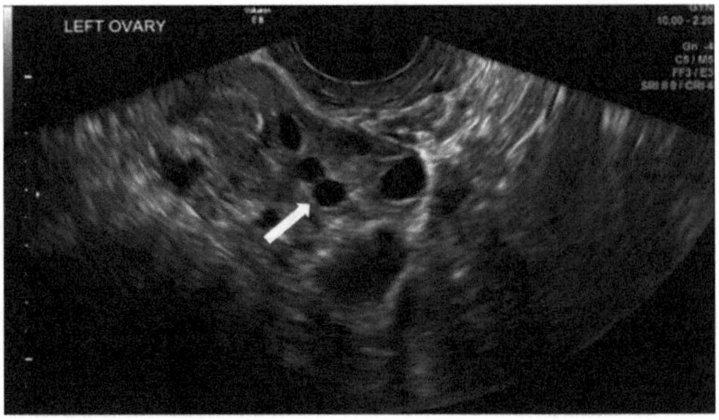

Fig. 6.1 Grey scale transvaginal ultrasound demonstrates several small follicles (*arrow*) at cortex of the left ovary

On MRI, ovarian follicles and follicular cysts may be seen rounded structures located at cortex of ovary. Signal characteristics within the follicles include T2 high signal intensity.

Pitfalls The presence of multiple peripheral small follicles on a background of ovarian enlargement and stromal hypertrophy should raise the suspicion of polycystic ovaries although polycystic ovarian syndrome is a clinical diagnosis.. Compared with polycystic ovaries, ovarian follicles tend to be fewer in number and larger, up to 10 mm in diameter.

Teaching Point Ovarian follicles are typically small, less than 1 cm in diameter, thin-walled, and anechoic on ultrasound and have high T2 signal intensity on MRI.

Case 6.2

Brief Case Summary 30-year-old female; check up, healthy

Imaging Findings Gray scale transvaginal US (arrow, Fig. 6.2) shows a thin-walled, unilocular well-defined anechoic cyst in right ovary. Transverse contrast-enhanced CT scan shows a well-circumscribed, low attenuation cyst (arrow, Fig. 6.3). Axial T2 MR image (arrow, Fig. 6.4) shows high signal intensity of the cyst.

Differential Diagnosis Surface epithelial tumor, Endometrioma, Ovarian dermoid

Diagnosis and Discussion: Follicular cyst

Occasionally the dominant maturing ovarian follicle fails to ovulate and does not involute. When the follicle is larger than 3 cm, it is considered an ovarian follicular cyst. They are typically 1–3 cm and rarely exceed 6 cm. Follicular cysts can have thin septations, focal thickening of the wall or increased attenuation. No solid nodular components should be present. On MRI, cysts are T1 hypointense, T2 hyperintense, however, the content may vary if complicated by hemorrhage. Spontaneous resolution of the follicular cysts is common.

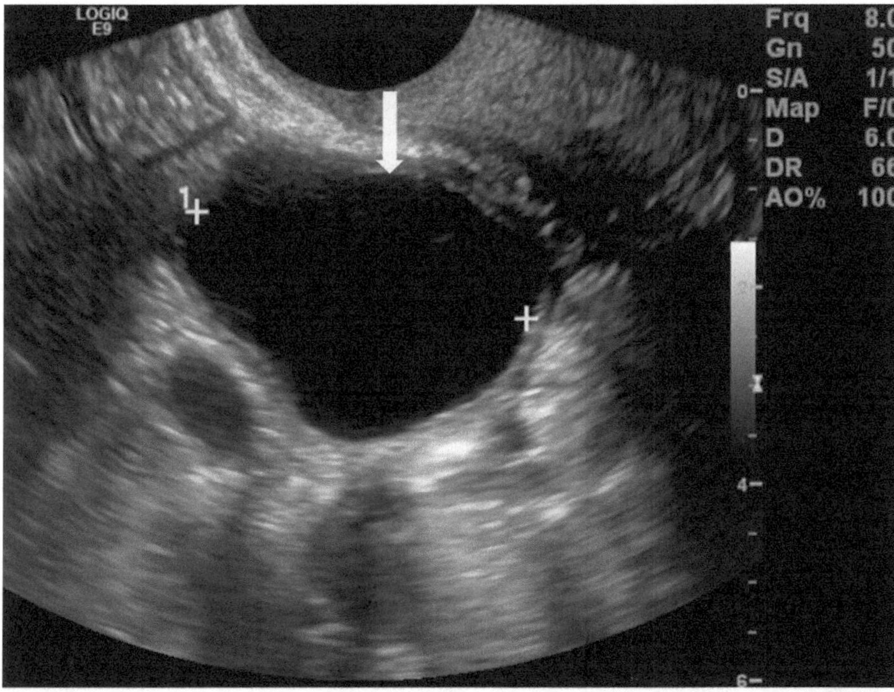

Fig. 6.2 Gray scale transvaginal US (*arrow*) shows a thin-walled, unilocular well-defined anechoic cyst in right ovary

Fig. 6.3 Transverse contrast-enhanced CT scan shows a well-circumscribed, low attenuation cyst (*arrow*)

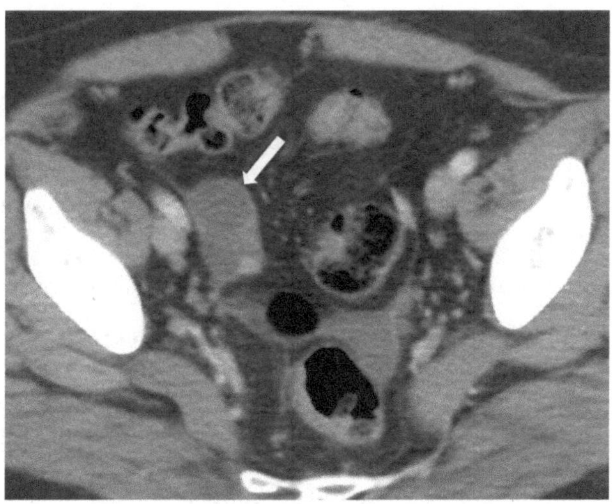

Pitfalls Clot in hemorrhagic cysts can mimic a solid nodule on US, but should not demonstrate flow on Doppler US.

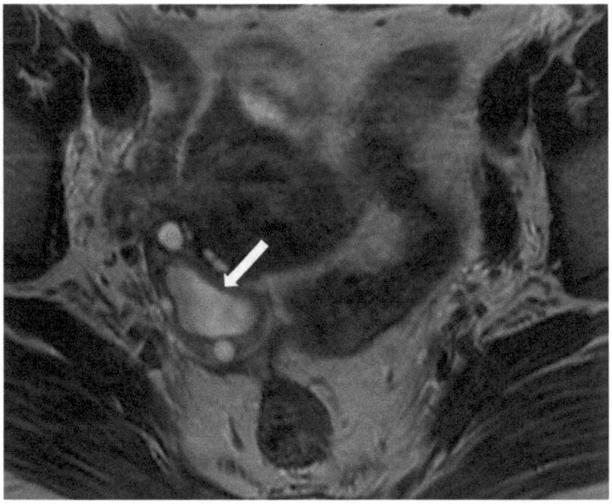

Fig. 6.4 Axial T2 MR image (*arrow*) shows high signal intensity of the cyst

Teaching Point

- Follow-up ultrasound in the premenopausal woman, should demonstrate resolution of follicular cysts after the next menstrual cycle.
- MRI is helpful in distinguishing hemorrhagic cystic from solid lesions.

Case 6.3

Brief Case Summary 25-year-old female with pelvic pain

Imaging Findings Gray scale transvaginal US shows a thick-walled ovary cyst (arrow, Fig. 6.5). Color Doppler US shows a "ring of fire" of increased vascularity of the thick-walled cyst with internal echogenic content (arrow, Fig. 6.6). Contrast-enhanced CT (Fig. 6.7) and MRI (Fig. 6.8) shows wall enhancement of the right ovarian cyst.

Differential Diagnosis Endometrioma, Ovarian abscess, Cystic ovarian tumors

Diagnosis and Discussion: Corpus lutein cyst

After ovulation and release of the oocyte, there is proliferation of the granulosa cells which are along the inner lining of the cyst. The dominant follicle collapses and the proliferation of the granuloma cells form the corpus luteum of menstruation.

The corpus luteum degenerates over 14 days and becomes a scarred corpus albicans. The corpus luteum can seal and contain fluid or blood and form a corpus luteum cyst. The corpus luteum cysts may grow to 1–10 cm in size but are usually less than 4 cm in size.

Corpus luteum cysts are often incidental findings and asymptomatic unless complicated by hemorrhagic or torsion. On US, the appearance varies but commonly

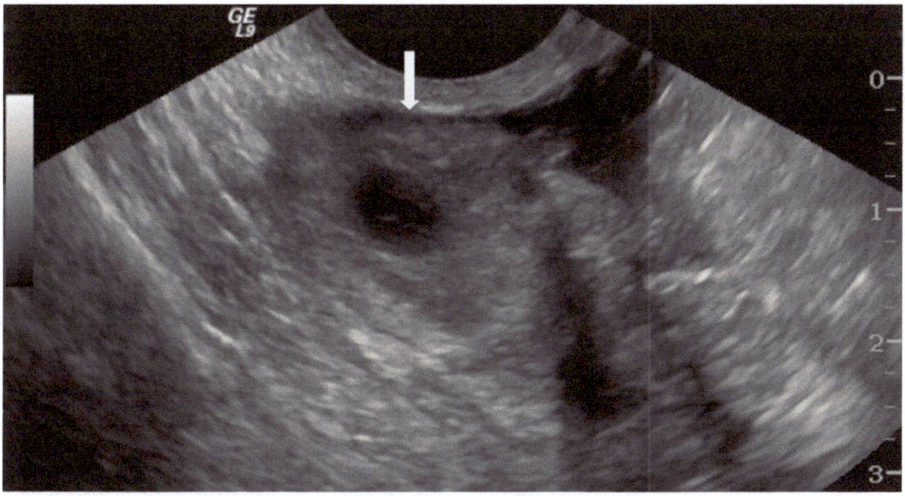

Fig. 6.5 Gray scale transvaginal US shows a thick-walled ovary cyst (*arrow*)

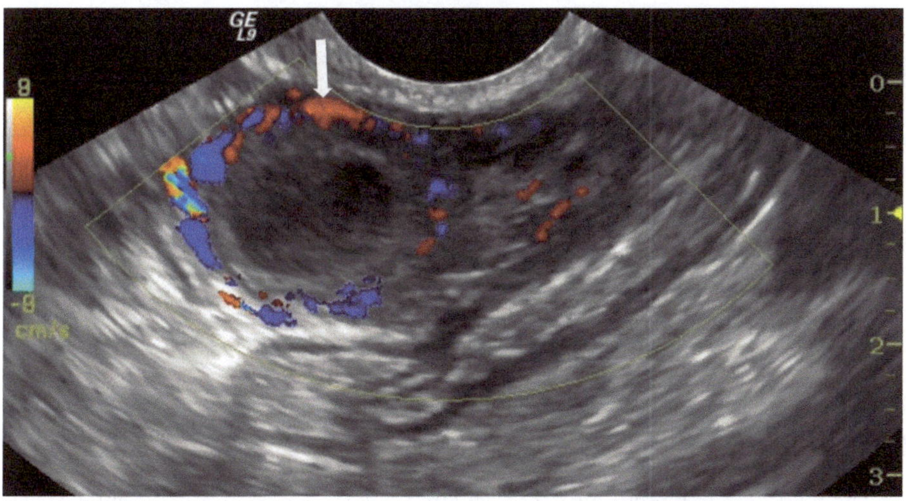

Fig. 6.6 Color Doppler US shows a "ring of fire" of increased vascularity of the thick-walled cyst with internal echogenic content (*arrow*)

they are typically small complex cysts and with color Doppler, the "ring of fire" sign can be seen in the cyst wall where there is increased vascularity. On MR, the cyst is T1 hypointense, T2 hyperintense with a thick wall but the signal can vary depending on the presence of hemorrhage.

Pitfalls The mural flow seen at Doppler ultrasound or contrast enhancement may overlap that of cystic ovarian tumors

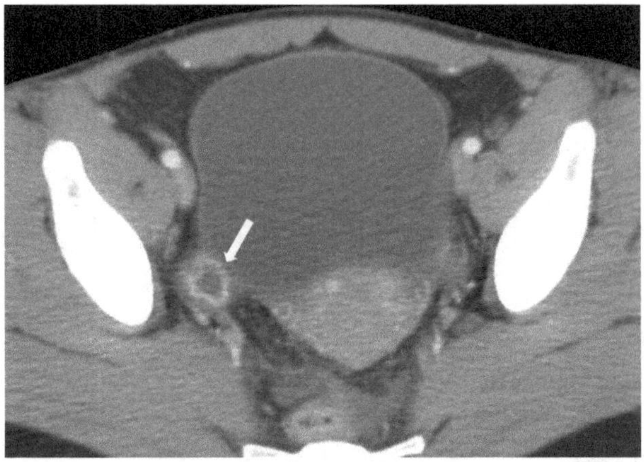

Fig. 6.7 Contrast-enhanced CT shows wall enhancement (*arrow*) of the right ovarian cyst

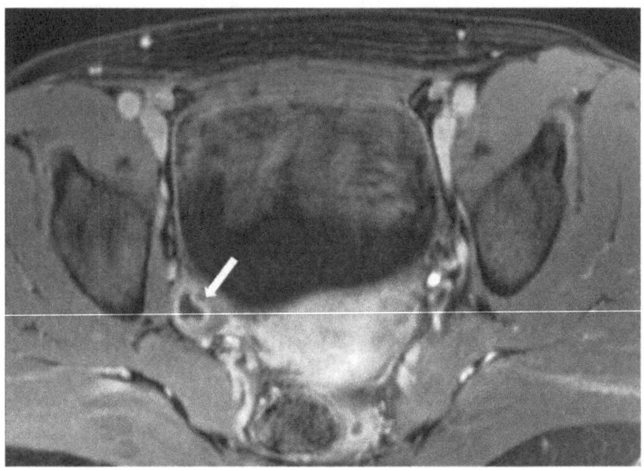

Fig. 6.8 MRI shows wall enhancement (*arrow*) of the right ovarian cyst

Teaching Point

- Most likely diagnosis when a vascular cyst or solid-appearing mass is present in premenopausal women
- The wall corpus luteum cysts are usually thicker than those of follicular cysts, a distinction that can be made by ultrasound.
- Hemorrhagic corpus luteum cysts may appear similar to the hemorrhagic cysts of endometriosis; on MRI, the older blood products within the more persistent endometriomas are more likely to produce the imaging finding of hemosiderin that shows low intensity in T2W images.

Case 6.4

Brief Case Summary A 13 week pregnant woman presents with upper quadrant abdominal pain.

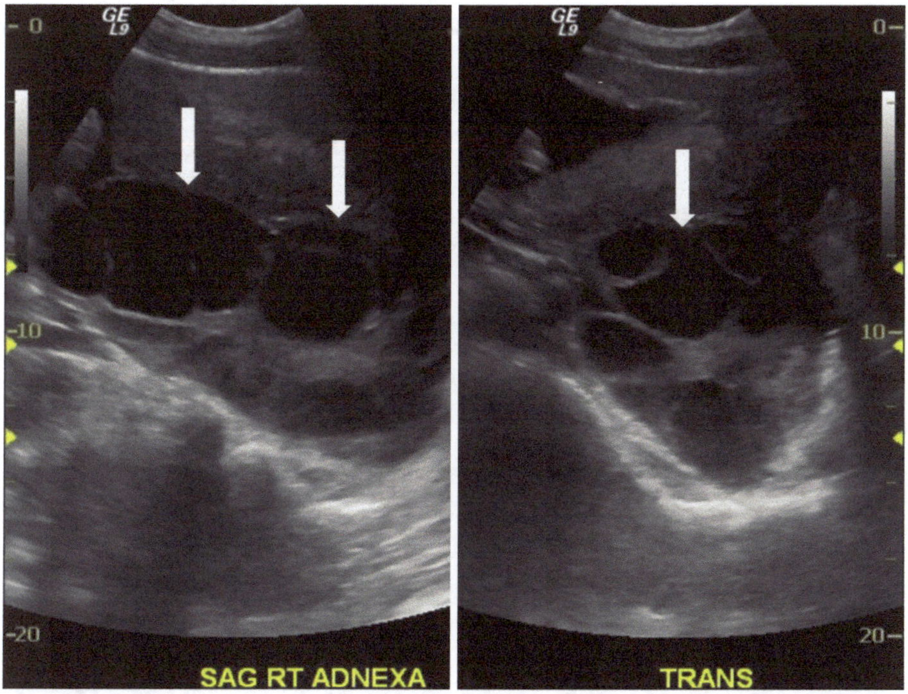

Fig. 6.9 Transverse transabdominal ultrasound shows bilateral enlarged multicystic ovaries (*arrows*)

Imaging Findings Transverse and sagittal transabdominal ultrasounds show bilateral enlarged multicystic ovaries (Figs. 6.9 and 6.10).

Differential Diagnosis Ovarian epithelial neoplasms, Luteoma of pregnancy, polycystic ovarian disease

Diagnosis and Discussion: Theca-lutein cysts

Theca lutein cysts are associated with disorders resulting in high levels of human chorionic gonadotropin (β-hCG) and are rarely seen in singleton pregnancies. Theses cysts may appear in patients with gestational trophoblastic disease, multiple gestations, and those undergoing infertility treatments that involve administration of ovarian stimulation agents. Theca-lutein cysts are usually asymptomatic. Abdominal pain if hemorrhage, rupture or torsion occurs.

On US, theca lutein cysts manifest as anechoic and multiloculated ovarian cysts in bilaterally enlarged ovaries. There may be thin intervening septations but no solid nodularity or papillary excrescences. The cysts may contain low level echoes if hemorrhage is present. MR findings mirror those on US and the cysts are simple T2 hyperintense lesions with possible thin internal septations. The central ovarian stroma may appear solid and a "spoke-wheel" appearance of the multiple cysts has been described.

Theca lutein cysts develop with complete hydatiform moles in approximately 14–30 % of cases. A uterus with a distended endometrium containing echogenic tissue is diagnostic. Partial molar pregnancies and complete molar pregnancies in the first trimester are not likely to be associated with theca lutein cysts as the β-hCG levels are relatively low.

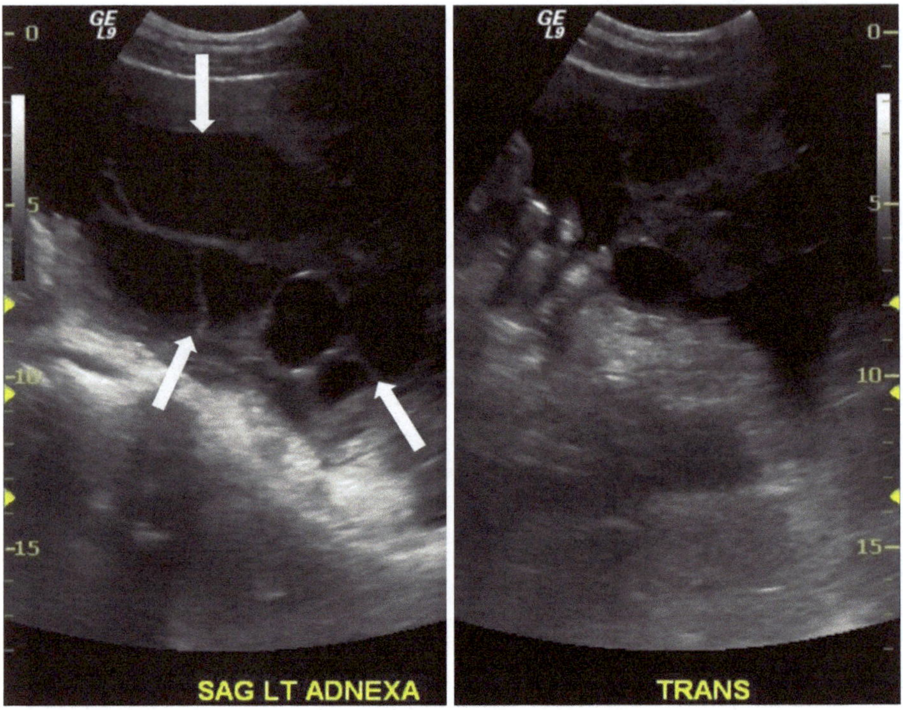

Fig. 6.10 Sagittal transabdominal ultrasound shows bilateral enlarged multicystic ovaries (*arrows*)

Pitfalls

- Misdiagnosis can result in unnecessary surgical removal of ovaries for suspected ovarian neoplasm

Teaching Point

- Presence of theca lutein cysts must be considered before ovarian neoplasm in the setting of a positive β-hCG or history of ovarian stimulation.
- They may be distinguished from bilateral ovarian carcinoma by the absence of solid-tissue components or papillary excrescences.
- May have hypervascular central uterine mass if associated with molar pregnancy.
- Typical regress after causative factor is removed.

Case 6.5

Brief Case Summary: 27 year old female with infertility.

Imaging Findings Gray scale US images of the adnexa demonstrate the presence of enlarged ovaries containing multiple peripherally oriented follicles (Fig. 6.11a, b). Axial T2 weighted MR image replicates the ultrasound findings with enlarged ovaries containing multiple peripheral follicles (Fig. 6.12).

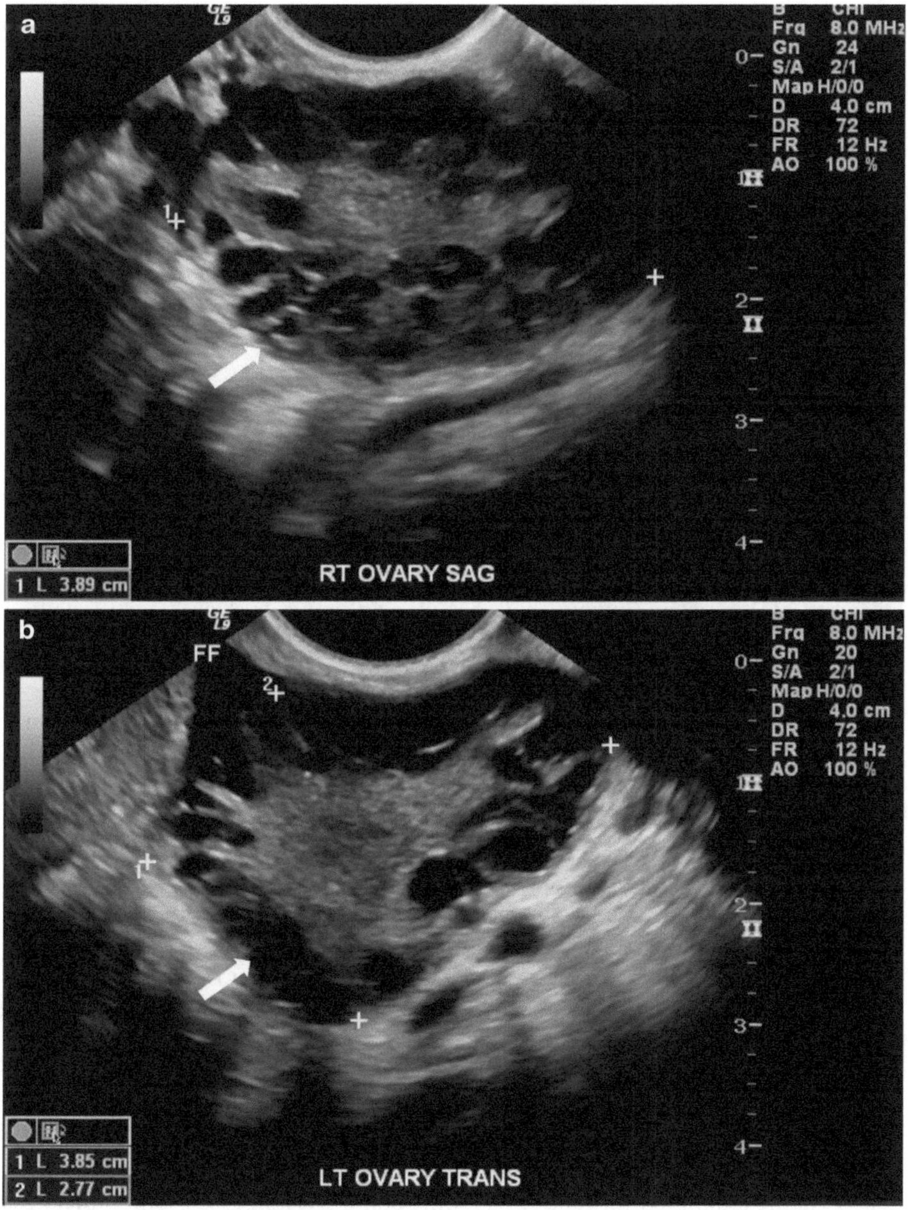

Fig. 6.11 (**a**, **b**). Gray scale US images of the adnexa demonstrate the presence of enlarged ovaries (*arrow*) containing multiple peripherally oriented follicles

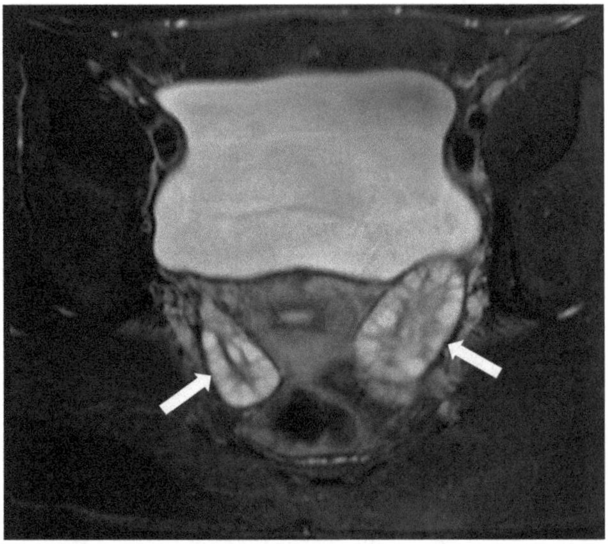

Fig. 6.12 Axial T2 weighted MR image replicates the ultrasound findings with enlarged ovaries (*arrow*) containing multiple peripheral follicles

Differential Diagnosis Polycystic ovaries, ovarian torsion, ovarian hyperstimulation syndrome, theca-lutein cysts.

Diagnosis and Discussion: Polycystic ovaries

Polycystic ovarian syndrome (PCOS, also known as Stein-Lenthal syndrome) represents the most common endocrine abnormality among women of reproductive age, with an incidence of approximately 5–10 %. The current diagnostic criteria for PCOS (Rotterdam criteria) involves having two of the following three conditions: (1) clinical or biochemical signs of hyperandrogenism, (2) oligo or anovulation and (3) polycystic ovaries by ultrasound. Clinically, patients often present with signs of hirsutism and irregular menstrual bleeding. In addition, patients are often overweight and have at an increased risk for hypertension, insulin-resistant diabetes mellitus and hyperlipidemia. There may also be an increased risk for endometrial hyperplasia and cancer.

The goal of transvaginal ultrasound is to diagnose the presence of polycystic ovaries as part of the clinical workup, though patients with normal ovaries may still have PCOS. The presence of an enlarged ovary (with volume exceeding 10 cm^3) and/or ovaries with 12 or more follicles measuring 2–9 mm in diameter is sufficient for the diagnosis of polycystic ovaries on imaging. Ovarian volumes may be estimated via the simplified formula for an ellipsoid: 0.5 x length x width x thickness of the ovary. The presence of multiple follicles has been classically termed the "string of pearls" sign, though adherence to a strict objective measurement is advocated. If ultrasound remains inconclusive, MR imaging may be performed. Findings on MRI reflect the sonographic criteria, with enlarged ovaries containing multiple subcentimeter follicles, which are hyperintense on T2 weighted images. The background ovarian stroma is generally of low signal on T2 weighted images.

The imaging findings can corroborate known or clinically suspected PCOS, however, the presence of normal ovaries does not exclude the syndrome. On the other hand, the presence of polycystic ovaries is not diagnostic of PCOS. Ultrasound may also be used to monitor ovarian volumes in patients with known PCOS being treated with ovulation induction agents, with decreased volumes on serial studies potentially predictive of improved fertility outcomes.

Pitfalls Enlarged ovaries may also be seen with other entities, including ovarian hyperstimulation syndrome (OHSS) and ovarian torsion. OHSS is most often seen in the setting of in-vitro fertilization and demonstrates variable sized cysts associated with signs of third spacing including ascites, pleural effusions. Torsion presents with pelvic pain with ultrasound demonstrating an enlarged ovary with a heterogeneous echotexture, peripherally displaced follicles and variable absence of flow. Theca-lutein cysts are typically seen in the setting of gestational trophoblastic disease and demonstrate multiple enlarged cysts on sonographic evaluation.

Teaching Points

1. Polycystic ovaries are enlarged ovaries with volume exceeding 10 cm^3 and/or ovaries with 12 or more follicles measuring 2–9 mm in diameter.
2. The current diagnostic criteria for PCOS (Rotterdam criteria) involves having two of the following three conditions: (1) clinical or biochemical signs of hyperandrogenism, (2) oligo or anovulation and (3) polycystic ovaries by ultrasound. Thus, the presence of normal ovaries by ultrasound does not exclude the presence of PCOS.
3. A combination of the clinical history and size of the follicles can allow confident differentiation from ovarian torsion, ovarian hyperstimulation syndrome and theca-lutein cysts.

Case 6.6

Brief Case Summary 35 year-old female with left adnexal mass

Imaging Findings Transvaginal ultrasound (Fig. 6.13) demonstrates a normal appearing left ovary (arrowhead) and a simple cystic lesion adjacent to the ovary (arrow). Axial T2W MR image (Fig. 6.14) show a simple extraovarian cystic lesion in the left adnexa (arrow) and a normal left ovary (arrowhead).

Differential Diagnosis Eccentric functional ovarian cysts, Peritoneal inclusion cysts, Hydrosalpinx

Diagnosis and Discussion: Paraovarian cyst

Paraovarian cysts arise from the broad ligament, typically from mesothelium of the peritoneum or paramesonephric elements and are covered by a single layer of cells. They account for approximately 10–20 % of all adnexal masses.

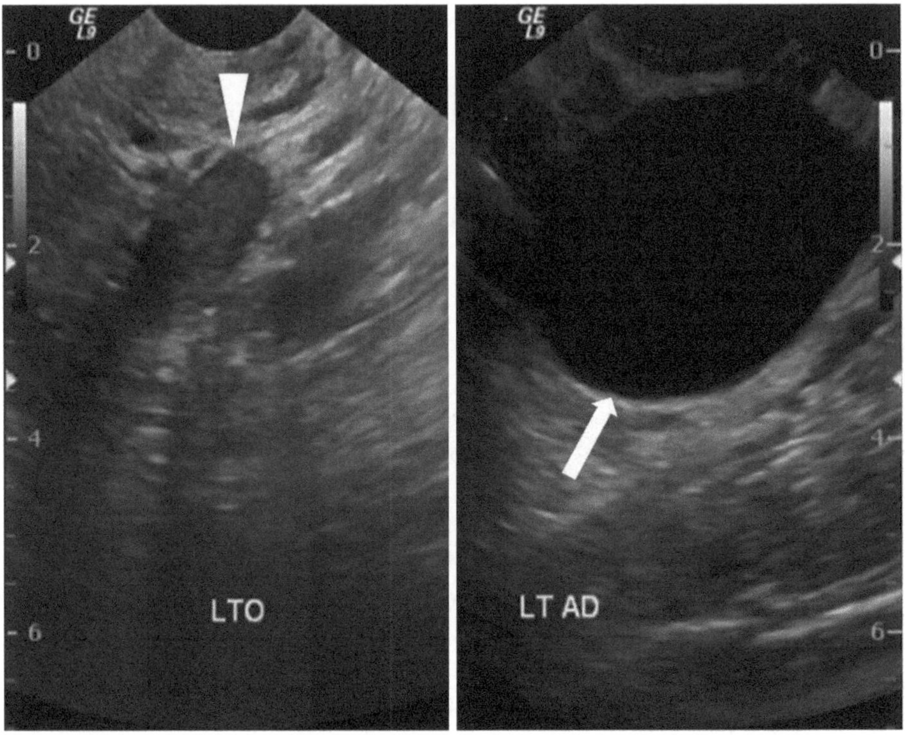

Fig. 6.13 Transvaginal ultrasound demonstrates a normal appearing left ovary (*arrowhead*) and a simple cystic lesion adjacent to the ovary (*arrow*)

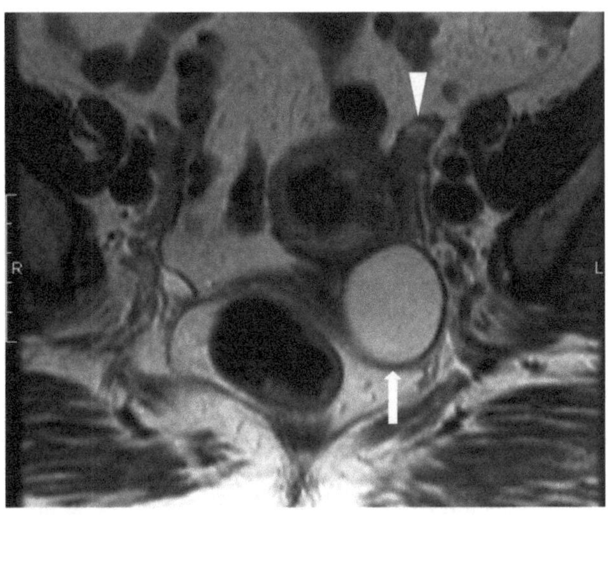

Fig. 6.14 Axial T2W MR image show a simple extraovarian cystic lesion in the left adnexa (*arrow*) and a normal left ovary (*arrowhead*)

Paraovarian cysts are located adjacent to but not originating from ipsilateral normal ovary. Differentiation between ovarian cysts and paraovarian cysts can be challenging but clear separation between the ovary and normal ovary is helpful in the diagnosis of paraovarian cysts. They are anechoic lesions of variable size, up to 20 cm in diameter and can be single or multicystic or unilateral or bilateral.

Malignant transformation has been reported in 2–3 % of paraovarian cysts and the presence of papillary projections growing from cyst wall are suspicious features.

Pitfalls Clear separation between the ovary and the cystic lesion is helpful in differentiating a paraovarian cyst from an ovarian cyst. An oval configuration of a hydrosalpinx can be confused with a paraovarian cyst. An MR of the pelvis can help in differentiating these diagnoses.

Teaching Point Dynamic evaluation with transvaginal ultrasound can show movement of cyst relative to other structures separate from the ovary. MR of the pelvis is helpful in ambiguous cases.

Case 6.7

Brief Case Summary 35 year-old female with cyclical pelvic pain.

Imaging Findings Axial T1 with fat saturation image of the pelvis (arrows, Fig. 6.15) demonstrates bilateral ovarian T1 hyperintense masses (arrows) which are less hyperintense on the T2 weighted images (arrows, Fig. 6.16) demonstrating the "T2 shading" sign.

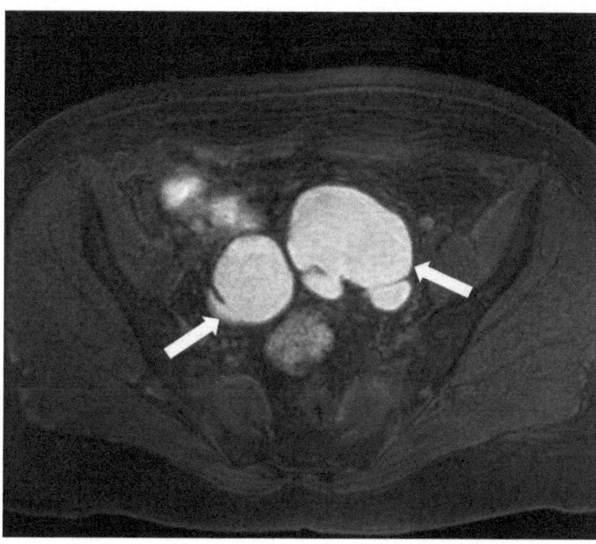

Fig. 6.15 Axial T1 with fat saturation image of the pelvis (*arrows*) demonstrates bilateral ovarian T1 hyperintense masses (*arrows*)

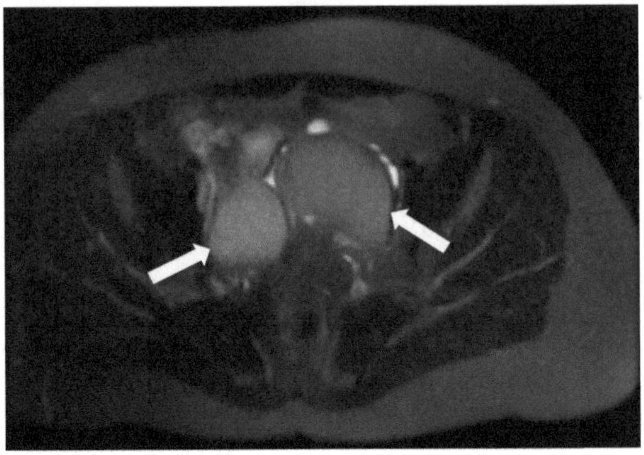

Fig. 6.16 T2 weighted images (*arrows*) demonstrating the "T2 shading" sign

Differential Diagnosis Hemorrhagic cysts, dermoid cysts, tubo-ovarian abscess, mucinous tumours.

Diagnosis and Discussion Endometriosis is defined as the presence of functional endometrial tissue outside the uterus. It occurs as small implants or cystic lesions called endometriomas on the serosal and peritoneal surfaces of the abdomen. The ovary is the most commonly involved structure, followed by the pelvic peritoneum. Extra-abdominal locations have also been described, the most frequent being the lungs and the central nervous system. The disease is more prevalent in childbearing age. It is diagnosed in 17–50 % of patients investigated for infertility and in 5–18 % of those with pelvic pain.

The etiopathogenesis is still controversial. The most accepted hypothesis is retrograde menstruation, with less popular theories being direct implantation after uterine surgical procedures and hematogenous dissemination.

A woman of childbearing age with chronic pelvic pain which may be cyclical in nature or a woman who presents with infertility must be evaluated for the presence of endometriosis given the morbidity associated with delayed diagnosis. Adhesions can lead to bowel obstruction. Patients can also present with extrabdominal manifestations which include catamenial pneumothorax or hemoptysis and recurrent subarachnoid hemorrhage.

The pathological lesions include implants, endometriotic cysts and adhesions. Implants can range from a few millimeters up to 2 cm. Endometriotic cysts, also known as "chocolate cysts", result from repeated hemorrhages in a deep implant, almost always in the ovaries. Imaging is less useful than diagnostic laparoscopy for diagnosis of this condition as there is no relation between the size of the implants and the nature and severity of the symptoms; small implants are often missed, which nonetheless may cause debilitating pain. Moreover, adhesions cannot be imaged but can be seen in a diagnostic laparoscopy.

Ultrasound, often the first modality to image a woman with pelvic pain, often detects the larger endometriomas, but is insensitive for the detection of implants and adhesions. The classic sonographic description of an endometrioma is a unilocular adnexal cystic lesion separate from the ovary with angular margins and homogenous low-level internal echoes. The lesions are often multiple and bilateral. The distribution pattern of the internal echoes has been termed as 'shading', which is a graduated change of increasing echogenicity from the non-dependent to the dependent area. Rarely, layering with fluid-fluid level may be seen. Echogenic foci may be noted in the wall of the endometrioma, hypothesised to be cholesterol resulting from breakdown of cell membranes. Mural nodules may be noted, which if vascular, should raise the suspicion of a secondary malignancy.

CT is not useful as a screening or diagnostic modality and findings are usually incidentally noted in the imaging workup of abdominal or pelvic pain. Mixed density adnexal masses, soft tissue nodules in the anterior abdominal wall, and adhesive bowel obstruction may be evident.

MRI is the imaging modality of choice in the workup of suspected endometriosis. T1 and T2 weighted sequences, with fat suppressed T1 sequence form the mainstay of the imaging protocol. Contrast imaging is not routinely required; it is performed in the evaluation of a mural nodule for malignancy, where subtraction imaging is useful.

MRI findings may be pathognomonic. The implants are hyperintense on T1 fat suppressed sequence. Endometriotic cysts exhibit signal characteristics consistent with hemorrhage, frequently hyperintense on both T1 and T2. "The T2 shading sign" is visualized on T2 sequence whereby the T1 hyperintense endometriomas show T2 shortening due to high concentration of protein and hemorrhage from recurrent hemorrhage. A T2 dark spot sign is more specific and is defined as discrete, well-defined markedly hypointense focus within the adnexal lesion on T2-weighted images. Hematosalphinx can be seen. Hemorrhagic foci and areas of scarring are noted in the rectovaginal septum, uterosacral ligaments and the pelvic floor muscles, seen as T2 hypointense foci. Distortion of normal anatomy is often seen with posterior displacement of the uterus and ovaries, angulation of bowel loops, and elevation of the posterior vaginal fornix. Rectal strictures may form and bladder or ureteric involvement can result in hydronephrosis.

Treatment is dependent on the desire for future fertility, stage of disease, symptoms and age. Medical management is reserved for the early stages with analgesics and hormonal therapy to suppress the cyclical hemorrhage. MRI is useful for assessment of treatment response. Laparoscopic adhesiolysis can be performed in case of bowel symptoms. If fertility is not desired, hysterectomy and bilateral salphingo-oopherectomy with attempt at excision of all implants are made.

Pitfalls Hemorrhagic ovarian cysts may mimic endometriomas; shading and a T2 dark spot are useful signs suggesting recurrent hemorrhage in an endometrioma, which are usually absent in the hemorrhagic cysts. Occasionally a 6 week follow up may be needed which will reveal change in morphology in a hemorrhagic cyst with retractile clot formation. A tubo-ovarian abscess, a mimic on ultrasound, can easily be distinguished clinically from endometrioma. Enhancing mural nodule, rapid growth of the endometrioma and disappearance of the T2 shading can portend a malignant change.

Teaching Points

1. Endometriosis is a disease of the young reproductive age group.
2. Diagnostic laparoscopy is the mainstay of diagnosis although imaging plays a crucial role in detection of endometriomas where MRI is the modality of choice.
3. Classic signs in US for an endometrioma are a cystic adnexal lesion, often multiple and bilateral, with diffuse low level internal echoes, hyperechoic wall foci and absence of neoplastic features.
4. Classic features in MRI for an endometrioma include T1 hyperintense adnexal cysts which have the "T2 shading sign" and "T2 dark spots".

Case 6.8

Brief Case Summary 33 year old female with an acute pelvic pain

Imaging Findings On CT (Fig. 6.17), there is an enlarged left ovary measuring 7.6 × 5.7 cm (arrow) containing a 3.6 cm cyst (asterisk) and follicles that is located to the right of midline, likely representing a torsed ovary. On an axial T2 weighted image (Fig. 6.18), a 8.3 × 6.1 × 6.3 cm cystic and solid adnexal lesion (arrow) superior to the bladder and anterior to the uterus but separate from the uterus is seen and contains multiple peripheral foci of T2 hyperintensity with a dominant 3.6 cm T2 hyperintense lesion (asterisk). On US with color Doppler (Fig. 6.19), the left ovary is enlarged with a twisted pedicle. Several follicles are seen in the ovary with a reticulated pattern (asterisk).

Differential Diagnosis Acute appendicitis, ureteric calculus, diverticulitis, colitis, mesenteric adenitis, ectopic pregnancy, pelvic inflammatory disease, ruptured ovarian cyst, infarcting broad ligament fibroid, ovarian hyperstimulation syndrome, and endometriosis.

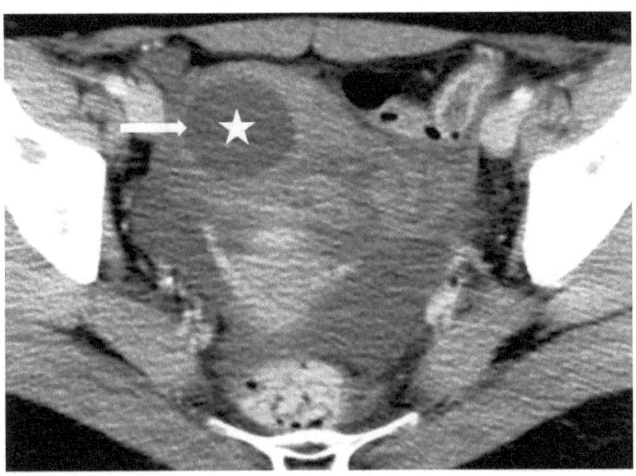

Fig. 6.17 CT showing an enlarged left ovary (*arrow*) containing a cyst (*asterisk*) and follicles that is located to the right of midline, likely representing a torsed ovary

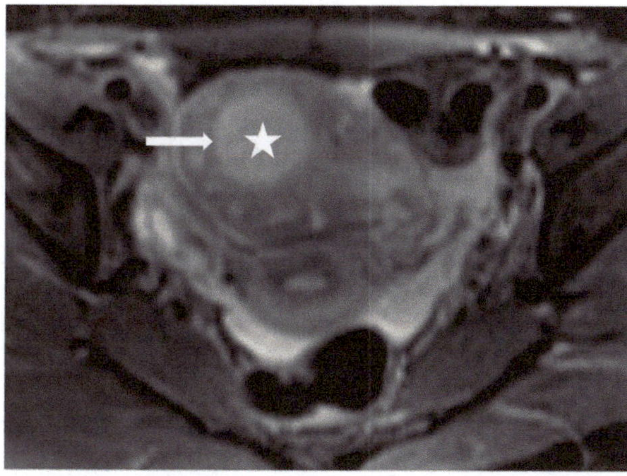

Fig. 6.18 Axial T2 weighted image showing a cystic and solid adnexal lesion (*arrow*) superior to the bladder and anterior to the uterus but separate from the uterus is seen and contains multiple peripheral foci of T2 hyperintensity with a dominant T2 hyperintense lesion (*asterisk*)

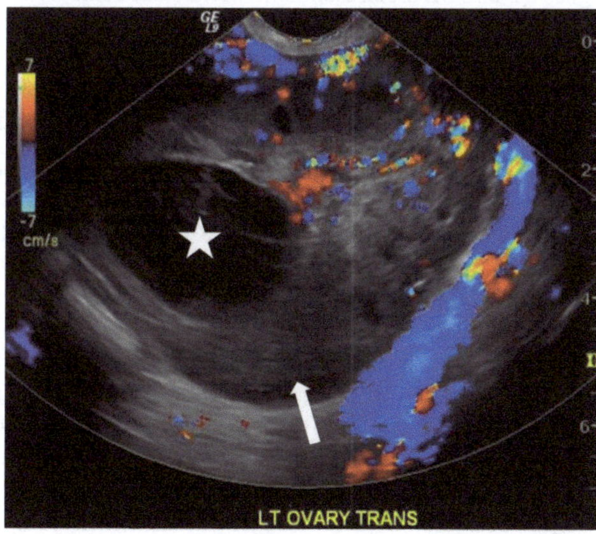

Fig. 6.19 US with color Doppler showing an enlarged left ovary (*arrow*) and is enlarged with a twisted pedicle. Several follicles are seen in the ovary with a reticulated pattern (*asterisk*)

Diagnosis and Discussion Ovarian torsion is the fifth most common gynecological emergency with an estimated prevalence of 2.7 % and 10–20 % cases occur during pregnancy. Ovarian torsion is frequently associated with ovarian stimulation treatment for IVF or ovarian masses. The most common lesion associated with a torsed ovary is a physiologic cyst, accounting for 17 % of lesions, and the most common tumor associated with a torsed ovary is a dermoid, accounting for 17 %. Ovarian torsion is defined as complete or partial rotation of the ovarian vascular pedicle on its long axis. Early and accurate diagnosis must be made to avoid interruption of venous and arterial flow which may lead to edema, ischemia and necrosis of ovary. If untreated, then peritonitis and death may ultimately result. Unfortunately, the clinical symptoms of ovarian torsion lack specificity and is often initially misdiagnosed as other acute abdominal diseases, and the rate of misdiagnosis varies from 23–66 %.

US is typically the first imaging modality and imaging features include an enlarged ovary, ovarian mass, free fluid, follicles at the periphery of an enlarged ovary, thickening of a cyst wall, and a twisted pedicle. The common finding found in 74 % cases is a unilaterally enlarged ovary (dimension more than 4.0 cm or volume greater than 20 cm^3 in a postmenopausal woman) with central afollicular stroma and multiple uniform 8–12-mm peripheral follicles. On Doppler US images in 35–93 % of patients with ovarian torsion, an abnormal venous blood flow is detected however altered arterial blood flow may not be seen. Additionally, color Doppler is helpful in looking for a "whirlpool sign" which denotes the twisted pedicle vessels which is the most specific feature of ovarian torsion. This sign also can be optimally showed on multiplanar CT and MRI images, especially after contrast administration. On enhanced images, heterogeneous minimal or absent enhancement of ovary may be identified due to ovarian ischemia to infarction. Besides displaying the above signs, CT and MRI can also demonstrate subacute ovarian hematoma and abnormal or absent ovarian enhancement. Subacute hemorrhage is best detected on unenhanced CT as an ovarian cyst with a layering hematocrit level or an ovarian high-density intraparenchymal hematoma, and on fat saturation T1-weighted MR images as a hematoma with hyperintense rim within an enlarged ovary.

Pitfalls Although twisting of the ovarian pedicle is a specific sign of ovary torsion, it is identified in less than one-third of patients on CT or MRI. Other signs such as enlarged ovary with multiple follicles and abnormal enhancement, are not specific and can be seen in many other female pelvic diseases. On CT, abnormal enhancement of a solid enlarged ovary can sometimes be difficult to distinguish from a nonenhancing cyst as well as an infarcted broad ligament fibroid. The prevalence of a normal ipsilateral ovary can aid to identify an infarcted fibroid. Some other pelvic diseases presenting as an enlarged ovarian or adnexal mass combined with acute pelvic pain can be confused with ovarian torsion, such as ectopic pregnancy, hemorrhagic corpus luteum cyst, and hypervascular nonepithelial primary ovarian tumors. The β-HCG test and enhanced CT or MRI scan may aid in the differential diagnosis. Polycystic ovarian hyperstimulation syndrome presents as massively enlarged ovaries which may also mimic ovarian torsion. The bilaterally enlarged ovaries and the clinical information with ovarian hyperstimulation are helpful in differentiating the two cases.

Teaching Point

1. A unilaterally enlarged ovary with central afollicular stroma and multiple uniform peripheral follicles is the most common sign of ovarian torsion and the "whirlpool sign" is the most specific feature.
2. Accurate and early detection of a torsed ovary can prevent ischemia and infarction of the ovary. CT and MRI images can aid to display the twisted pedicle vessels, abnormal blood supply of ovary, and subacute ovarian hematoma.
3. Ovarian cysts and dermoids are commonly seen lesions associated with ovarian torsion.

Case 6.9

Brief Case Summary 42 year old woman with fullness in pelvis.

Imaging Findings Color Doppler ultrasound (Fig. 6.20) image shows a large well defined heterogeneous lesion posterior to the uterus with numerous floating echogenic spherical globules.

Axial MRI in-phase (Fig. 6.21a) and opposed phase (Fig. 6.21b) images confirmed the presence of spherical globules within the lesion which are hyperintense on T1 weighted image (Fig. 6.21a) with signal loss on an opposed phase sequence (Fig. 6.21b) consistent with intralesional fat.

Differential Diagnosis Malignant ovarian tumor.

Diagnosis and Discussion Mature cystic ovarian teratoma.

Mature cystic teratoma is the commonest germ cell tumor, it comprises 10–15 % of ovarian neoplasms. It is a benign tumor comprised of derivatives of all 3 germ cell layers, although ectodermal elements predominate, hence the term dermoid cyst.

Sonography is usually sufficient for diagnosis showing cystic lesions with fat-fluid levels, internal echogenic elements, and calcifications. The finding of multiple intracystic echogenic globules is less common but there is sufficient literature to suggest this as a pathognomonic appearance, owing to their low density they tend to float within the cyst. In equivocal cases CT or MRI show these findings to better

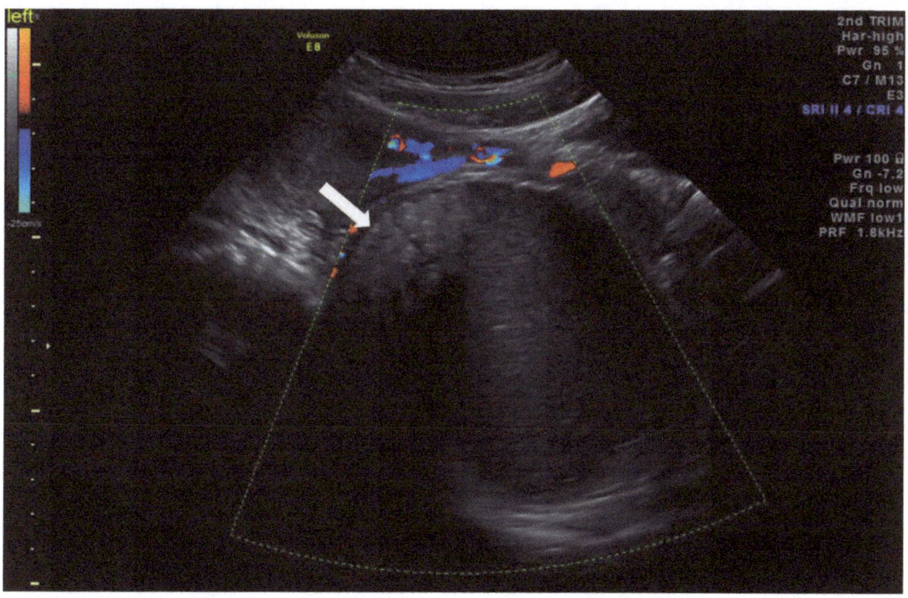

Fig. 6.20 Color Doppler ultrasound image shows a large well defined heterogeneous lesion (*arrow*) posterior to the uterus with numerous floating echogenic spherical globules

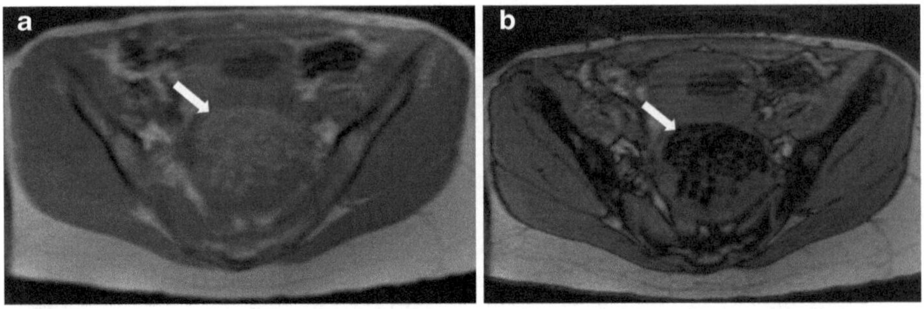

Fig. 6.21 (**a**) Axial MRI in-phase and (**b**) opposed phase images confirmed the presence of spherical globules (*arrow*) within the lesion which are hyperintense on in-phase T1 weighted image (**a**) with signal loss on an opposed phase sequence (**b**) consistent with intralesional fat

advantage. Almost all of the case with this appearance have been large cysts suggesting that these globules form when there is sufficient space available for them to act as a nidus with surrounding deposition of sebaceous material and fat. The fat content of these globules can be proven by in and opposed phase images on MRI, with signal dropout in opposed phase images.

Other germ cell tumors of the ovary include embryonal carcinoma, choriocarcinoma, and endodermal sinus tumor.

Pitfalls

- These fat globules if few in number can be confused for a mural nodule of ovarian malignancy. Application of Doppler color flow will aid in differentiation as teratoma fat globules do not show vascularity.

Teaching Point

- The finding of floating lipid spherules within a large cyst is pathognomonic for a mature cystic teratoma.
- Floating fat globules, no color flow on Doppler ultrasound, and loss of signal on opposed-phase MR images confirm the diagnosis of dermoid and should help in avoiding misdiagnosis.

Case 6.10

Brief Case Summary 52 years old female with clinical stage IIB clear cell adenocarcinoma of cervix.

Imaging Findings Axial T2 MR image (Fig. 6.22) demonstrates a right ovarian hypointense lesion (arrow) with homogeneous enhancement, on the axial T1 postgadolinium image (Fig. 6.23). In the left adnexa, a 2.8 cm T2 hyperintense nonenhancing lesion is seen in the ovary (asterisk) consistent with a benign cyst.

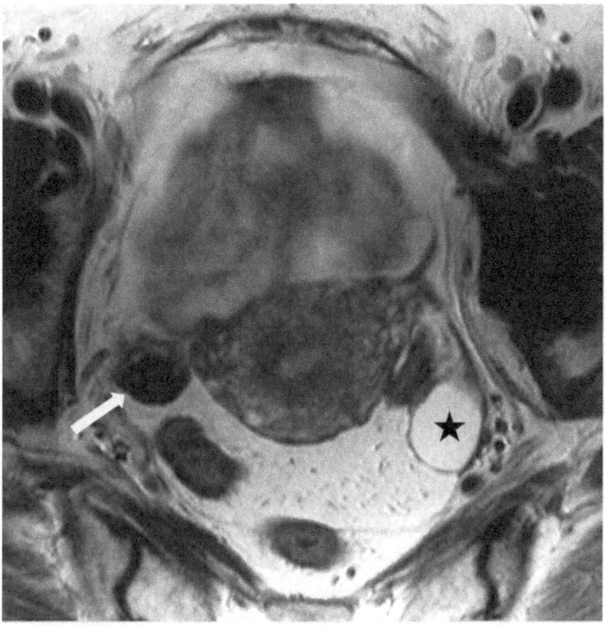

Fig. 6.22 Axial T2 MR image demonstrates a right ovarian hypointense lesion (*arrow*). In the left adnexa, a T2 hyperintense lesion is seen in the ovary (*asterisk*) consistent with a benign cyst

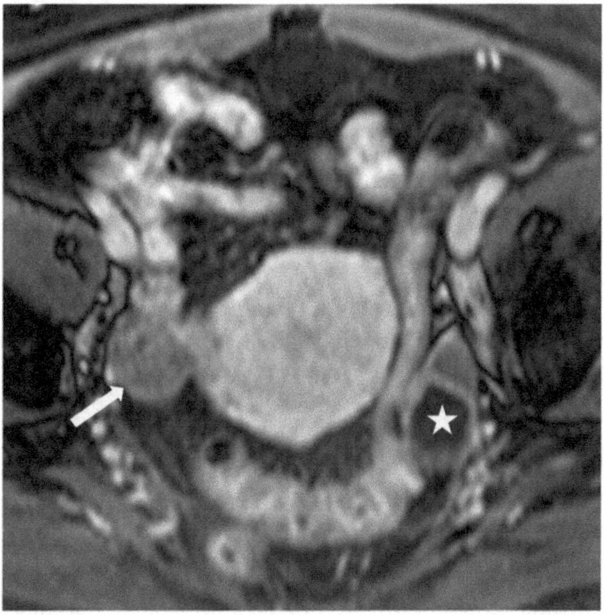

Fig. 6.23 Axial T1 postgadolinium image. In the left adnexa, T2 hyperintense nonenhancing lesion is seen in the ovary (*asterisk*) consistent with a benign cyst

Differential Diagnosis Thecomas, fibrosed thecomas, fibrothecomas, cystadenofibroma, pedunculated uterine fibroids and broad ligament

Diagnosis and Discussion Fibromas account for approximately 4 % of all ovarian tumors and represent the most commonly encountered subtype of sex cord-stromal tumors. They occur at all ages but are most frequently seen in perimenopausal and postmenopausal women. Fibromas are usually asymptomatic and typically found incidentally. They are rarely associated with hormone production, but not infrequently connected with increased ascites and elevation of CA 125 levels, although Meig's syndrome (ascites, ovarian tumor, and pleural effusion) only occurs in a small percentage of cases. Pathologically, fibromas are of stromal derivation and have no epithelial component. They are composed of whorled fascicles of cytologically bland spindle cells forming variable amounts of collagen. Fibromas typically reveal a firm, encapsulated, chalky-white, whorled mass with smooth contour, mimicking fibroids. Some of fibromas also contain both solid and cystic (usually only a few) parts, occasionally completely cystic pattern. The appearance of ascites, increased CA 125 levels, and solid components of fibromas can make differentiation from ovarian malignant tumors difficult. Calcifications and bilaterality are seldomly observed in fibromas.

On ultrasound, solid fibromas most commonly manifest as solid hypoechoic masses. The presence of striped shadows is typical of benign fibromas, which possibly can be explained by the cellular bundles and intersecting strips of hyaline-appearing collagen and fibrous tissue. However, owning to the varying degrees of cellularity, collagen content and stromal edema, the US appearance of fibromas is variable, and hyperechoic masses with increased through-transmission may be seen. About 75 % of fibromas manifest minimal or moderate amount of color Doppler signal, but fibromas can show either no vascularity or abundant vascularization. On CT, fibromas manifest as diffuse, slightly hypoattenuating masses, with poor and delayed enhancement on CT scan, which is unlike most other solid masses. Typical fibromas demonstrate homogeneous, isointense to hypointense to uterine myometrium on T1-weighted MR images and well-circumscribed masses with low signal intensity compared with myometrium on T2-weighted images. This low signal intensity results from the abundant collagen content of the tumors. Some cases may contain scattered high-signal-intensity areas representing edema or cystic degeneration, which are more common in the larger tumors (>6 cm). A T2-hypointense capsule can also be noted in about 60 % of cases, especially the larger ones. In premenopausal women, the residual ovary can be seen on MR imaging where 54 % of the remaining ovary shows a crescent configuration along the periphery of the fibroma (i.e., the "ovarian crescent sign"), as well as the others show a preserved, normal-appearing ovoid shape, suggesting exophytic growth of the fibroma from the periphery of the ovary. To the former growth pattern, the presence of peripheral small follicles or cortical inclusion cysts can be noted on T2-weighted images, which can help in differentiation from fibroids.

Pitfalls Some fibromas are sonographically atypical with a cystic appearance and may be confused with ovarian cystadenofibromas or mucinous cystadenomas coexisting with benign Brenner tumors. Pedunculated uterine fibroids and broad ligament fibroids frequently appear as adnexal or ovarian masses with low signal intensity on T2-weighted images, similar to fibromas. The presence of peripheral follicles and the weak enhancement help differentiate fibromas from fibroids. But in patients with a solid-appearing ovary without visible follicles, the different diagnosis might be difficult.

Teaching Point

1. A solid, well-circumscribed ovarian mass with striped shadows on ultrasound, homogeneously hypointense on T2-weighted MR images should be highly suspicious as fibroma, especially with delayed enhancement and the presence of ascites.
2. Compared to ultrasonography and CT, MRI is more useful to display the structural characteristics of fibroma and its relationship with remaining ovary.
3. The presence of peripheral follicles and the weak enhancement aid in differentiating fibromas from pedunculated uterine fibroids and broad ligament fibroids.

Case 6.11

Brief Case Summary 63-year-old woman with left lower extremity deep vein thrombosis and large right ovarian mass.

Imaging Findings There is a 31 × 31 × 20 cm T2 hyperintense cystic lesion (Fig. 6.24, arrow) of the right ovary. This is multiloculated (arrowhead) with a predominantly large single cystic component. On a postgadolinium T1 weighted image (Fig. 6.25), the mass has a stained-glass appearance (asterisk) with areas of solid nodules (arrowheads). Dependently there is some layering sediment (filled asterisk).

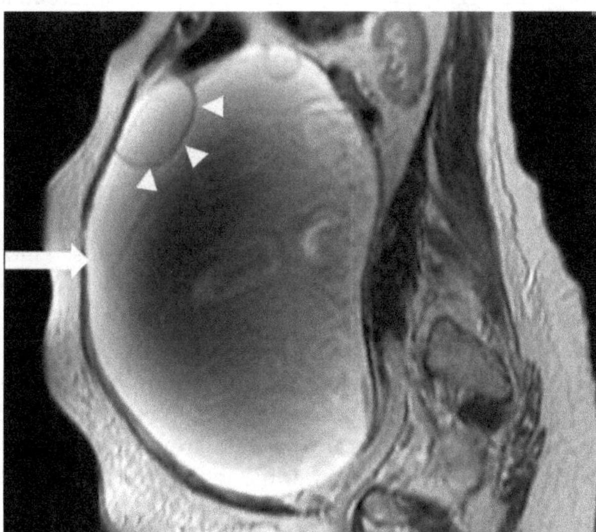

Fig. 6.24 A 31 × 31 × 20 cm T2 hyperintense cystic lesion (*arrow*) of the right ovary. This is multiloculated (*arrowhead*) with a predominantly large single cystic component

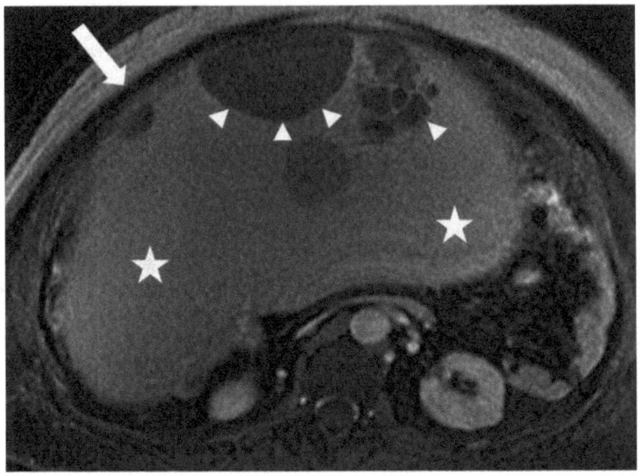

Fig. 6.25 A postgadolinium T1 weighted image; the mass has a stained-glass appearance (*asterisk*) with areas of solid nodules (*arrowheads*). Dependently there is some layering sediment (*filled asterisk*)

Differential Diagnosis Adenofibroma, serous cystadenoma, mucinous borderline cystadenoma, mucinous cystadenocarcinoma, cystic teratoma, endometrioma, endometrioid ovarian carcinoma, cystic metastases.

Diagnosis and Discussion Ovarian mucinous cystadenoma is a type of epithelial ovarian tumor, accounting for approximately 80 % of mucinous ovarian tumors and 20–25 % of all benign ovarian tumors. In contrast to serous cystadenomas of the ovary, mucinous cystadenomas are less common and less likely to be bilateral with only 2–5 % of cases being bilateral. Pathologically, mucinous cystadenoma is composed of a single layer of columnar cells with abundant intracellular mucin and small basilar nuclei lining the cysts. Papillae are unusual, except in occasional examples of mucinous and seromucinous cystadenomas of endocervical-like type, which are highly papillary. Gastrointestinal differentiation is more often noted in borderline tumors and carcinomas than cystadenomas. Typical mucinous cystadenomas are large, multilocular masses with numerous smooth, thin-walled cysts containing proteinaceous or mucus and hemorrhage.

On the ultrasound, mucinous cystadenomas demonstrate low-level internal echoes with multiple thin septa. CT may demonstrate high attenuation in some loculations due to the high protein content of the mucoid material. On the MR and CT images, due to complex contents in the loculations, the tumors often present with various attenuations or signal intensities, which is called as "stained-glass appearances". The signal intensity of mucin depends on the degree of mucin concentration. On T1-weighted images, loculations with watery mucin have lower signal intensity than loculations with thicker mucin, whereas on T2-weighted images, the loculations with watery mucin have high signal intensity whereas loculations with thicker mucin appear slightly hypointense. Contrast-enhanced images help to distinguish septal wall thickness from cysts. The presence of a thick wall or septation may suggest borderline lesions while the presence of solid components suggests carcinoma.

Pitfalls Other cystic ovarian benign lesions and neoplasms with hemorrhage or mucus in the cystic portions broaden the differential diagnosis of mucinous cystadenoma based on imaging. As the most representative one of them, borderline mucinous cystadenoma has a multilocular appearance at MR imaging and are indistinguishable from mucinous cystadenomas. Because of overlapping appearances, serous and mucinous cystadenomas are difficult to accurately differentiate on ultrasound alone. Fortunately, T1-and T2-weighted MR images can readily discriminate the "stained glass appearance" loculations of mucinous cystadenomas from water signal loculations of serous cystasenomas . Furthermore, high-signal-intensity loculations may influence the enhancement assessment on precontrast images. Subtraction postprocessing may aid in identifying true enhancement.

Teaching Point

1. A multilocular cystic mass of the ovary with a thin regular walls and septa, the "stained glass appearance" on MRI, and without endocystic or exocystic vegetations, should be considered to be a benign mucinous cystadenoma.
2. Comparing with ultrasonography and CT, MRI is superior in differentiating the heterogeneity of the loculations in mucinous cystadenomas.
3. Borderline tumor and carcinoma should be considered in the differential diagnosis when a thick wall or septation is present.

Case 6.12

Brief Case Summary 20-year-old woman with abdominal pain.

Imaging Findings There is a large unilocular cyst that crosses the midline and extends up to approximately the liver, measuring approximately 20 cm×5 cm. There is no evidence of wall thickening of the cyst and there are no septations.

On the sagittal T2 image (Fig. 6.26), a large T2 hyperintense cystic lesion measuring 20×5 cm is seen (asterisks) arising from the pelvis extending into the abdomen. On the T1 post gadolinium image with fat saturation (Fig. 6.27), no enhancement or solid enhancing components are visualized in the cystic lesion.

Differential Diagnosis Ovarian functional cysts, ovarian inflammatory cystic lesions, mucinous cystadenoma

Diagnosis and Discussion Serous cystadenoma accounts for approximately 60 % of all the serous benign ovarian neoplasms and is more common than mucinous cystadenoma. It predominantly affects women between 40 and 50 years old. Bilaterality is frequent, occurring in 12–23 % of cases. Serous cystadenomas usually appear as uni- or bilocular cystic masses. Grossly, the tumors consist of a thin-walled unilocular cyst with smooth inner and outer surfaces. Microscopically, the lining of the cyst is flat or may contain small papillary projections. Psammoma

Fig. 6.26 Sagittal T2 image of a large T2 hyperintense cystic lesion measuring 20×5 cm is seen (*asterisks*) arising from the pelvis extending into the abdomen (*asterisks*)

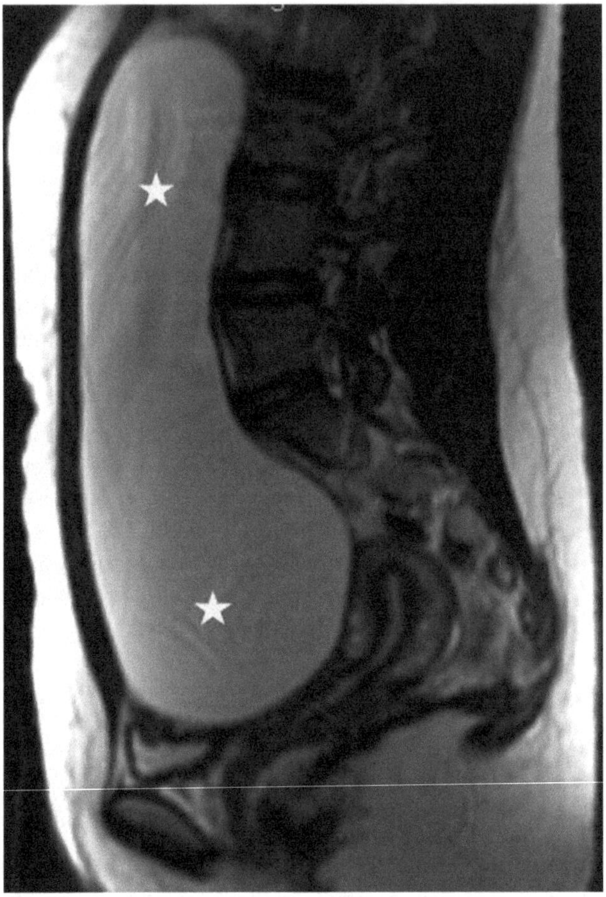

bodies (microscopic calcifications) occasionally can be seen at histologic analysis and proved on CT images.

On ultrasonography, serous cystadenomas are usually seen as an anechogenic to homogenously hypoechogenic unilocular cyst that are larger than typical functional cysts. Papillary projections are rare but tend to be thin with a regular surface forming an acute angle with the cyst wall. Some lesions may contain sonographically detectable septations. The typical CT appearance of serous cystadenoma is a thin wall cystic lesion, without soft tissue components or papillary projections. Due to the serous nature of the fluid, CT density of the cysts assume homogeneous low intensity as pure water, except for companying with high-density hemorrhage. In uncomplicated cases, serous cystadenomas show low signal intensity on T1-weighted images and high signal intensity on T2-weighted images. Hemorrhage within the cysts can be depicted as iso to hyperintense signal intensity on both T1- and T2-weighted images. Additionally, regular thin walls, minimal septa, and

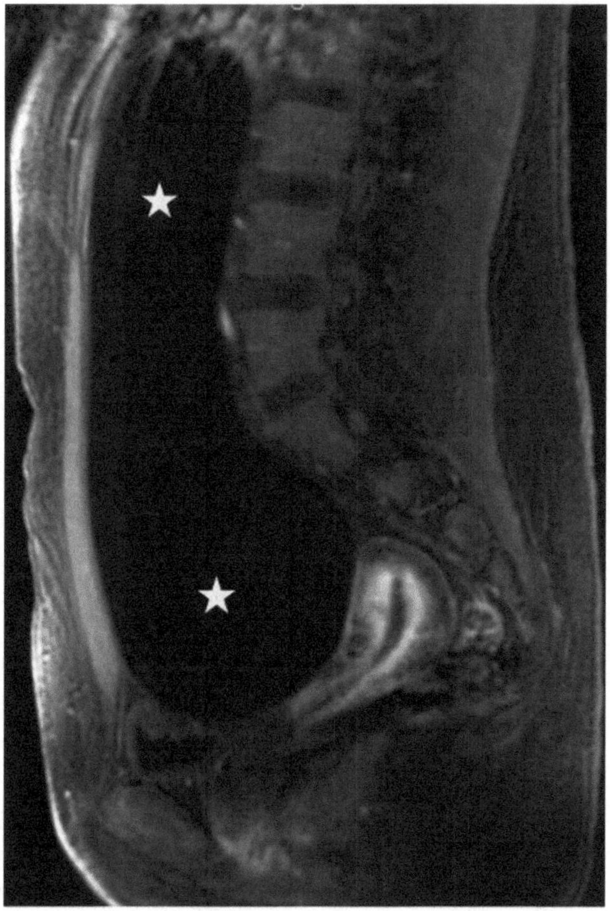

Fig. 6.27 T1 post gadolinium image showing fat saturation, no enhancement or solid enhancing components are visualized in the cystic lesion (*asterisks*)

small papillary projections of the tumors can be depicted better with enhanced CT or MR images.

Pitfalls Serous and mucinous cystadenomas are the two most common types of epithelial neoplasms and have a lot of overlapping pathology, disease course, as well as imaging features. However, some features are helpful to differentiate the two types (see Table 6.1).

Similar imaging characteristics, such as unilocular pattern, anechoic on US or low intensity on MR, thin and smooth walls, absence of papillary projections, may appear in both ovarian functional cysts and serous cystadenomas. Complex functional cysts, for example, hemorrhagic corpus luteum cyst, also make accurate diagnosis difficult. Follow-up US or further assessment of cyst walls and septa with contrast enhanced MR imaging might help. In addition, when cyst wall thickness greater than 3 mm and/or vegetations are noted, serous malignant neoplasms should be included in differential diagnosis.

Table 6.1 Features that help differentiate serous from mucinous tumors

	Tumor type	
Feature	Serous	Mucinous
Clinical findings		
Benign ovarian tumors	25 %	20 %
Malignant ovarian tumors	50 %	10 %
Proportion of malignant cases	60 % benign, 15 % low malignant potential, 25 % malignant	80 % benign, 10–15 % low malignant potential, 5–10 % malignant
Imaging findings		
Size	Smaller than mucinous tumors	Often large; may be enormous
Wall, locule	Thin-walled cyst, usually unilocular	Multilocular, small cystic component, honeycomb-like locules
Opacity or signal intensity of locule	Stable	Variable
Papillary projections	Often seen	Rare
Calcification	Psammomatous, common	Linear, rare
Bilaterality	Frequent	Rare
Carcinomatosis	More common	Pseudomyxoma peritonei

Teaching Point

1. A unilocular or bilocular cystic ovarian mass with a thin regular wall and septa, homogeneous CT attenuation or MR imaging signal intensity of the loculations, and without endocystic or exocystic vegetations, is considered to be a benign serous cystadenoma.
2. Serous cystadenomas need to be carefully distinguished from complex functional cysts and mucinous cystadenomas based on imaging features.
3. Owing to its relative high bilateral incidence (approximately 12–23 %), when a serous cystadenoma is suspected, it is of increased importance to evaluate the contralateral ovary.

Case 6.13

Brief Case Summary 35 year old female with complaint of bloating and gastrointestinal issues.

Imaging Findings Axial CT (Fig. 6.28) shows a complex cystic-solid $10.5 \times 10.4 \times 13$ cm lesion (arrow) located at right adnexal area, with irregular nodular solid enhancing component (asterisk).

Differential Diagnosis Serous cystadenoma, serous cystadenocarcinoma, ovarian endometriosis, endometrioid tumors

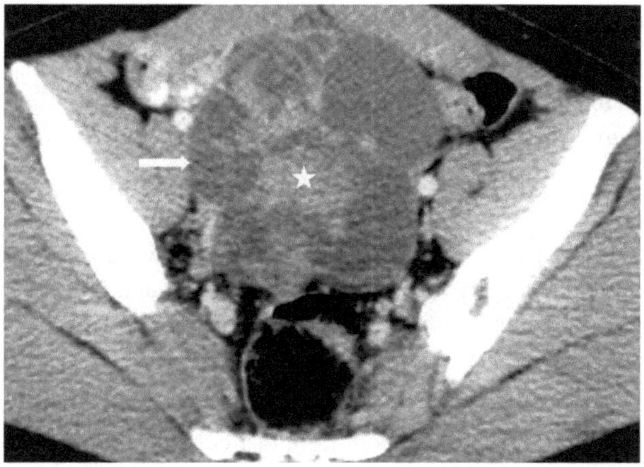

Fig. 6.28 Axial CT shows a complex cystic-solid 10.5×10.4×13 cm lesion (*arrow*) located at right adnexal area, with irregular nodular solid enhancing component (*asterisk*)

Diagnosis and Discussion Clear cell carcinoma (CCC) is a less common surface epithelial carcinoma, constituting up to 10 % of ovarian cancers and are similar to clear cell carcinomas of the endometrium, cervix, or vagina. The mean age of patients presenting with CCC is approximately 50 years. About 10 % of patients are still associated with hypercalcemia and about 25–50 % of patients are associated with endometriosis. Synchronous carcinoma of the uterus and pelvic endometriosis commonly occur with CCC. As with endometrioid tumors, nearly all clear cell tumors are invasive carcinomas. Kaku et al. reported the prognosis of CCC was despite a majority, approximately 82.6 % of patients with CCC presenting with stage I disease. Both distant organ involvement (40 %) and lymph node involvement (40 %) are frequent in patients with recurrent CCC.

CCCs are more frequently seen as unilocular smooth cystic masses associated with irregular walls, thick septa (>3 cm), solid protrusions on US, CT and MR images. The cystic masses are usually larger than 4 cm. MR is sensitive in differentiating the various cystic contents, such as protein and hemorrhage. The signal intensities of cystic contents vary from low to very high on T1WI, while high on T2WI in all cases. Both US and MR images can clearly display the solid protrusions based on superior contrast between cystic contents and solid protrusions. The solid protrusions are either single or few in number and include round, papillary and irregular shapes, with the round shape being more common. On enhanced CT and MR images, the solid parts homogeneously or heterogeneously enhance.

Pitfalls The imaging characteristics of ovarian CCC lack specificity when compared to other cystic tumors of ovary, such as serous cystadenoma and cystadenocarcinoma. CCCs also may be misdiagnosed as ovarian chocolate cysts.

Teaching Point

1. CCCs are often associated with hypercalcemia, endometriosis, and endometrioid tumors.
2. A greater than 4 cm unilocular smooth cystic mass associated with one or a few solid protrusions should raise suspicious for a CCC, but these signs lack specificity.

Case 6.14

Brief Case Summary 16-year-old woman with right ovarian mass and clinical symptoms of polycystic ovarian syndrome.

Imaging Findings There is a complex multiloculated cystic lesion (arrow) in the right adnexa measuring 8.6 × 8.0 × 9.6 cm. A normal right ovary cannot be identified separate from this lesion. The lesion contains multiple cysts of varying sizes, some of which demonstrate intrinsic T1 signal that could represent blood or proteinaceous products (not shown). Along the superior margin of the lesion is a solid enhancing component on the postgadolinium image (Fig. 6.29, asterisk) that shows low signal intensity on T2-weighted image (Fig. 6.30, asterisk).

Differential Diagnosis Granulosa cell tumor, endometrioma, fibrothecoma, cystadenoma, and cystadenoma.

Diagnosis and Discussion Sertoli-Leydig cell tumor (SLCT) of the ovary is a rare sex cord stromal tumor, accounting for less than 0.5 % of all ovarian tumors. Its histopathological characteristics are the biphasic proliferation of Sertoli and Leydig cells with varying degrees of differentiation. The prognosis of Sertoli-Leydig cell tumor is closely associated with the stage and degree of tumor differentiation. Pathologically, SLCT are divided into four subtypes: I. well- (11 %); II.

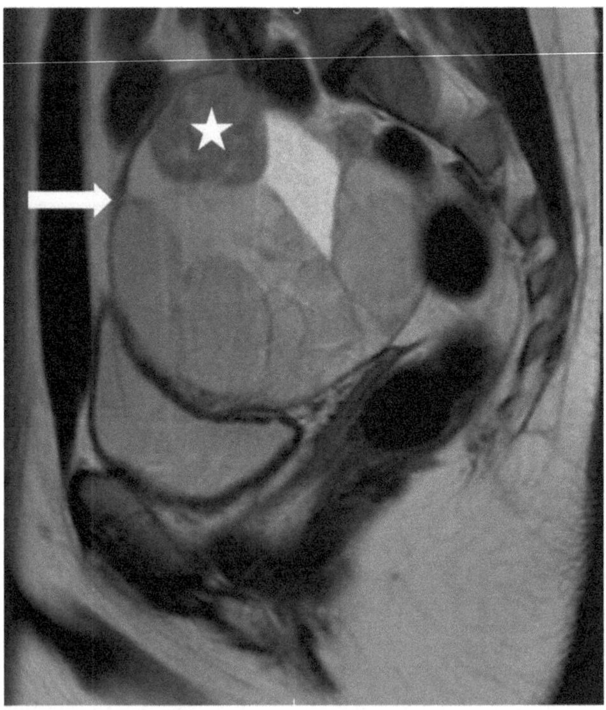

Fig. 6.29 T2-weighted image showing heterogenous multiloculated lesion (*arrow*) with low signal intensity (*asterisk*) and high signal intensity components

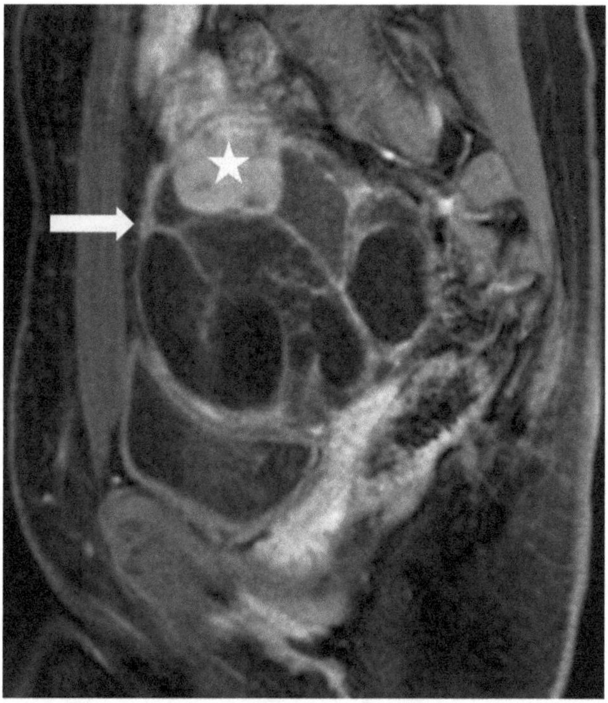

Fig. 6.30 T1 weighted Postgadolinium image showing a complex multiloculated cystic lesion (*arrow*) in the right adnexa measuring 8.6 × 8.0 × 9.6 cm, and a solid enhancing component along the superior margin of the lesion (*asterisk*)

intermediately- (54 %); III poorly differentiated (13 %); and IV. containing heterologous elements (22 %). The majority of SLCTs behave in a benign fashion, and 92 % of the tumors are stage I at presentation. Only 10–18 % of SLCTs with subtype III can behave in a malignant fashion. SLCTs commonly affect young females, and approximately 75 % of the patients are less than 30 years old. Most SLCTs (approximately 62.5 %) show endocrine functions (producing androgen or estrogen) and related clinical symptoms, in which virilization is the most common manifestation. In the patients with non-functional SLCTs, the higher proportions of large tumors, tumor rupture, and tumors of poor differentiation may indicate more aggressive biological behaviors.

SLCTs are typically unilateral tumors with 5–15 cm in diameter and can be solid (38 %), solid and cystic (58 %), and cystic (4 %). SLCTs with subtype III tend to contain areas of hemorrhage and necrosis more frequently than tumors with subtype I. SLCTs generally show a solid or solid and cystic appearance on sonography. The masses are often richly vascularized with a lower vascular resistive index. MR features of solid SLCTs include a predominantly solid mass of low signal intensity on T2 weighted images. The solid and cystic SLCTs show the irregularly thickened wall and septa, the moderate signal intensity in the solid components on T2 weighted images, and the obvious enhancement of the solid components on enhanced images. The low to moderate signal feature of solid components on T2 weighted images may represent abundant stroma in the tumors.

Pitfalls Although the majority of SLCTs present with an elevation of androgen and related symptoms, some SLCTs are nonfunctional with nonspecific presenting symptoms. Approximately 15 % of SLCTs can present with estrogenic manifestations, such as postmenopausal hemorrhage, which make them more difficult to be differentiated from granulosa cell tumors. In contrast to granulosa cell tumors, SLCTs tend to recur relatively soon after initial diagnosis. Additionally, coexisting with other types of ovarian tumors further increases the diagnostic difficulty of ovarian SLCTs. Measuring the androgen level is recommended as a routine diagnostic procedure in addition to imaging examinations in cases of SLCTs. In the setting of elevated androgen levels, SLCTs can be diagnosed only by eliminating other possible causes of hyperandrogenemia, including Cushing syndrome, adrenal hyperplasia, pituitary adenoma, other causes of ovarian and adrenal androgen hypersecretion, intersexuality, and medically induced androgenization. Sometimes the solid and cystic type of SLCTs can mimic an ovarian cystadenoma due in part to the mucinous heterologous elements. However, the signal intensity in different loculations of cystadenoma is frequently heterogeneous.

Teaching Point

1. A young female patient with an elevation of androgen and related symptoms with a unilateral ovarian solid or solid-cystic mass should be raise the suspicion of SLCT, especially when solid components of the mass show low or moderate signal intensity on T2 weighted images.
2. Even in the absence of elevated androgen levels or associated symptoms, the diagnosis of SLCT cannot be excluded and should be differentiated from other ovarian solid-cystic tumors, such as granulosa cell tumors and cystadenomas. Moreover, other causes of hyperandrogenemia must be excluded.

Case 6.15

Brief Case Summary 43 year old female with abnormal premenopausal vaginal bleeding.

Imaging Findings Coronal T2 weighted MR image shows a 6.2×5.1 cm heterogeneous left adnexal mass which abuts the uterus and left ovary (Fig. 6.31, arrow) with diffusely distributed T2 hyperintense foci. After administration of gadolinium, there is mild enhancement (Fig. 6.32, arrow). The lesion is a heterogeneous solid mass with internal vascularity on US (Fig. 6.33, arrow).

Differential Diagnosis Malignant germ cell tumors (yolk sac tumor, etc.), serous carcinoma, and endometrioid carcinoma, mucinous or serous cystadenoma or cystadenocarcinoma, dermoid cyst, Krukenberg's tumor, hemorrhagic ovarian cyst, endometriosis, hematosalpinges, and tuboovarian abscess ,fibroma, thecoma, uterine myoma, Brenner tumor, and dysgerminoma

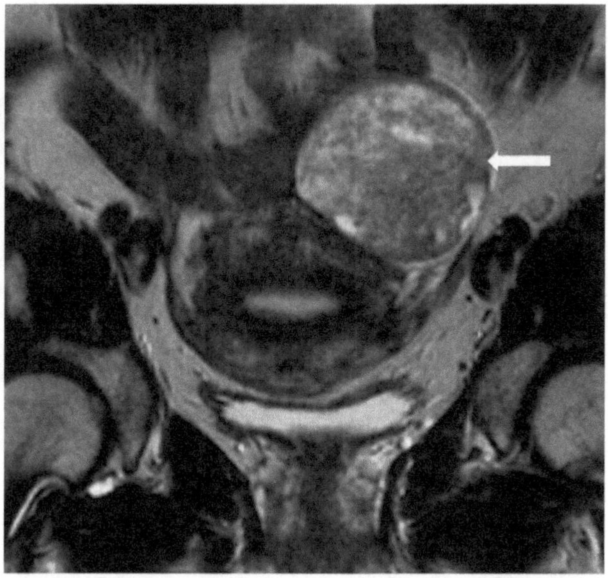

Fig. 6.31 Coronal T2 weighted MR image shows a 6.2×5.1 cm heterogeneous left adnexal mass which abuts the uterus and left ovary (*arrow*) with diffusely distributed T2 hyperintense foci

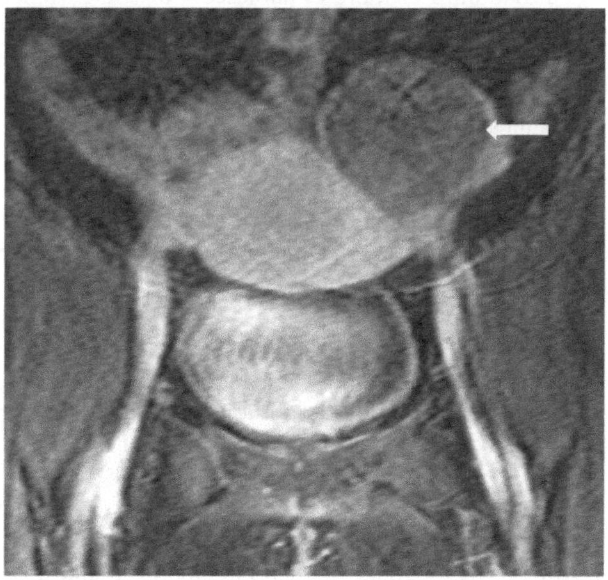

Fig. 6.32 After administration of gadolinium, there is mild enhancement (*arrow*)

Diagnosis and Discussion The granulosa cell tumor (GCT) of ovary is a rare sex cord stromal cell tumor, which accounts for <2 % of all ovarian tumors and approximately 70 % of sex cord stromal tumors. GCT is divided into two types, the adult and the juvenile types. The juvenile type presents mainly in children whereas the adult type commonly occurs in premenopausal and postmenopausal women. Both types show different histologic and clinical features. As the most common

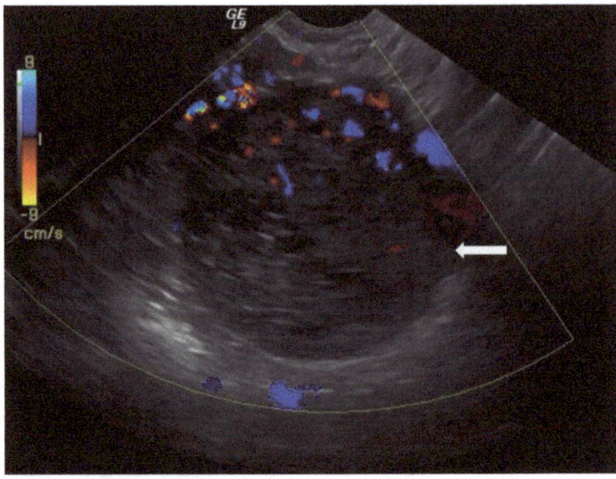

Fig. 6.33 The lesion is a heterogeneous solid mass with internal vascularity on US (*arrow*)

hormone-producing tumor, the clinical manifestations mainly depend on the estrogen activity of the tumor, age of the patient, and size of the tumor. Children usually present with precocious puberty, breast enlargement or occasionally galactorrhea. About one-third or more of adolescent or adult women with GCTs have endometrial hyperplasia or endometrial carcinoma related to estrogen production and present with abnormal vaginal bleeding. GCT is considered a low malignant potential tumor with a favorable prognosis. The local spread of GCT is usually within the pelvis and lower abdomen and recurs seldom or very late, sometimes as long as 30–40 years later and distant metastasis is rare.

GCTs are unilateral in 90–95 % of patients. GCTs have varied histologic patterns, including microfollicular, macrofollicular, trabecular, insula, water-silk, solid-tubular, diffuse, and luteinized patterns. The tumor forms of adult ovarian GCTs also vary from solid masses to tumors with variable degrees of hemorrhagic or fibrotic changes to multilocular cystic lesions to completely cystic tumors. Solid adult ovarian GCTs are usually small, whereas cystic masses are larger. The common manifestations of GCTs include two patterns. One is that of unlobulated solid masses with internal cystic portions and the other is that of a large multilocular–solid mass with mixed intensity of the cyst fluid. The later pattern is also called as "swiss cheese" or "sponge-like" sign. The typical presentations of GCTs are well-defined solid masses with scattered cystic portions or echogenic or septated cystic masses on US, solid masses with low attenuation on CT, and solid masses with a various amount of cystic components and hemorrhage on MRI. The solid component of the GCTs displays low signal intensity on T1-weighted images and increased signal intensity on T2-weighted images. A hemorrhagic component may show high signal intensity on both T1- and T2-weighted images. Foci of low signal intensity on both T1- and T2-weighted images may indicate fibrotic tissue or hemosiderin from an prior hemorrhage. The most important differences between GCTs and epithelial ovarian carcinomas are that a smaller proportion of GCTs have papillary projections, a greater proportion is vascularized and the echogenicity or intensity of the cyst fluid is more often mixed. Some patients with GCTs also present enlarged uterus or thickened endometrium, but these changes are difficult to evaluate on CT images.

Pitfalls Besides two common types mentioned above, GCTs have many "unusual appearances", such as a unilocular cystic form, an entirely solid form, a lobulated solid mass with internal nonhemorrhagic cysts, and so on. These unusual appearances should be differentiated from other ovarian cystic lesions, including mucinous or serous cystadenoma, dermoid cyst, hemorrhagic ovarian cyst, endometriosis, tuboovarian abscess and other ovarian solid tumors, including fibroma, thecoma, uterine myoma, Brenner tumor, and dysgerminoma. Particularly regarding patients with GCT but without elevating estrogen level, lack of hormone-related clinical manifestations may make the differential diagnosis more difficult.

Teaching Point

1. GCTs of the ovary usually appear as large multiseptated cystic mass ("swiss cheese" sign) or medium solid mass with internal cysts.
2. Estrogen-related clinical manifestations and characteristic MR features including hemorrhagic cysts and endometrial hyperplasia should raise the suspicion of a GCT.

Case 6.16

Brief Case Summary 62 year old woman with abdominal pain and distention.

Imaging Findings Coronal reformatted image (Fig. 6.34) of an abdominal CT with oral and IV contrast shows bilateral solid ovarian masses (arrows) with heterogeneous enhancement. Note the nodular thickening in the body of the stomach (arrowhead) and associated mild ascites.

Differential Diagnosis primary ovarian tumor

Diagnosis and Discussion Krukenberg tumor

About 7 % of all ovarian tumors are metastatic. The term krukenberg tumor refers to metastases to ovaries from either a colon or gastric primary malignancy. The other common primary sites are the breast and genitourinary system. Hematologic malignancies such as lymphoma may also display secondary ovarian involvement. Recognition of secondary tumors of the ovary is important as these patients have a poorer prognosis compared to their counterparts with primary tumors. Most patients with gastric malignancy and metastases to ovaries succumb within 1 year.

One of the important features of metastases to ovaries are bilateral masses. However, bilaterality alone is not reliable as primary malignancies such as endometroid carcinoma and papillary adenocarcinoma can be bilateral.

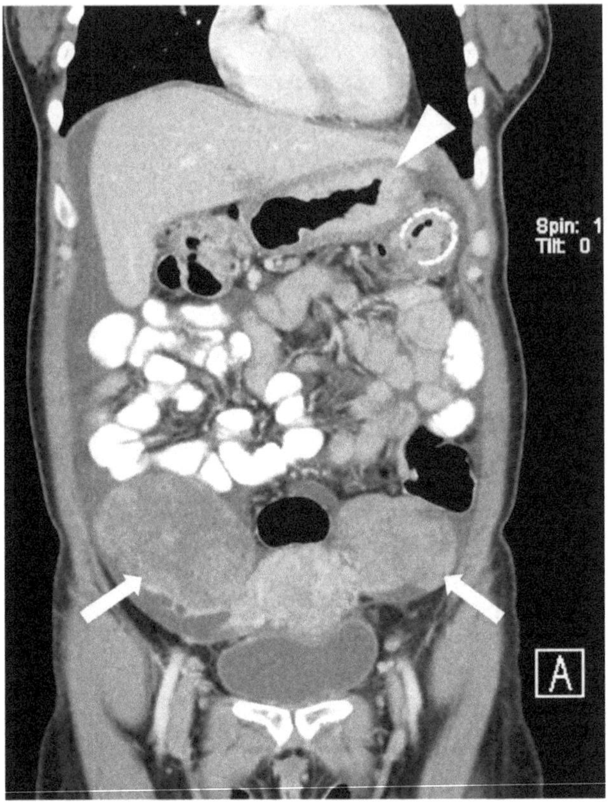

Fig. 6.34 Coronal reformatted image of an abdominal CT with oral and IV contrast shows bilateral solid ovarian masses (*arrows*) with heterogeneous enhancement. Note the nodular thickening in the body of the stomach (*arrowhead*) and associated mild ascites

Metastases to ovaries should be suspected if encountered with a finding of bilateral solid or predominantly solid masses. Some authors have suggested that finding intramural cysts is associated with a high likelihood that the lesion is a krukenberg tumor. Further, solid masses tend to be from primaries in stomach, breast, or uterus and secondary lymphomatous involvement whereas cystic heterogeneous lesions with irregular borders tend to metastasis from colon, biliary tract or rectum.

Ultrasound reveals bilateral solid homogenous ovarian masses usually accompanied by ascites. Few cystic components may be seen. CT allows for complete imaging evaluation in the search for the primary malignancy. The bilateral ovarian masses usually show homogenous moderate enhancement. MRI may show intramural cysts to better advantage in cases of metastases from mucinous tumors of colon/rectum and septal enhancement in the cysts may be better depicted. Solid lesions usually show low to intermediate T2 intensity and moderate post contrast enhancement is seen.

Imaging Pitfalls

- Confusion with ovarian primary tumor is to be avoided and a meticulous search for the primary lesion should be performed. In contrast primary ovarian tumors usually have a mixed solid and cystic appearance.

- Metastastic colonic tumors in particular can closely resemble mucinous adenocarcinoma of ovaries with a "stained glass" appearance on MRI, however, mucinous adenocarcinoma are rarely bilateral.

Teaching Points

- Bilateral purely/predominantly solid ovarian masses should trigger a search for a primary malignancy.
- Most common primary sites are stomach, colon, breast and genitourinary system.
- Metastases from colonic primary can resemble mucinous adenocarcinoma ovary.

Uterus

Case 6.17

Brief Case Summary 18 year old female with amenorrhea.

Imaging Findings Sagittal T2 MR image shows absence of a uterus but demonstrates the presence of the lower third of the vagina (Fig. 6.35, arrow). The right ovary (Fig. 6.36, arrow) and left ovary (Fig. 6.37, arrow) are normal.

Differential Diagnosis Turner's syndrome, isolated vaginal atresia, androgen insensitivity syndrome, congenital adrenal hyperplasia

Diagnosis and Discussion Mayer Rokitansky Kuster Hauser Syndrome

Mayer Rokitansky Küster Hauser Syndrome belongs to class I Müllerian duct anomalies and is a rare congenital disorder affecting the female genital tract.

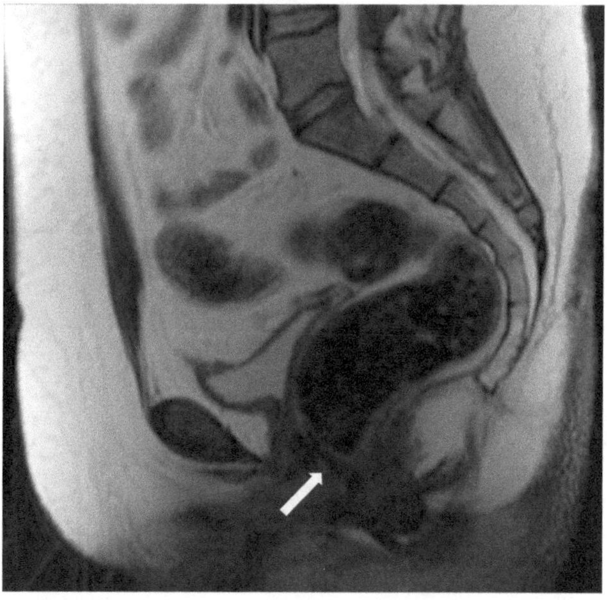

Fig. 6.35 Sagittal T2 MR image shows absence of a uterus but demonstrates the presence of the lower third of the vagina (*arrow*)

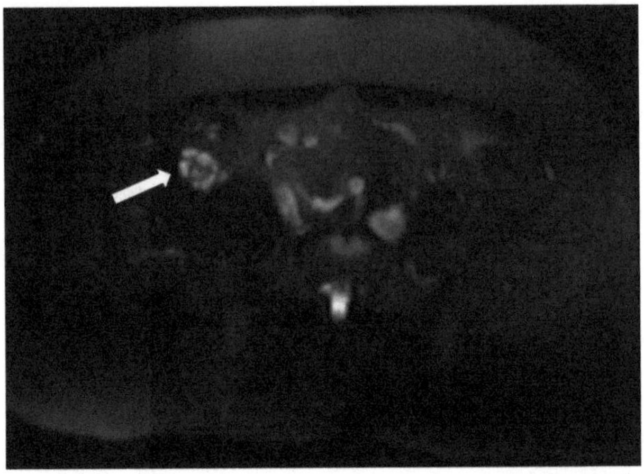

Fig. 6.36 Normal right ovary (*arrow*)

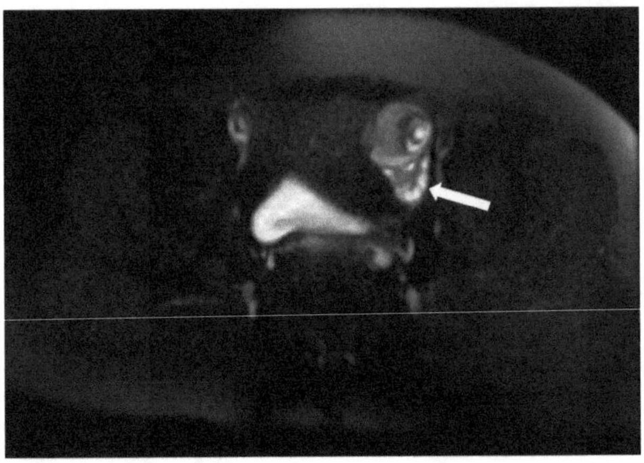

Fig. 6.37 Normal left ovary (*arrow*)

It is characterized by absent or hypoplastic uterus and vagina with normal ovaries, fallopian tubes, external genitalia and secondary sexual characteristics. The patients are phenotypically females with normal 46XX karyotype. Associated renal and skeletal anomalies are common. Cardiac and anorectal anomalies may also rarely be seen. Based on the presence or absence of associated anomalies, it can be divided into a typical form, characterized only by absence of uterus and upper vagina and an atypical form which is associated with systemic anomalies.

MRKH syndrome results from arrested development of paramesonephric duct during the 7th week of gestation. Usual age of presentation is 15–18 years with primary amenorrhea being the commonest presenting feature. Uncommonly patients may also present with cyclical abdominal pain owing to presence of endometrial tissue in the rudimentary uterus, inability to have intercourse or dyspareunia due to dysplastic vagina and later with infertility.

Ultrasound can show the upper level of vagina with level of obstruction, uterine duplication anomalies and associated renal/bladder anomalies, if present. CT due to ionizing radiation is not a commonly used modality.

MRI due to multiplanar capability and excellent soft tissue resolution is the mainstay of imaging. Not only does it allow for the diagnosis of müllerian anomalies but also shows the degree of dysgenesis and associated anomalies. Sagittal T2W images are best to evaluate the uterus, cervix and vagina. Uterine hypoplasia is diagnosed when there is a small uterus with a intercornual distance of less than 2 cm. Associated uterine findings such as reduced endometrial and myometrial widths and poor zonal differentiation may be seen. Axial images are used to evaluate vaginal agenesis (seen in 95 % of patients) where there is no soft tissue between the rectum and urethra. 5 % of patients have a blind ending lower 1/3rd of vaginal tissue, the extent of which can be accurately determined on MRI. Visualization of normal ovaries is a crucial factor in diagnosis of MRKH syndrome and can be easily assessed on axial MRI images. Associated anorectal and renal anomalies like renal agenesis, ectopic kidney or horseshoe kidney can be visualized on a combination of axial and coronal images. Spinal MRI may be required to rule out vertebral anomalies.

Imaging Pitfalls Turner's syndrome can be differentiated from MRKH syndrome as patients with Turner's syndrome have an abnormal karyotype and present with gonadal dysgenesis with nondevelopment of secondary sexual characteristics. The uterus and vagina are structurally normal in cases of Turner's syndrome.

Androgen insensitivity syndrome is male pseudohermaphroditism wherein phenotypical females present with rudimentary uterus and vagina along with cryptorchidism.

Congenital adrenal hyperplasia usually presents with ambiguous genitalia and features of virilization.

Teaching Point Mayer Rokitansky Küster Hauser Syndrome presents with a spectrum of abnormalities, the hallmark being the absence or hypoplasia of uterus and vagina with an otherwise normal external genitalia and secondary sexual characteristics.

Case 6.18

Brief Case Summary 16-year-old woman with dysmenorrhea

Imaging Findings Gray scale ultrasonography (arrows, Fig. 6.38a, b) shows two separate and widely divergent uterine horns with two distinct cervices. Coronal T2 weighted MR images (arrows, Fig. 6.39a, b) in the same patient show uterine didelphys with complete separate uterine horns and complete duplication of the cervices. Note the presence of blood products in both dilated horns.

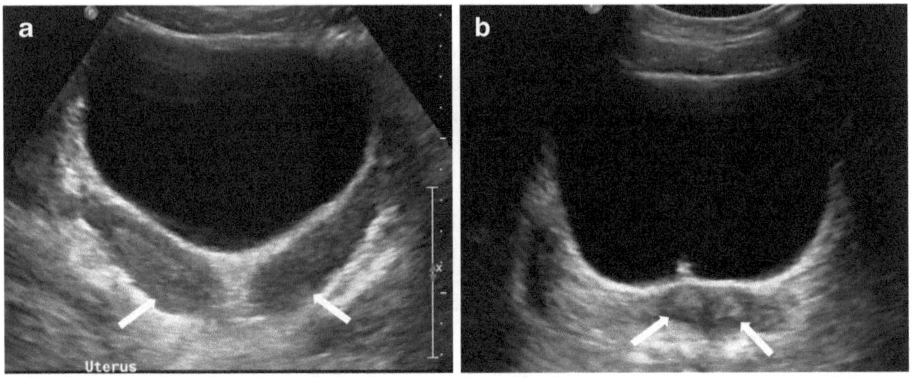

Fig. 6.38 Gray scale ultrasonography (*arrows*, **a**, **b**) shows two separate and widely divergent uterine horns with two distinct cervices

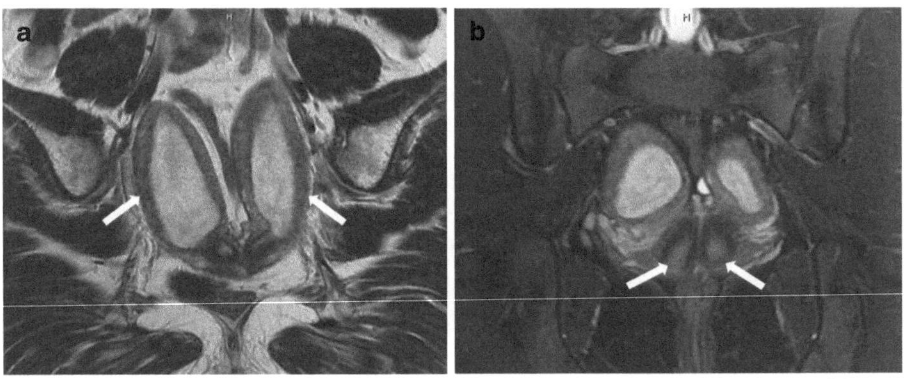

Fig. 6.39 Coronal T2 weighted MR images (*arrows*, **a**, **b**) in the same patient show uterine didelphys with complete separate uterine horns and complete duplication of the cervices. Note the presence of blood products in both dilated horns

Differential Diagnosis Bicornuate bicollis uterus, septate uterus

Diagnosis and Discussion Uterus didelphys.

Uterine didelphys is a Müllerian type III class anomaly which results from nondevelopment or non-fusion of müllerian ducts or failed resorption of uterine septum. It accounts for about 8 % of Müllerian anomalies and is characterized by complete duplication of uterus and cervix with no visible communication of endometrial cavities. Each of the uteri has a single horn pointing towards its respective fallopian tube. There is an associated longitudinal vaginal septum, seen in 75 % of cases.

The patients are usually asymptomatic unless a transverse vaginal septum is present which causes obstruction and thus hematometrocolpos. There are instances of preterm abortions, preterm labor and fetal malpresentation, although reports of full term normal pregnancies have also been recorded.

Diagnosis is made by hysterosalpingography (HSG), sonohysterography, transvaginal/3D ultrasound or pelvic MRI. CT due to its ionizing radiations is not a preferred modality.

HSG shows two separate endocervical canals opening into two separate endometrial cavities each continuing into their respective fallopian tubes. No communication is seen between the two cavities. When a longitudinal vaginal septum is present, there may be visualization of only one cervical canal and endometrial cavity which then may simulate a unicornuate uterus. Pelvic ultrasound and MRI also depict similar features of two separate though normal sized endometrial cavities and cervices with a large fundal cleft and no communication. The extent of duplication is better visualized on MRI due to its excellent soft tissue resolution. The vaginal septum and obstruction, if any, is also well seen on MRI. The uterine endometrial and myometrial zonal anatomy is otherwise maintained. 3D ultrasound forms an important and indispensible diagnostic tool in evaluation of uterine malformations. It is useful to demonstrate the outer uterine contour as well as the endometrial cavities.

Imaging Pitfalls Unlike in uterus didelphys, the uterine horns in bicornuate bicollis uterus are caudally fused with some degree of communication between the endometrial cavities usually at uterine isthmus.

The septated uterus shows normal intercornual distance and normal fundal contour. There is a septum separating the two endometrial cavities which appear smaller in size. The degree of separation of uterine horns is less compared to bicornuate and didelphys uteri (less than 75°). The septa when fibrous will show hypointense signal on MRI.

Teaching Point Uterine didelphys is characterized by two entirely and widely separate uterine horns and cervices. There may be vaginal duplication. A large fundal cleft is noted with no communication between the two uterine horns.

Case 6.19

Brief Case Summary 20 year-old woman with prior pregnancy loss.

Imaging Findings Oblique axial T2 weighted image shows divergent uterine horns with an increased intercornual distance (Fig. 6.40).

Differential Diagnosis Septate uterus, uterus didelphys, intrauterine synechiae

Diagnosis and Discussion Bicornuate uterus.

Bicornuate uterus is a type IV Mullerian duct anomaly which involves duplication of uterus. It results from partial failure of fusion of two uterine horns during development of paramesonephric duct and accounts for about 25 % of Mullerian anomalies. Based on the involvement of the cervical canal it can be divided into bicornuate bicollis with two cervical canals and bicornuate unicollis with one cervical canal. Twenty-five percent of cases may also show a longitudinal vaginal

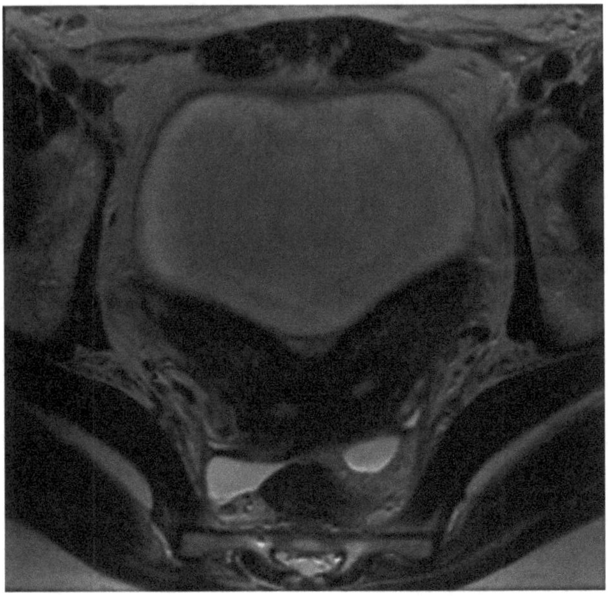

Fig. 6.40 Oblique axial T2 weighted image shows divergent uterine horns with an increased intercornual distance

septum. Associated renal abnormalities may be seen as well. The patients are generally asymptomatic and the condition is diagnosed incidentally on pelvic imaging. When symptomatic, patients may present with early pregnancy loss, preterm labor, malpresentations or cervical incompetence.

Imaging modalities comprise of ultrasound, hysterosalpingogram and MRI. Ultrasound and MRI are helpful to show the external uterine contour which is concave and shows a characteristic deep fundal cleft (more than 1 cm deep). The intercornual distance is increased, >4 cm. Two uterine horns, separated by a muscular or mixed muscular and fibrous septum, are seen with at least some degree of communication generally at the isthmus. A nonspecific but helpful finding is the angle between the two uterine horns which measures more than 105°. MRI shows the extent of cervical duplication; if the failure of fusion extends to the internal os, then it is considered unicollis and similarly if the fusion failure extends to the external os, then it is considered bicollis. A vaginal septum, if present, can also be well evaluated on MR.

Imaging Pitfalls Unlike in uterus didelphys, the uterine horns in bicornuate bicollis uterus are caudally fused with some degree of communication between the endometrial cavities usually at the uterine isthmus. Also the two uterine horns may appear smaller in size with smaller endometrial cavities due to nonfusion.

The septated uterus shows normal intercornual distance and a normal fundal contour, which may be convex, flattened or slightly concave (less than 1 cm deep) unlike bicornuate uterus. The degree of separation of uterine horns is less as compared to a bicornuate uterus (less than 75°). The latter finding being nonspecific because a majority of the uterine angles fall between 75 and 105° resulting in overlap.

Intrauterine synechiae are seen as irregular bands within the endometrial cavity which are hypointense on MRI.

Teaching Points

1. The differentiation between bicornuate and septate uterus is important as it carries significant management implications with surgical treatment as a treatment option in septate uterus.
2. MRI forms the mainstay of imaging of Mullerian anomalies, particularly with differentiation between septate and bicornuate uterus

Case 6.20

Brief Case Summary A 39-year-old woman with pelvic pain.

Imaging Findings Axial T2 weighted MR image (Fig. 6.41) shows the uterus measuring 9 cm in length and deviating towards the right with a single uterine horn (arrow). A second uterine horn is not seen. On US (Fig. 6.42), the uterus demonstrates unicornuate configuration (arrow).

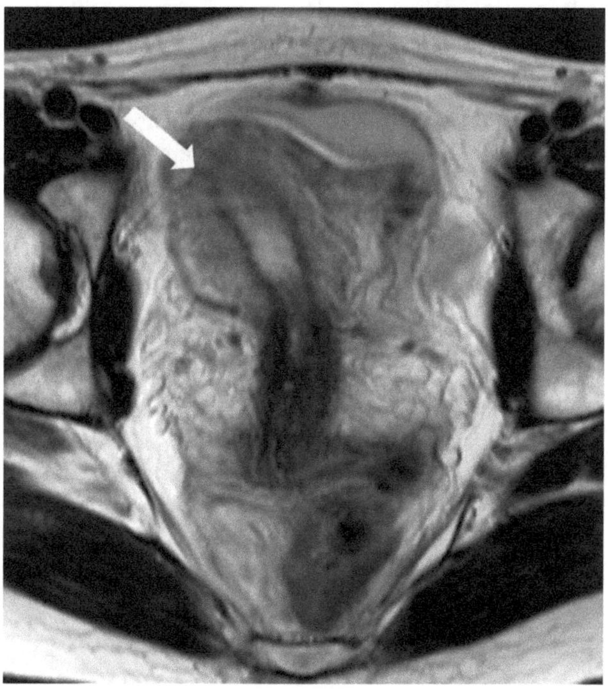

Fig. 6.41 Axial T2 weighted MR image shows the uterus measuring 9 cm in length and deviating towards the right with a single uterine horn (*arrow*). A second uterine horn is not seen

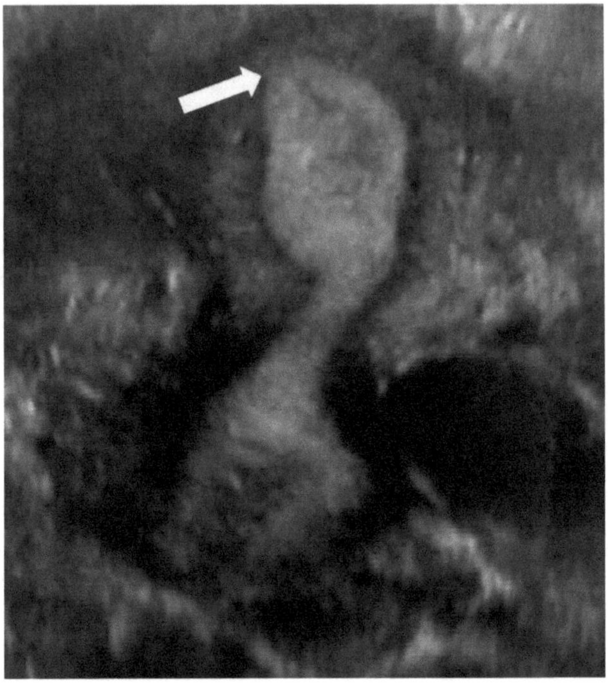

Fig. 6.42 US of the uterus demonstrating unicornuate configuration (*arrow*)

Differential Diagnosis Bicornuate uterus, uterus didelphys with unilateral obstructed cavity, endometriosis, ovarian tumors.

Diagnosis and Discussion Unicornuate uterus, the Class II malformation of Müllerian duct anomalies (MDAs), results from nondevelopment or incomplete development of one of the paramesonephric ducts. It accounts for 13 % of MDAs and is much less common than these other uterine malformations. Four subgroups were classified by the American Society for Reproductive Medicine: a. type A1a, unicornuate uterus with communicating rudimentary horn, accounting for 10 %; b. type A1b, unicornuate uterus with non-communicating rudimentary horn, accounting for 22 %; c. type A2, rudimentary horn without a cavity, accounting for 33 %; d. type B, an isolated unicornuate uterus with no contralateral structure, accounting for 35 %. Women with a unicornuate uterus are often asymptomatic and have higher term pregnancy rate of approximately 47 %. Unfortunately, the pregnancy loss and obstetrical complications caused by this anomaly cannot be corrected by surgery. Patients may feel pain or palpable pelvic mass if the non-communicating rudimentary horns with functional endometrium develop hematometros. Surgical resection is the treatment of choice in these cases. Of all MDAs, unicornuate uterus has the highest incidence of associated renal anomalies, in which ipsilateral renal agenesis is most common.

The endometrial cavity is usually towards to one side and represents a fusiform shape, tapering at the apex and draining into a single fallopian tube on hysterosalpingography. A unicornuate uterus may be difficult to identify with 2D ultrasound but US has a sensitivity of 85 % and specificity of 100 % in detecting the presence of a rudimentary horn. Coronal images of 3D sonography and MRI can clearly show the asymmetric laterally deviated uterine corpus and noncommunicating rudimentary horn. The remaining single horn typically appears as a "banana or cigar-shaped" endometrial cavity with normal myometrial zonal anatomy and only one fallopian tube. The uterus is usually laterally deviated and has a reduced volume. The rudimentary horn, which is best seen on coronal and axis T2-weighted images, can be either solid or have a small cavity with functioning endometrium and may or may not communicate with the main uterine cavity. The rudimentary horn demonstrates similar signal intensities to that of myometrium on MRI, while the noncommunicating horn with hematometra may show high signal intensity on T1 and low signal intensity on T2-weighted images. In addition, MRI can provide a field of view large enough to evaluate for the associated renal anomalies.

Imaging Pitfalls Owing to lack of the precise clinical and imaging criteria to define specific categorization of MDAs, there exist some disagreements among various radiologists and clinicians. For example, unicornuate uterus with a large communicating rudimentary horn also can be diagnosed as a bicornuate uterus with an asymmetric horn. Occasionally, a noncommunicating rudimentary horn containing hematometra can be mistaken for a unilateral obstructed cavity of uterus didelphys. In this case, the assessment of cervix and fallopian tube may be helpful in the differentiation. Additionally, due to the small size and lack of specific tissue characteristics, small uterine remnants may not be seen on MRI or may be seen only retrospectively.

Teaching Point

1. A smaller uterus with a "banana or cigar" shape, normal myometrial zonal anatomy, and a single fallopian tube is highly suspicious for a unicornuate uterus, especially when a rudimentary horn is confirmed.
2. MRI is superior to ultrasonography in identifying hematometra in the rudimentary horn and its large field of view provides additional information in detecting associated renal anomalies.

Case 6.21

Brief Case Summary 33-year-old woman with pelvic pain.

Imaging Findings The 3-D US reconstructed image (Fig. 6.43) demonstrates 2 endometrial cavities (asterisk) divided by a septum (arrow). On the T2 weighted oblique coronal plane of the uterus (Fig. 6.44), 2 well formed endometrial cavities (asterisks) are seen, with a broad septum (arrow), dividing the endometrial cavity centrally. The septum extends approximately 2.9 cm from the external contour of the uterine fundus and 2.2 cm from the intra cornual line. There is a single cervix (hollow asterisk).

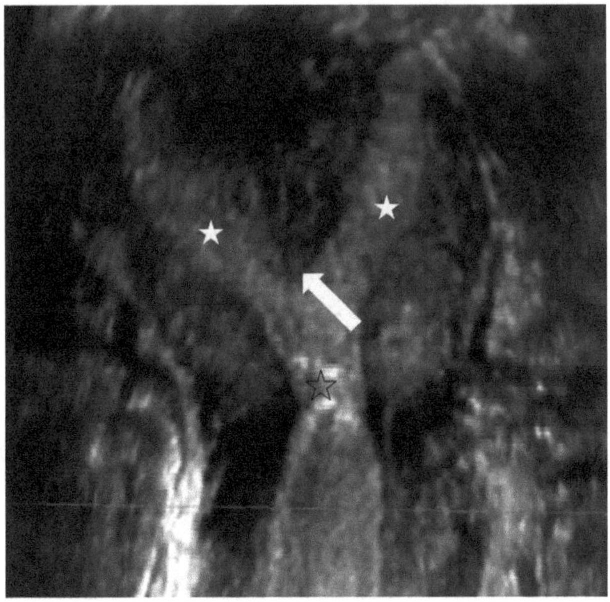

Fig. 6.43 3-D US reconstructed image demonstrating 2 endometrial cavities (*asterisk*) divided by a septum (*arrow*)

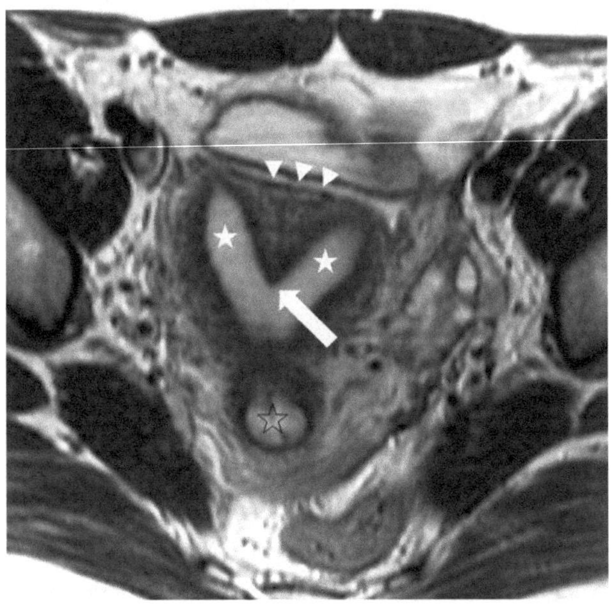

Fig. 6.44 T2 weighted oblique coronal plane of the uterus (Fig. 6.44), showing 2 well-formed endometrial cavities (*asterisks*) are seen, with a broad septum (*arrow*), dividing the endometrial cavity centrally. The septum extends approximately 2.9 cm from the external contour of the uterine fundus and 2.2 cm from the intra cornual line. There is a single cervix (*hollow asterisk*)

Differential Diagnosis Bicornuate uterus, uterus didelphys, arcuate uterus

Diagnosis and Discussion Septate uterus, or class V anomaly of Müllerian duct anomalies (MDAs) according to the classification by the American Fertility Society, is the result of complete fusion of the paramesonephric ducts but failure of septal resorption. It is the most common uterine anomaly (accounting for 55 %) and is also the most common anomaly associated with reproductive failure (up to 67 %), probably due to placental implantation on the septum. It is important to comment on placental location when a septate uterus is confirmed or suspected. A septate uterus has a normal outer fundal contour which is convex or flat or has a slight indentation less than 1 cm deep. The intercornual distance is within the normal range and the intercornual angle is less than 75°. The septum could be partial or complete and its compositions include myometrium, fibrous tissue, or variable amounts of both. There are two subtypes of septate uterus: A. complete, septum reaches down to the internal os (uterus biseptus, bicollis); B. incomplete, a partial septum ends above it (uterus biseptus, unicollis).

Hysterosalpingography (HSG), MRI and sonography are main imaging diagnostic methods for MDAs. HSG can display the divided cavities but cannot detect the external fundal contour of the uterus and tissue compositions of the septum, which severely impairs its accuracy in differentiating a septate from a bicornuate uterus. Both for MRI and sonography, the coronal image of the uterus is the best plane to accurately diagnose MDAs as it allows for simultaneous visualization of both the internal and external contours. Two divided cavities with high signal intensity are clearly displayed on oblique T2-weighted image, as well as a normal fundal contour with an outward fundal convexity or flat may be noted. Additionally, MRI can accurately differentiate a fibrous composition of the septum in septate uterus from a well-vascularized myometrial septum in bicornuate uterus. A myometrial septum is typically isointense to myometrium whereas a fibrous septum usually shows low signal intensity in both sequences. In contrast to MRI, 3D ultrasonography has the benefit of characterizing small anatomic structures, such as a thin and linear fibrous septum. In the diagnosis of septate uterus, MRI has a specificity of 66–100 % and sensitivity of 73–100 %, whereas 3D ultrasonography had sensitivity of 98–99 % and specificity of 100 %.

Pitfalls Of all MDA, bicornuate and septate uterus are the most difficult to differentiate and are often confused. The distinction is essential because of their different prognoses and treatment options. Septate uterus is associated with a high spontaneous abortion rate, but it can be treated by hysteroscopy metroplasty with resection of the septum. A bicornuate uterus has a much lower spontaneous abortion rate but unlike septate uterus, treatment requires a transabdominal surgical approach. As mentioned above, MRI can distinguish the fibrous septum of septate uterus from myometrial septum of bicornuate uterus. However, myometrial or mixed septum of septate uterus can pose a diagnostic challenge. The shape of outer fundal contour may help to the differentiation. In addition, the intermediate and incomplete forms of bicornuate and septate uteri, due to simultaneous lack of fusion and reabsorption of Müllerian ducts, may lead to an inaccurate diagnosis. In this case, 3D ultrasonography accompanied by complete gynecological examination and the assessment of the cervix and vagina on MRI should be performed. Moreover, the longitudinal fold of the cervical mucosa needs to be carefully differentiated from a fibrous septum on axial views of the cervix and by following any septum to its proximal attachment.

Sometimes, poor signal-to-noise ratio (SNR) of T2-weighted image also influences the identification of a thin uterine septum.

Teaching Point

1. A uterus characterized by a normal outer fundal contour, two divided uterine cavities with a normal intercornual distance and a intercornual angle less than 75°, and a septum with low or intermediate signal intensity on T 2-weighted image should be highly suspected as septate uterus;
2. Identification of the outer fundal contour, the compositions of septum and assessment of the cervix and vagina may help the differential diagnosis between septate uterus and other MDAs;
3. Based on its high spatial resolution, 3D ultrasonography seems more accurate than MRI on the differentiation of bicornuate and septate uteri.

Case 6.22

Brief Case Summary 31-year-old woman with history of infertility and DES exposure in utero.

Imaging Findings Hysterosalpingography shows a T- shape uterus with a small endometrial cavity. Bilateral intraluminal cornual filling defects, suggestive of polyps are also noted (Fig. 6.45).

Differential Diagnosis Infantile pre pubertal uterus

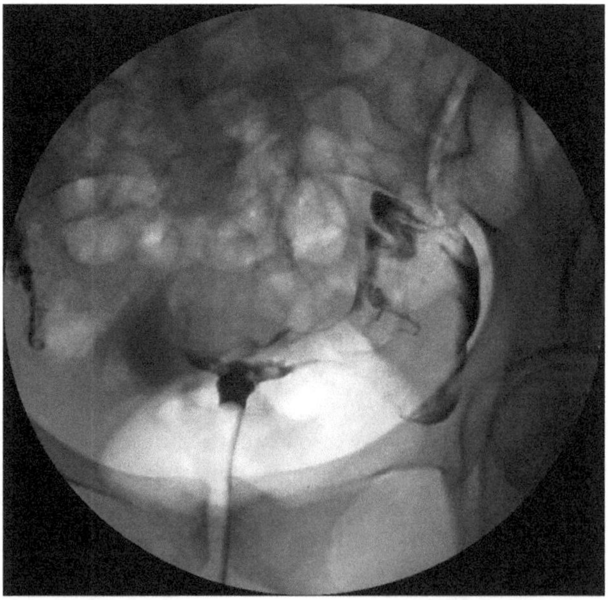

Fig. 6.45 Hysterosalpingography shows a T-shape uterus with a small endometrial cavity. Bilateral intraluminal cornual filling defects, suggestive of polyps are also noted

Diagnosis and Discussion Diethylstilbestrol Related Mullerian Anomalies

In utero exposure to diethylstilbestrol, a synthetic estrogen prescribed to prevent miscarriages between 1945 and 1971, is responsible for abnormalities of both the male and female genital tract. The abnormalities were seen in female offsprings in about 15 % of women exposed to DES during pregnancy. It is categorized as type VII Müllerian anomaly, the hallmark being a characteristic T shaped uterus. Also noted are histological changes in the cervical and vaginal tissues with increased risk of clear cell carcinoma of vagina and cervix. Other complications noted are infertility, high incidence of ectopic pregnancy, and early pregnancy loss due to cervical incompetence.

Diagnostic modalities include hysterosalpingography (HSG), ultrasound (3D) and MRI.

HSG is useful to provide confident diagnosis of DES-related anomaly. It shows a narrow irregular or malformed vagina and endocervical canal. Other findings seen involving the cervix and vagina are hoods or ridges, protuberances (called Cock's combs), sulci, pseudopolyps or cervical stenosis. The endometrial cavity appears small with a shortened upper uterine segment leading to a T shape. The shape and width of body and arms of T can vary widely. The endometrium may also show constrictions or irregular margins, synechiae, or polypoidal defects. The fallopian tubes show dilatation of their interstitial and isthmic parts, irregular inner margins, hydrosalpinx or diverticuli.

Ultrasound and MRI show hypoplasia of uterus. There is myometrial hypertrophy causing thinning and irregularity of endometrial cavity.

Pitfalls An infantile prepubertal uterus may simulate DES related hypoplastic uterus in cases of severe estrogen deficiency or prolonged OCP use. The mucosal changes seen on HSG along with cervicovaginal dysplasia, however, may point towards the correct diagnosis.

Teaching Point

1. In utero exposure to DES leads to a spectrum of anomalies in male and female genital tracts with increased risk of clear cell carcinoma of cervix and vagina.
2. HSG is sufficient to provide a confident diagnosis of DES related uterine anomalies.

Case 6.23

Brief Case Summary 30 year old woman with prior history of IUD placement, now with bleeding per vagina and pelvic pain.

Imaging Findings 3D ultrasound images (Fig. 6.46) reveal a displaced IUD in the lower uterine segment and cervical canal (arrow) in a morphologically normal uterus. The left arm appears to be embedded in the myometrium. No evidence of perforation is noted.

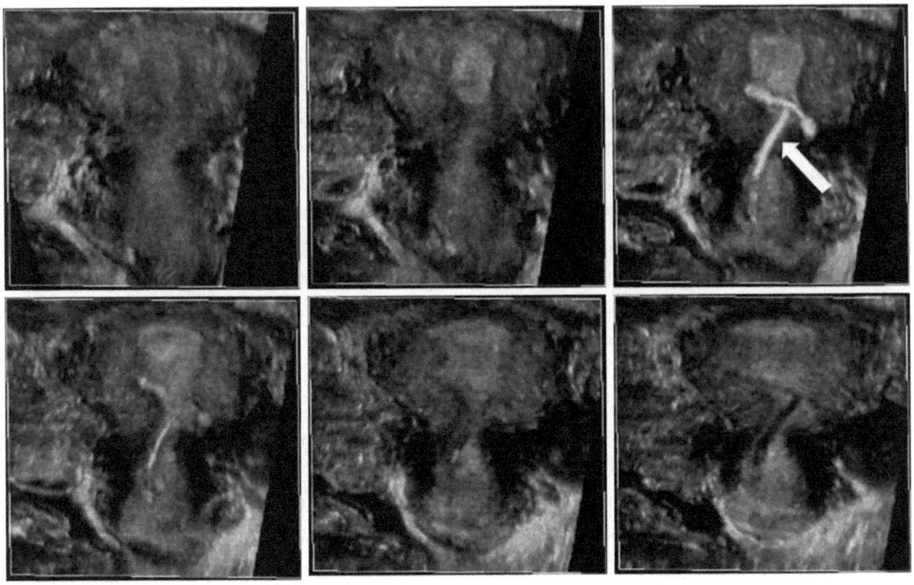

Fig. 6.46 3D ultrasound images reveal a displaced IUD in the lower uterine segment and cervical canal (*arrow*) in a morphologically normal uterus. The left arm appears to be embedded in the myometrium. No evidence of perforation is noted

Differential Diagnosis None.

Diagnosis and Discussion Displaced IUD.

Intrauterine devices (IUD) are used as a rapid, safe, and reversible form of contraception. Two types of IUD are available, a copper IUD (Paraguard; Barr Pharmaceuticals, Pomona, NY) and a plastic (Mirena; Bayer Health-care Pharmaceuticals, Wayne, NJ)

A basic IUD consists of a T shaped frame with copper or levonorgestrel impregnated into the stem and a polyethylene string at its bottom. The copper IUD is hyperechoic on US and are radiopaque. The levonorgestrel IUD in contrast have some amount of barium sulfate and are easily visualized on radiography but poorly seen on US.

Expulsion can occur in up to 10 % of patients. Insertion early in the menstrual cycle, nulliparity, severe uterine anatomic deformation, and immediate postpartum insertion are known risk factors. Contrary to popular belief, position of the uterus (anteverted or retroverted) does seem to affect incidence of expulsion.

Radiography or CT is the imaging of choice if uterine perforation is suspected as it allows rapid localization of the IUD. Once perforation is excluded, an ultrasound is performed to evaluate the positioning of the IUD. On US, an IUD in situ has an echogenic stem and two perpendicular arms extending laterally at the uterine fundus. The distance from the device to the top of the fundus should be 3 mm or less and a distance of >4 mm is associated with a higher risk of displacement and expulsion.

The string can be visualized by US but not by radiography. A 2D ultrasound suffices for locating the IUD within the uterine cavity due to its echogenic stem but the arms however are less clearly seen. 3D US is usually performed to assess the position of the device. Both the copper and levonorgestrel impregnated devices are more conspicuous on a 3D scan and are best seen in coronal and sagittal views.

Embedment refers to extension of the IUD into the myometrium. These patients are usually symptomatic. A 3D ultrasound is particularity useful to demonstrate embedment.

Management of a displaced IUD depends on its location. A cervical IUD can be removed using an IUD hook or hysteroscopic removal. Cervical IUD in particular are associated with accidental pregnancies. A serosal perforation resulting in a peritoneal IUD causes an inflammatory reaction and associated adhesions mandating surgical management. The formation of adhesions appears to be related to the delay in treatment and the WHO recommends perforated IUD's be removed as soon as possible.

Pitfalls

- Knowledge of the type of IUD is important, as the copper IUD is readily visualized on US but radiopaque whereas the Mirena IUD is well visualized on radiography and CT but poorly seen on US.
- Careful assessment of the IUD location is imperative as expulsion, embedment, and uterine perforation are risks of an IUD.

Teaching Points

- An IUD not visualized on clinical examination, radiography or USG can be assumed to have been expelled.
- Scanning the adnexa is crucial as patients with malpositioned IUD are at increased risk for ectopic pregnancies.

Case 6.24

Brief Case Summary 35 year-old woman with pelvic pain.

Imaging Findings Sagittal (Fig. 6.47) and axial (Fig. 6.48) demonstrate a thickened junctional zone (JZ) measuring >12 mm, most prominent in the posterior junctional zone. Also note small foci of T2 hyperintensity within the thickened junctional zone.

Differential Diagnosis Leiomyoma, physiologic contraction.

Diagnosis and Discussion Adenomyosis

Adenomyosis refers to heterotopic endometrial tissue within the myometrium with resulting smooth muscle hypertrophy. It usually occurs in women over the age of 30, multiparity being a major risk factor. Clinically 1/3rd of patients are asymptomatic, the remaining present with menorrhagia and chronic pelvic pain.

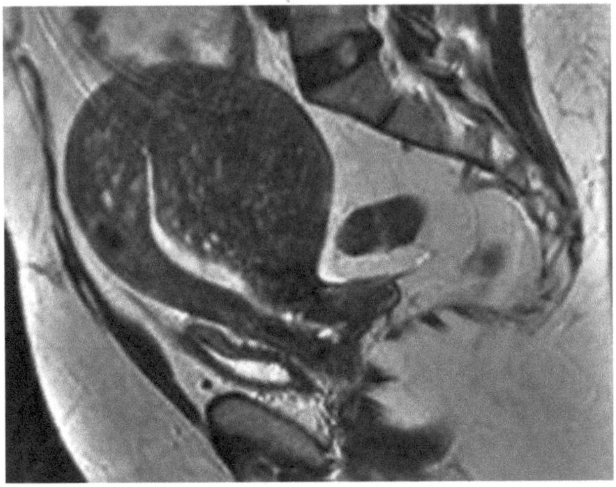

Fig. 6.47 Sagittal image demonstrating a thickened junctional zone (JZ) measuring >12 mm, most prominent in the posterior junctional zone. Also note small foci of T2 hyperintensity within the thickened junctional zone

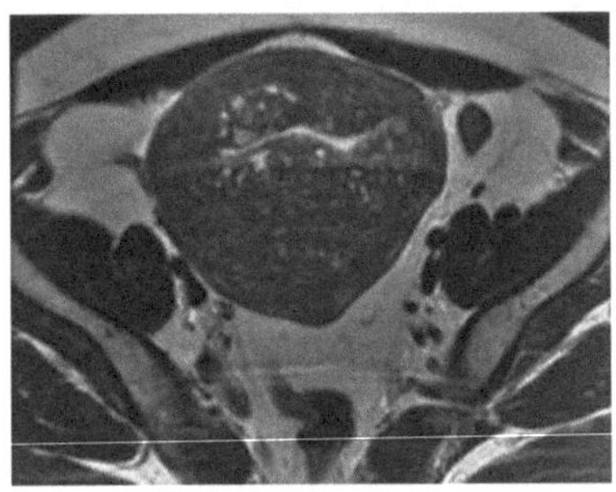

Fig. 6.48 Axial image demonstrating a thickened junctional zone (JZ) measuring >12 mm, most prominent in the posterior junctional zone. Also note small foci of T2 hyperintensity within the thickened junctional zone

Imaging is usually done by ultrasound initially. Direct signs of adenomyosis include diffuse uterine enlargement with heterogeneous appearance and thickening of myometrium, subendometrial cysts and a poorly defined endo-myometrial junction. A transvaginal approach provides optimal visualization of the sonographic findings.

On MRI the characteristic feature is thickening of JZ with a thickness greater than 12 mm. The JZ is typically ill-defined and small foci of T2 hyperintensity can be seen within thickened JZ. In some cases T1 and T2 high signal intensity foci are seen in a subendometrial location which correspond to cystic/hemorrhagic ectopic endometrial glands. The use of diffusion weighted imaging may aid in detection of small hemorrhagic foci as adenomyosis displays intermediate ADC values in contradistinction to very low ADC values that may be seen in coexistent endometrial carcinoma.

Pitfalls

- Differentiation from leiomyoma is possible as the former is well defined and exerts mass effect on surrounding structures.

- Imaging during the early proliferative phase of menstruation may mimic adenomyosis as the myometrial signal is low. Imaging is best carried out in the secretory phase of the cycle.
- Mimics of adenomyosis include physiologic uterine contraction and malignant tumors.
  - Physiologic contraction- T2 weighted cine images are helpful in demonstrating the transient nature of a contraction.
  - Malignant tumors including both primary and metastatic tend to be of low T2 signal and have ill defined infiltrative margins. They also have high signal on DWI and a low ADC coupled with elevated choline on MR spectroscopy which may aid in detection of these lesions.

Teaching Points

- US is the initial imaging study and MRI is the modality of choice for problem solving in suspected cases of adenomyosis.
- A thickened junctional zone with subendometrial high T1 and T2 foci are typical imaging characteristics of adenomyosis.
- Imaging is best carried out in the secretory phase of the cycle to provide maximum lesion to myometrium contrast.

Case 6.25

Brief Case Summary 50 year-old woman with vaginal bleeding.

Imaging Findings Sagittal US (Fig. 6.49) illustrates a thickened endometrium measuring 20 mm.

Differential Diagnosis secretory phase endometrium, endometrial carcinoma, endometrial polyp, submucosal fibroid.

Diagnosis and Discussion Endometrial hyperplasia is defined pathologically as a spectrum of proliferative disorders of the endometrium, generally under the influence of unopposed estrogenic stimulation. It can range from simple hyperplasia without cellular atypia at one end to complex hyperplasia with cellular atypia at the other. The former carries a 2 % risk of malignant transformation whereas the latter has a 23 % risk. It occurs with anovulatory cycles in premenopausal women and usually with exogenous estrogen in postmenopausal women.

The majority of patients with endometrial hyperplasia present with abnormal uterine bleeding (AUB). In premenopausal women, AUB is defined as either excessive bleeding (menorrhagia) or intermenstrual bleeding (metrorrhagia). In postmenopausal women, any bleeding is considered abnormal.

In premenopausal women, imaging with pelvic ultrasound is the first-line of investigation in the workup of AUB. It is ideally performed on days 4–10 of the

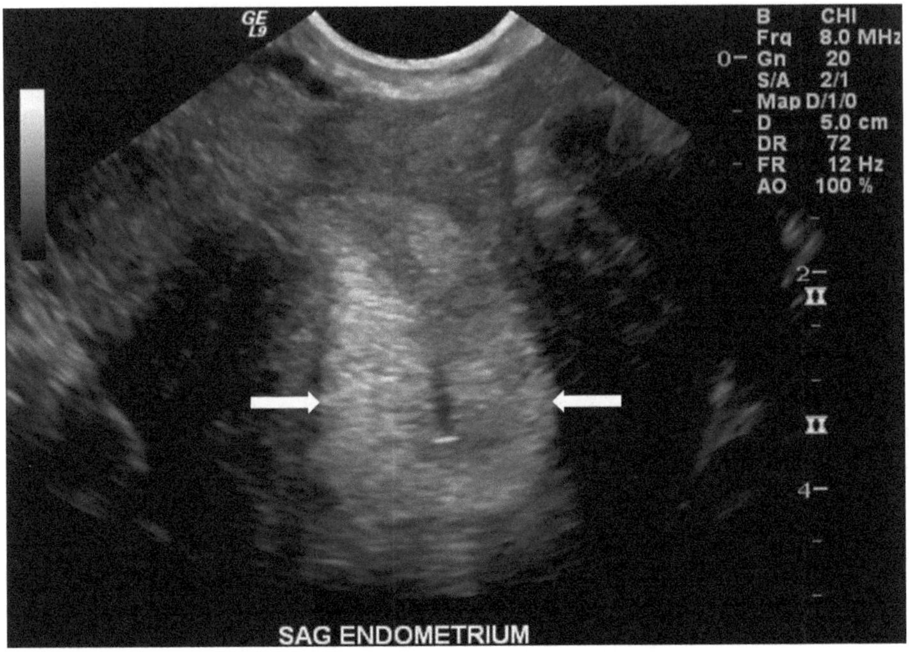

Fig. 6.49 Sagittal US illustrates a thickened endometrium (*arrows*) measuring 20 mm

menstrual cycle. In postmenopausal women, most gynecologists prefer non-focal endometrial sampling without initial imaging, whereas others start with transvaginal sonography. In the case of a diffuse abnormality, endometrial sampling is performed and if a focal abnormality is suggested, then a hysterosonography (saline infusion sonography) is performed to better characterize and to guide hysteroscopy.

Transabdominal ultrasound is useful in measuring the size of the uterus and to evaluate for leiomyomas. Transvaginal ultrasound (TVUS) is the best method to measure the endometrial thickness which is the critical parameter to suggest endometrial hyperplasia. Assessment of the echotexture and presence of irregularities can also be performed. The endometrium should be measured in a sagittal image of the uterus at its thickest point (double-thickness measurement), with exclusion of any fluid in the endometrial canal. Hyperplasia may be a focal or diffuse process manifesting as echogenic thickening with or without small intrinsic cystic spaces.

In premenopausal women, the normal endometrial thickness and echotexture vary with the phase of the menstrual cycle. During the follicular phase, the endometrium is hypoechoic and thin, permitting improved detection of endometrial polyps which tend to be echogenic; hence the optimal timing of a TVUS in the first week after the menses. During the secretory phase, the endometrium is thicker and more echogenic. Overall, a thickness >16 mm in a symptomatic premenopausal patient may be considered abnormal but with a sensitivity of 67 % and a specificity of 75 %. A cutoff of 8 mm yields a higher sensitivity of 84 % but with a lower specificity of 56 %. In the postmenopausal patient, an endometrial thickness cutoff of 5 mm is concerning and should initiate further workup. In both group of patients, any focal abnormality or thickening warrants further workup.

Hysterosonography is useful for differentiating focal from diffuse hyperplasia and endometrial hyperplasia from polyps. MRI of the pelvis may be a useful problem-solving tool when US evaluation of the endometrium is suboptimal, due to uterine orientation or coexisting abnormalities such as adenomyosis or leiomyomas. The normal endometrium is hyperintense on T2 and isointense on T1 to the myometrium. Hyperplastic endometrium is iso or slightly hypointense on T2 to the normal endometrium.

Pitfalls Timing of the TVUS is of prime importance to avoid a secretory phase study which may show a false positive result. If no fluid is present in the endometrial canal, a polyp may mimic hyperplastic endometrium. Doppler US imaging helps to detect the feeding vessel and vascular stalk in a polyp. Hysterosonography can be used to differentiate focal and diffuse hyperplasia and endometrial hyperplasia from polyps. Endometrial carcinoma cannot be reliably differentiated from hyperplasia on imaging unless signs of frank myometrial invasion are present.

Teaching Points

1. Endometrial hyperplasia is defined as proliferation of the endometrium under the influence of unopposed estrogenic stimulation.
2. In premenopausal women, timing of the TVUS in the early proliferative phase is important. A thickness of >16 mm may be considered pathological. In postmenopausal women, a thickness of >5 mm warrants endometrial sampling.
3. Hysterosonography and MRI can be problem solving tools.

Case 6.26

Brief Case Summary 65 year-old woman with a history of breast cancer, currently being treated with tamoxifen.

Imaging Findings Two coronal US views of the uterus (Figs. 6.50 and 6.51) demonstrate a thickened hyperechoic endometrium (arrows) with cystic spaces.

Differential Diagnosis Endometrial polyp, endometrial cystic atrophy, endometrial carcinoma

Diagnosis and Discussion Tamoxifen is a selective estrogen receptor modulator which is prescribed as part of adjuvant chemotherapy of breast cancer, mainly in the postmenopausal age group. Along with the desired anti-estrogen effect on the breast, it carries with it the unwanted property of a weak estrogen agonist in the postmenopausal endometrial tissue. This side-effect becomes manifest in more than one way, of which, endometrial carcinoma and uterine sarcoma are the most dreaded.

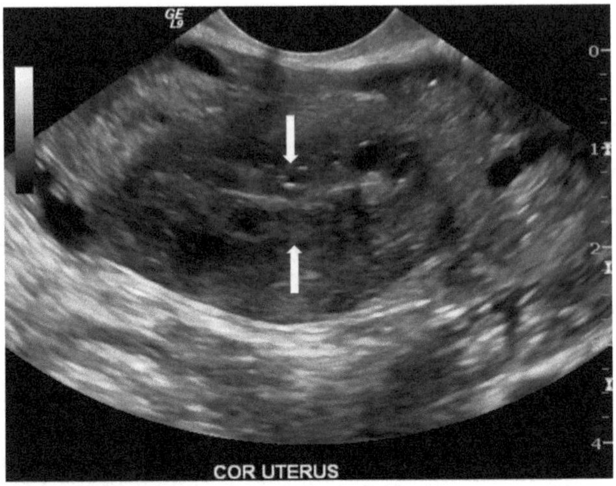

Fig. 6.50 Coronal US view of the uterus demonstrating a thickened hyperechoic endometrium (*arrows*) with cystic spaces

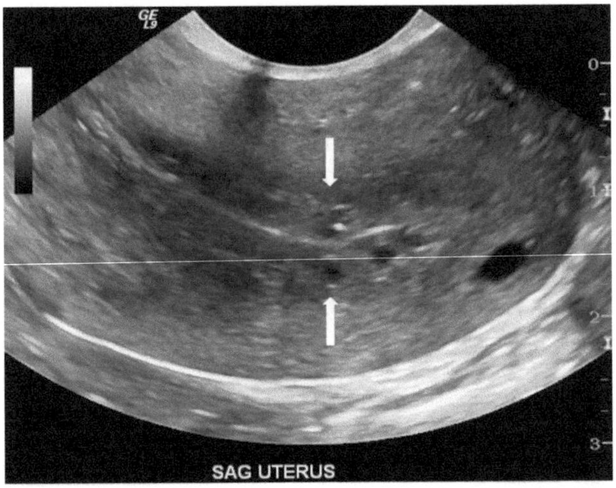

Fig. 6.51 Another coronal US view of the uterus demonstrating a thickened hyperechoic endometrium (*arrows*) with cystic spaces

Tamoxifen-induced endometrial changes include cystic atrophy, polyps, hyperplasia, adenomyosis, and carcinoma. One of the less concerning manifestations is endometrial hyperplasia, which has a higher incidence in patients treated with tamoxifen. The pathology may reveal a simple or complex morphology, with or without cytological atypia, and findings are indistinguishable from endometrial hyperplasia of other causes.

The presentation is similar to that of endometrial hyperplasia from other causes with abnormal uterine bleeding. A postmenopausal woman on Tamoxifen is closely monitored for abnormal bleeding, which if develops, needs an aggressive workup to exclude malignancy including imaging and histopathogical investigations.

Transvaginal ultrasound (TVUS) is the first-line investigation and has good sensitivity but moderate specificity. A normal postmenopausal endometrium is not more than 5 mm in bilayer thickness. In patients on Tamoxifen, the endometrium is thicker compared with control subjects (9–13 mm versus 4.0–5.4 mm). Hence there is controversy regarding the upper limit of normal endometrial thickness in asymptomatic patients receiving Tamoxifen. Some advocate 8 mm as the upper limit, while others consider the 5 mm to be the upper limit.

The most common TVUS pattern seen in women treated with tamoxifen is a thickened endometrium with cystic spaces described as a 'Swiss cheese' pattern. There is controversy regarding the location of these cysts but are likely subendometrial in location. Hysterosonography is a very useful adjunct in that it has proven to downgrade a very concerning endometrial appearance on TVUS, thus preventing invasive investigation. MRI may be appropriate in patients with an equivocal or abnormal TVUS who are unable to undergo hysterosonography due to cervical stenosis. A heterogenous T2 signal intensity with lace-like enhancement in the endometrial canal correlates with a pathological endometrium at biopsy.

The ACOG guidelines for gynecological management of breast cancer patients on Tamoxifen recommend close monitoring for symptoms but there is no role for routine surveillance with TVUS. Patients with a pretreatment benign endometrial polyp are at increased risk for endometrial hyperplasia and may benefit from surveillance with TVUS. Hence a pretreatment imaging with TVUS is essential, preferably supplemented with a hysterosonography.

Once atypical endometrial hyperplasia develops, appropriate gynecological management has to be instituted and the tamoxifen administration reassessed. If Tamoxifen use is deemed essential, then a hysterectomy is performed after which the drug can be reinstated.

Pitfalls Endometrial polyps require hysterosonography to be reliably differentiated from endometrial hyperplasia. Cystic endometrial atrophy is diagnosed histologically when multiple cystic spaces lined by atrophic endometrium are present within a dense fibrous stroma and this cannot be reliably distinguished from tamoxifen induced endometrial hyperplasia on imaging.

Teaching Points

1. Tamoxifen is an adjuvant chemotherapeutic drug for breast cancer, which has adverse weak estrogenic effect on the endometrium.
2. Cystic atrophy, polyps, hyperplasia, adenomyosis, and carcinoma are the effects of the drug on the endometrium.
3. Endometrial hyperplasia is suggested by an abnormally thickened endometrium with subendometrial cysts. The upper limit of normal endometrial thickness in patients taking tamoxifen ranges from 5 to 8 mm.

Case 6.27

Brief Case Summary 48 years old woman with menorrhagia and pelvic pain.

Imaging Findings Axial T1W MR postgadolinium image (arrow, Fig. 6.52) shows a bulky uterus containing multiple enhancing intramural fibroids which are T2 hypointense (arrows, Figs. 6.53 and 6.54) with the largest intramural fibroid located in the anterior myometrium measuring 5.8 cm.

Differential Diagnosis Leiomyosarcoma, Adenomyosis, lipoleiomyoma, ovarian masses and transient myometrial contraction.

Diagnosis and Discussion: Uterine leiomyoma

Uterine leiomyomas (fibroids) are benign tumors of the uterine smooth muscles and are the most common benign uterine tumors in women of reproductive age. They usually affect 30–40 % of women older than the age of 35 years and there is an increase incidence in African American women. Majority of the cases are

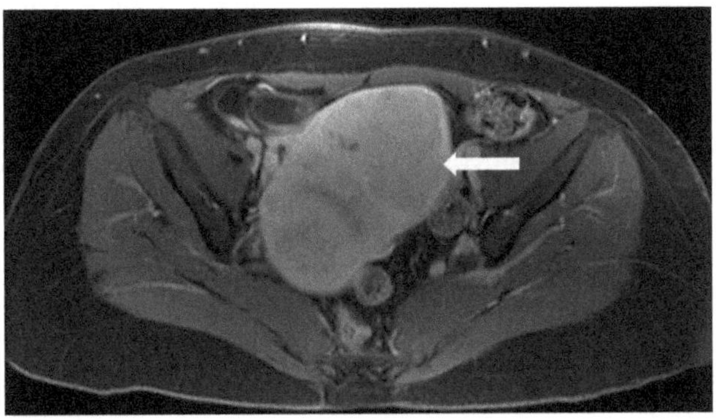

Fig. 6.52 Axial T1W MR postgadolinium image (*arrow*) shows a bulky uterus containing multiple enhancing intramural fibroids

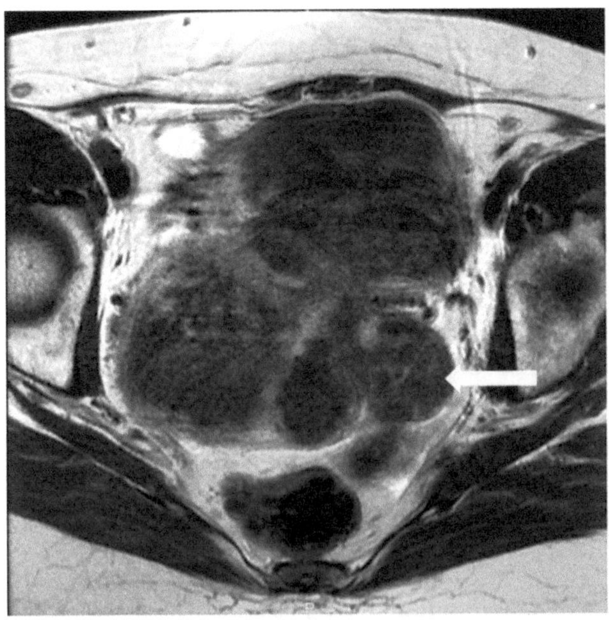

Fig. 6.53 Image showing T2 hypointense fibroids (*arrows*) with the largest intramural fibroid located in the anterior myometrium measuring 5.8 cm

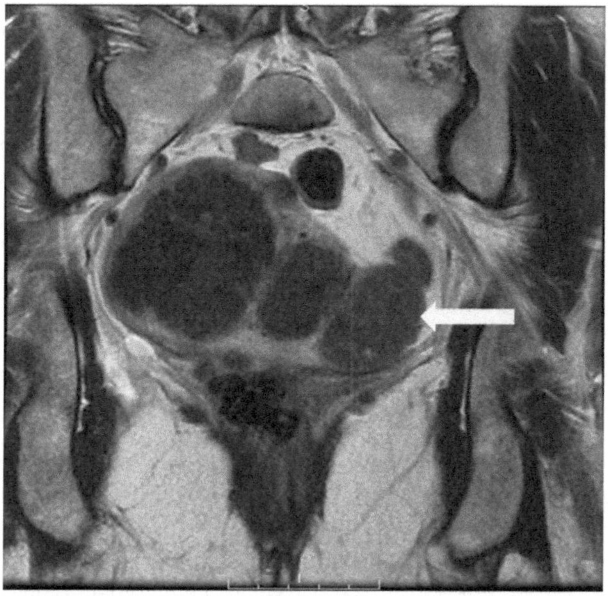

Fig. 6.54 Another image showing T2 hypointense fibroids (*arrow*) with the largest intramural fibroid located in the anterior myometrium measuring 5.8 cm

asymptomatic while symptoms are present in approximately 25–30 % of cases of which most present with menorrhagia and other symptoms ranging from pressure affect to severe pelvic pain. In addition to menorrhagia, fibroids can cause dysmenorrhea and infertility. The mechanism of leiomyoma associated menorrhagia is unknown; however possible vascular defects or impaired endometrial hemostasis have been suggested as an underlying cause.

Uterine leiomyomas are classified into three subtypes based on their locations. The most common type is intramural leiomyoma followed by subserosal leiomyoma (sessile or pedunculated) and submucosal leiomyoma which is the least common.

Uterine leiomyomas typically appear as well-defined, rounded, homogenous myometrial masses. Their sizes range from few millimeters to several centimeters. Uterine leiomyomas are prone to calcification and can also undergo degeneration (hyaline, cystic, or red). Ultrasound of the pelvis is usually the initial investigation to rule out the underlying cause of menorrhagia or pelvic related symptoms, however, US is not as sensitive as other modalities. Transabdominal and transvaginal scans are often preformed and the sonographic findings of uterine leiomyomas vary from being isoechoic to hypoechoic relative to the myometrium and show peripheral vascularity on color Doppler ultrasound. Uncomplicated leiomyomas usually have the same density as myometrium on noncontrast CT images and show less enhancement than myometrium on post contrast CT images. MR is a more accurate modality in diagnosing and describing leiomyomas where they appear isointense as compared to the myometrium on T1W images and hypointense on T2W images.

Common treatment options include hysterectomy (total or supracervical), myomectomy, hysteroscopic removal, uterine artery embolization and thermo ablative procedures. Medical options are of limited and mostly short term use which includes GnRH agonists.

Pitfalls

- Transformation of uterine leiomyomas into leiomyosarcomas is rare, however, no pelvic imaging modality can reliably differentiate between benign leiomyomas and uterine sarcomas.
- Focal uterine adenomyosis is often differentiated from leiomyoma by the ill-defined oval shape. Lipo leiomyomas is differentiated from leiomyomas based on their fatty contents.
- Transient myometrial contraction could be mistaken with leiomyomas as it will appear as a focal lesion on MR which disappears in subsequent images.

Teaching Point

- Most uterine leiomyomas cases are asymptomatic. Symptomatic cases have variable presentations including pelvic pain, menorrhagia, dysmenorrhea and/or infertility.
- Uterine leiomyomas are classified into three subtypes based on their locations: Intramural, subserosal (sessile or pedunculated) and submucosal leiomyoma.
- Uterine leiomyomas are prone to calcification and could also undergo degeneration (hyaline, cystic, or red).
- MR is more accurate modality in diagnosing and describing endometrium leiomyomas where they appear isointense as compared to the myometrium on T1W images and hypointense on T2W images.

Case 6.28

Brief Case Summary 56 year old post-menopausal female presenting with bleed and history of intermittent hematuria and altered bowel habits.

Imaging Findings Sagittal (Fig. 6.55) and axial (Fig. 6.56) CT images of the abdomen and pelvis with IV and oral contrast demonstrate a large moderately enhancing cervical mass with an endometrial collection (asterisk, Fig. 6.55). There is effacement of perirectal fat plane posteriorly and perivesical fat plane anteriorly (arrows, Fig. 6.55). Soft tissue density in the adnexa (arrows, Fig. 6.56) is seen suggestive of adnexal and peri-ureteric fat plane involvement. Coronal image of the kidneys (Fig. 6.57) show mild hydronephrosis bilaterally.

Differential Diagnosis Endometrial carcinoma, Ano-rectal Carcinoma

Diagnosis and Discussion Cervical cancer is a malignant neoplasm arising from cells originating in the cervix. One of the most common symptoms of cervical cancer is abnormal vaginal bleeding, but in some cases there may be no symptoms until the cancer has progressed to an advanced stage. Human papillomavirus (HPV)

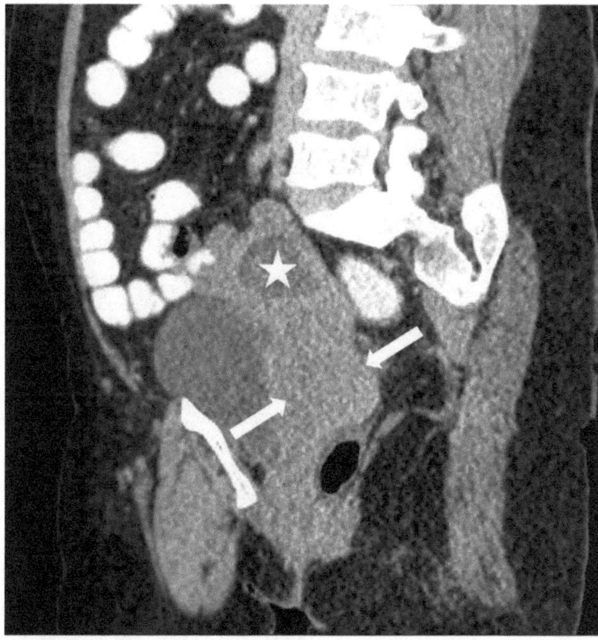

Fig. 6.55 Sagittal CT image of the abdomen and pelvis with IV and oral contrast demonstrate a large moderately enhancing cervical mass with an endometrial collection (*asterisk*). There is effacement of perirectal fat plane posteriorly and perivesical fat plane anteriorly (*arrows*)

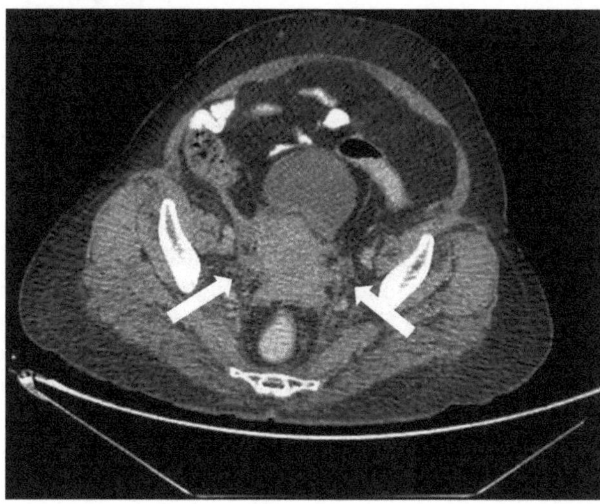

Fig. 6.56 Axial CT image of the abdomen and pelvis with IV and oral contrast demonstrate a large moderately enhancing cervical mass. Soft tissue density in the adnexa (*arrows*) is seen suggestive of adnexal and peri-ureteric fat plane involvement

infection appears to be involved in the development of more than 90 % of cases. HPV vaccines are effective against two to four of the high risk strains of this family of viruses. Since the vaccines only cover some types of HPV, guidelines still recommend that women have regular Pap smear screening, even after vaccination. Cancer screening using the Pap smear can identify precancerous changes in cervical cells. Treatment of high-grade changes can prevent the development of cancer

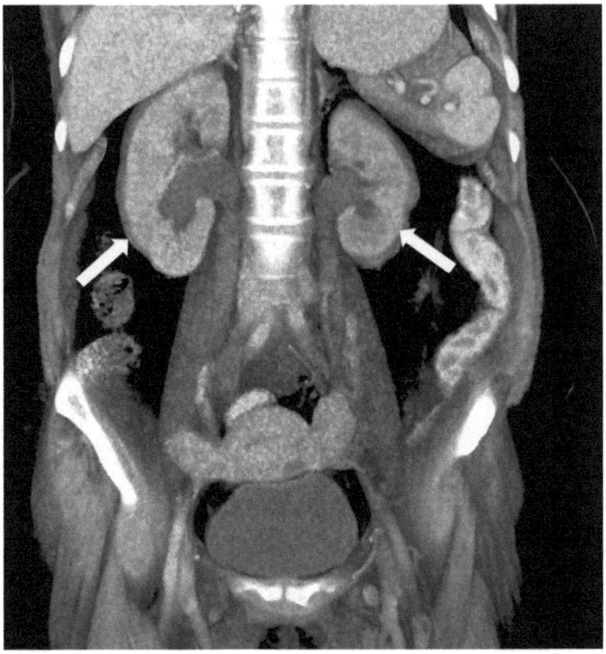

Fig. 6.57 Coronal image of the kidneys show mild hydronephrosis (*arrows*) bilaterally

in many cases. In developed countries, the widespread use of cervical screening programs has dramatically reduced the incidence of invasive cervical cancer. Treatment usually consists of surgery (including local excision) in early stages, and chemotherapy and/or radiotherapy in more advanced stages of the disease. Worldwide, cervical cancer is second most common and the fifth deadliest cancer in women. Approximately 80 % of cervical cancers occur in developing countries. The Pap smear can be used as a screening test, but has a false negative rate up to 50 %. Confirmation of the diagnosis of cervical cancer or pre-cancer requires a biopsy of the cervix. This is often done through colposcopy, a magnified visual inspection of the cervix aided by using a dilute acetic acid (e.g. vinegar) solution to highlight abnormal cells on the surface of the cervix. Further treatment options include loop electrical excision procedure (LEEP) and conization, in which the inner lining of the cervix is removed and examined pathologically. These are carried out if the biopsy confirms severe cervical intraepithelial neoplasia. Cervical cancer is staged by the International Federation of Gynecology and Obstetrics (FIGO) staging system, which is based on clinical examination, rather than surgical findings. It allows only the following diagnostic tests to be used in determining the stage: palpation, inspection, colposcopy, endocervical curettage, hysteroscopy, cystoscopy, proctoscopy, intravenous urography, and X-ray examination of the lungs and skeleton, and cervical conization.

The pretreatment evaluation of patients with cervical cancer includes physical examination, chest radiography, and intravenous urography (IVU) or cross-sectional imaging (computed tomography [CT] or magnetic resonance imaging [MRI]).

In early stage disease with a small tumor confined to the cervix, IVU and cross-sectional imaging are not routinely performed because of their relatively low yield.

IVU is not needed when cross-sectional imaging is performed. Barium enema examination, radioisotope bone scanning, cystoscopy, and proctosigmoidoscopy have a low yield, particularly in early disease, and these procedures are performed for only specific indications that are based on the symptoms or clinical findings.

MRI has excellent soft-tissue contrast resolution, which exceeds that of CT and ultrasonography (US). Consequently, MRI is significantly more valuable than CT and US in the assessment of the size of the tumor, the depth of the cervical invasion, and the locoregional extent of the disease (direct invasion of the parametrium, pelvic sidewall, bladder, or rectum).

CT and MRI are approximately equivalent, and both are significantly superior to US, in the detection of enlarged lymph nodes. Overall, CT and MRI are more accurate staging modalities than US. Furthermore, US is not suited for staging of the full extent of the tumor spread because of the inability to adequately depict all potential sites of metastasis or the anatomic regions that contain lymph nodes.

Despite the advantages of MRI, the gynecology literature mostly recommends the use of CT scanning for the pretreatment evaluation of cervical cancer. Reportedly, the additional information provided with the excellent soft-tissue contrast resolution of MRI often has no significant effect on clinical or therapeutic decision making.

In general, CT and MRI are not warranted in patients with small-volume, early disease (stage Ib disease and a cervical tumor diameter less than 2.0 cm) because of the low probability of parametrial invasion and nodal metastasis. Imaging with CT or MRI is appropriate when the cervical tumor is larger than 2.0 cm, when the size of the tumor cannot be adequately evaluated during the clinical examination, or when the tumor is endocervical.

Pitfalls Imaging is not the gold standard for staging cervical carcinoma, however, laparoscopic evaluation or examination under anaesthesia is the definitive method of staging.

Teaching Point

1. Cervical carcinoma is a very common malignancy in developing countries and its incidence is higher in women in south Asia.
2. Imaging is a complimentary tool to clinical staging and cystoscopy and other ancillary investigations.

Case 6.29

Brief Case Summary 55-year-old woman with postmenopausal bleeding

Imaging Findings Sagittal transvaginal ultrasound (TVUS) image of the uterus (Fig. 6.58) demonstrates a thickened and heterogeneous endometrium (arrow). Axial (Fig. 6.59) and sagittal (Fig. 6.60) T2W image shows heterogeneously high

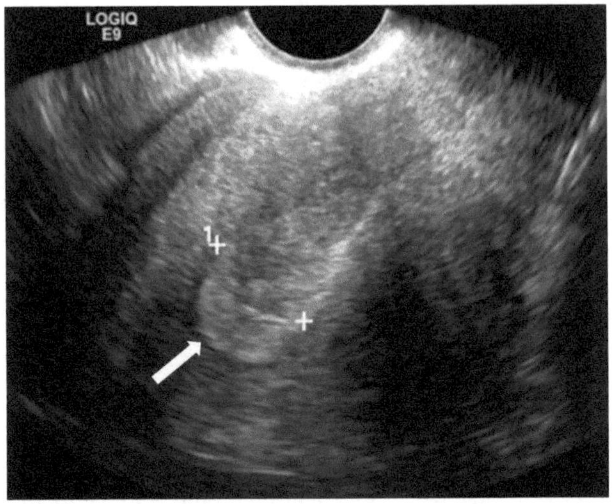

Fig. 6.58 Sagittal transvaginal ultrasound (TVUS) image of the uterus demonstrates a thickened and heterogeneous endometrium (*arrow*)

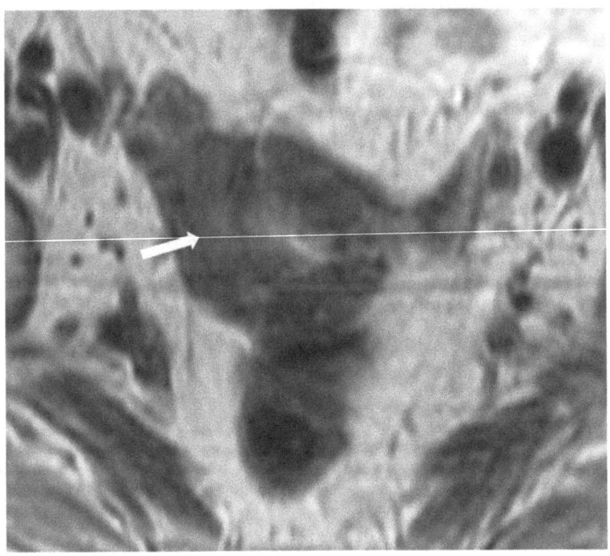

Fig. 6.59 Axial T2W image show heterogeneously high signal intensity T2W lesion (*arrow*) which show lower signal than the surrounding brightly enhancing myometrium on contrast-enhanced MR images (Figs. 6.61 and 6.62)

signal intensity T2W lesion which shows lower signal than the surrounding brightly enhancing myometrium on contrast-enhanced MR images (Figs. 6.61 and 6.62).

Differential Diagnosis Endometrial hyperplasia, Endometrial polyps, Hormonal therapy/ Tamoxifen

Diagnosis and Discussion: Endometrial carcinoma

Endometrial cancer is a malignant neoplasm of the endometrium typically occurring in women in the sixth to seventh decades of life. Endometrial cancer can arise

Fig. 6.60 Sagittal T2W image show heterogeneously high signal intensity T2W lesion (*arrow*)

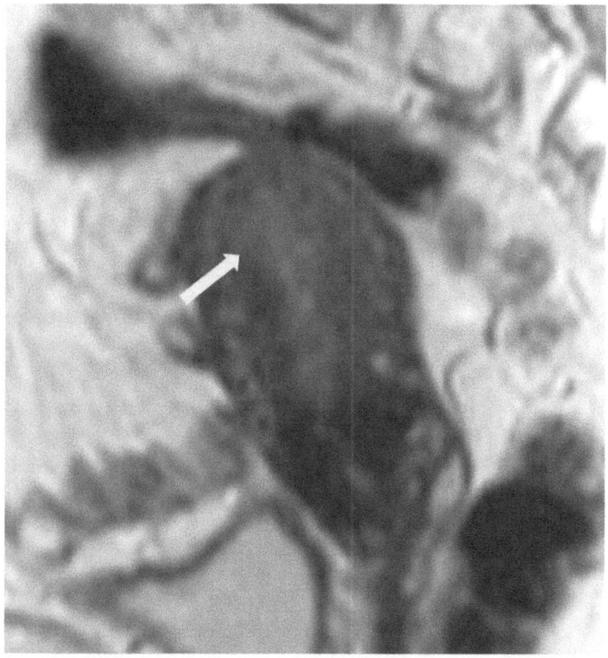

Fig. 6.61 Contrast-enhanced MR image showing lower signal (*arrow*) than the surrounding brightly enhancing myometrium

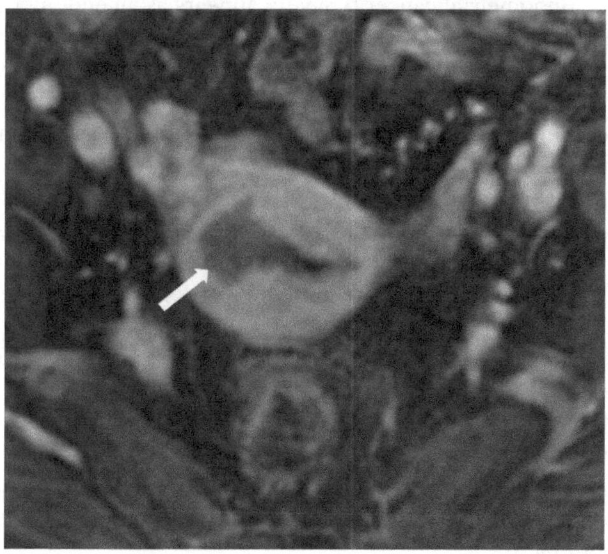

spontaneously from atrophic or inert endometrium or can arise from unopposed estrogen stimulation. Most common presentation of endometrial carcinoma is a postmenopausal woman with abnormal vaginal bleeding.

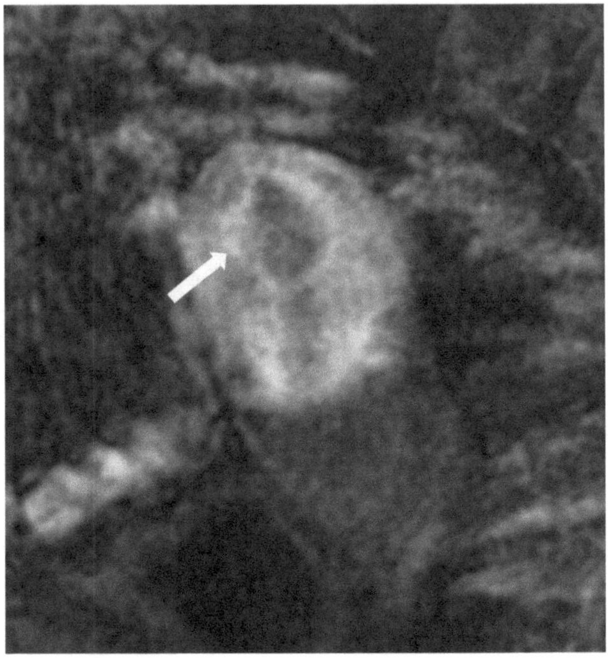

Fig. 6.62 Another contrast-enhanced MR image showing lower signal (*arrow*) than the surrounding brightly enhancing myometrium

Endometrial cancer typically appears as an endometrial mass resulting in expansion of the endometrial cavity. The tumor can appear as a localized or diffuse mass with the localized tumor manifesting as a polypoid mass whereas the diffuse tumor is extensive invasion of the endometrium. Transvaginal ultrasound is often the initial imaging examination for women with uterine bleeding. CT and MRI are important tools in accurate pre-treatment assessment of endometrial cancer and may affect treatment planning. MRI is the most accurate imaging technique for local staging whereas CT and PET/CT are useful for detecting metastasis and for detecting recurrent disease on surveillance. More recently lymph node specific contrast agents have emerged as useful tools in determining metastatic involvement of lymph nodes.

Staging in endometrial cancer is surgical–pathological based on the FIGO (International Federation of Gynecology and Obstetrics) system. Prognosis depends on the age of patient, histological grade, depth of myometrial invasion and cervical invasion and lymph node metastases. Myometrial invasion and accurate cervical involvement cannot be predicted clinically. There is no consensus on the role of imaging in the routine preoperative assessment of endometrial carcinoma.

Pitfalls Adenomyosis, leiomyomas, and large tumors can interfere with assessment of myometrial invasion. Bullous edema of the bladder wall does not indicate bladder invasion.

Teaching Point

- The key MR imaging sequences required for optimal staging of endometrial cancer are high-resolution T2-weighted images, which depict the zonal anatomy of the uterus, and dynamic contrast-enhanced MR, which identifies viable tumor, enabling accurate assessment of myometrial invasion and nodal disease.
- Use sagittal and axial oblique MR images for assessing myometrial invasion and cervical invasion.

Case 6.30

Brief Case Summary 51 year old woman with abnormal vaginal bleeding and pelvic pain.

Imaging Findings Axial T1W MR image (Fig. 6.63) shows an irregular well defined uterine mass demonstrating multiple areas of low signal intensity surrounded with high signal intensity regions (arrow) representing hemorrhagic areas. Axial fat saturated, post-gadolinium T1W MR image (Fig. 6.64) shows heterogeneous enhancement of the uterine mass.

Coronal (Fig. 6.65) and sagittal (Fig. 6.66) T2W MR images of the same patient demonstrate a uterine mass causing distortion of the endometrial canal. The superior

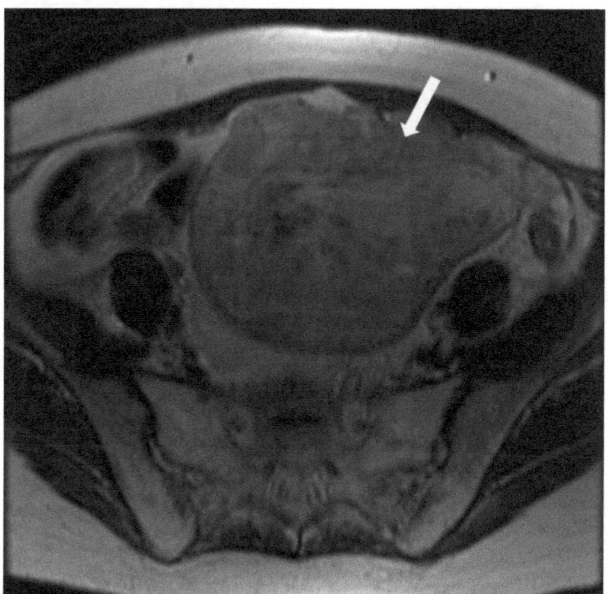

Fig. 6.63 Axial T1W MR image shows an irregular well defined uterine mass demonstrating multiple areas of low signal intensity surrounded with high signal intensity regions (*arrow*) representing hemorrhagic areas

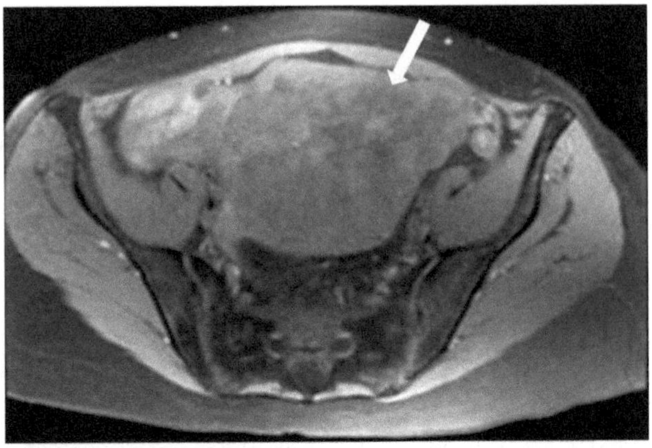

Fig. 6.64 Axial fat saturated, post-gadolinium T1W MR image shows heterogeneous enhancement (*arrow*) of the uterine mass

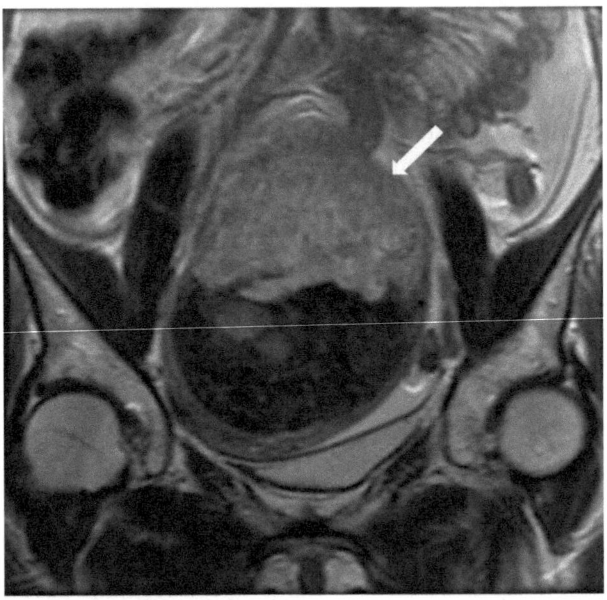

Fig. 6.65 Coronal T2W MR image of the same patient demonstrate a uterine mass causing distortion of the endometrial canal. The superior part of the mass is extensively irregular and heterogeneous (*arrow*) whereas the inferior half of the mass demonstrates T2 hypointensity consistent with a fibroid

part of the mass is extensively irregular and heterogeneous (arrows) whereas the inferior half of the mass demonstrates T2 hypointensity consistent with a fibroid.

Differential Diagnosis Leiomyoma, adenomyosis, endometrial carcinoma and other malignant uterine tumors.

Diagnosis and Discussion: Uterine leiomyosarcoma

Uterine leiomyosarcoma is a rare gynecological malignant mesenchymal tumor arising from the smooth muscle connective tissue of the myometrium and/or myometrium vessels. It is usually diagnosed incidentally in postmenopausal women.

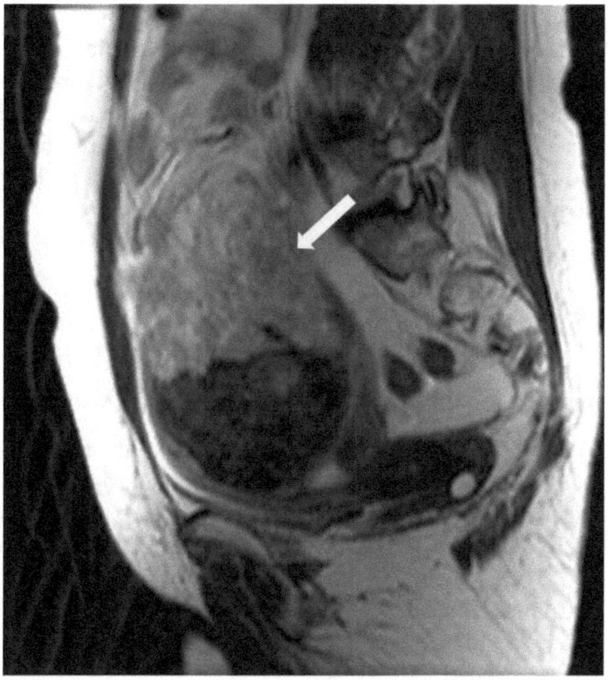

Fig. 6.66 Sagittal T2W MR image of the same patient demonstrate a uterine mass causing distortion of the endometrial canal. The superior part of the mass is extensively irregular and heterogeneous (*arrow*) whereas the inferior half of the mass demonstrates T2 hypointensity consistent with a fibroid

The most common presentations of uterine leiomyosarcoma are abnormal vaginal bleeding, pelvic pain and/or palpable pelvic mass.

Uterine leiomyosarcoma typically appear as fairly defined, heterogeneous solitary lesion surrounded by necrotic and hemorrhagic areas. Uterine leiomyosarcoma ranges in size from few to several centimeters.

Ultrasound usually is the initial imaging modality used. It shows an ill-defined heterogeneous mass with increased vascularity on colored Doppler ultrasound. Uterine leiomyosarcoma often has a similar density to the myometrium on non-enhanced CT images making it almost undifferentiated from the normal uterus, however, the presence of low attenuation areas within the uterus is an alarming sign. The low attenuation areas are often indicative of hemorrhagic and necrotic regions surrounding a mass. Contrast enhanced CT images add more valuable information where a leiomyosarcoma appears as an enhancing, well defined heterogeneous low density mass surrounded with areas of non enhancement indicative of the necrotic tissues. MR imaging is the best modality used for characterization of the lesion. Uterine leiomyosarcoma shows low signal intensities with areas of high signal representing hemorrhagic regions on T1W images and heterogeneous signal intensities on T2W images.

Pitfalls Differentiating between leiomyosarcoma and degenerated leiomyoma by using the current modalities remains very challenging. A rapidly growing pelvic mass along with signs suggesting malignancy will help in such a dilemma.

Teaching Points Uterine leiomyosarcoma is a rare malignant mesenchymal tumor of the uterine smooth muscles and vessels. Patients usually present with complaints of abnormal vaginal bleeding, pelvic pain and/or palpable pelvic mass. Uterine leiomyosarcoma appears heterogeneous with vascularity on ultrasound images, heterogeneously enhanced with areas of low densities on contrast enhanced CT images and heterogeneous on MRI images with areas of high signal intensities representing the hemorrhagic regions.

Case 6.31

Brief Case Summary A 58 year old female with vaginal bleeding

Imaging Findings A large mass is seen in the uterus (arrows, Figs. 6.67, 6.68, and 6.69) which is markedly distended with heterogeneous signal intensity on both sagittal T2 (Fig. 6.67) and axial T1 fat saturated, postgadolinium image (Fig. 6.68) and likely representing both necrotic and viable tissue as well as hemorrhage (asterisk, Fig. 6.68).The mass is highly vascular with areas of irregular enhancement and a central nonenhancing region (arrow, Fig. 6.69). Additionally, there are two fibroids (asterisks, Figs. 6.67 and 6.69) in the anterior and posterior fundus.

Differential Diagnosis Invasive mole, placental site trophoblastic tumor, retained products of conception.

Diagnosis and Discussion Choriocarcinoma is a malignant gestational trophoblastic tumor (GTN) characterized by abnormal proliferation of trophoblastic tissue. Only about half of the cases arise from a complete hydatiform mole. An additional 25 % of cases occur after normal pregnancies and 25 % arise after spontaneous

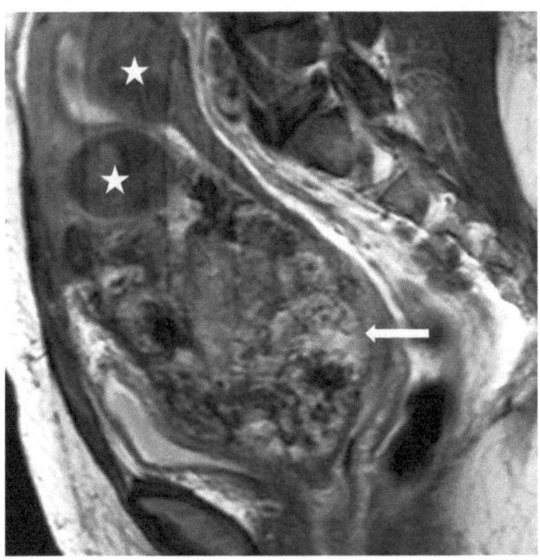

Fig. 6.67 A large mass is seen in the uterus (*arrow*) which is markedly distended with heterogeneous signal intensity on sagittal T2 fat saturated, postgadolinium image. There are two fibroids (*asterisks*) in the anterior and posterior fundus

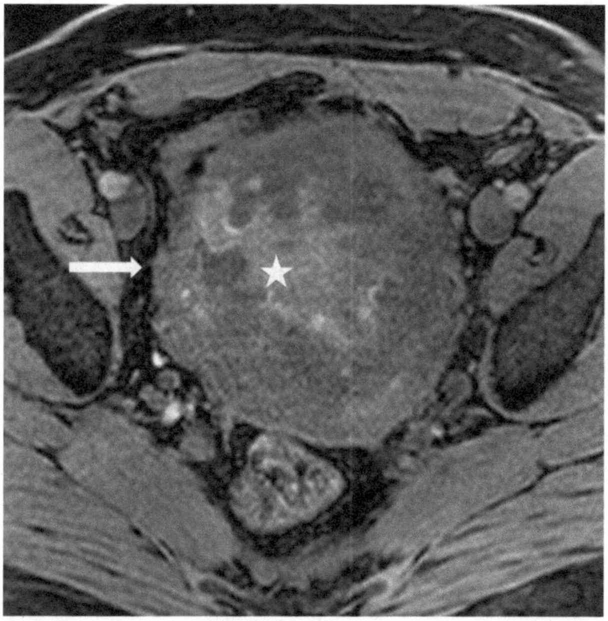

Fig. 6.68 A large mass is seen in the uterus (*arrow*) on postgadolinium image, likely representing both necrotic and viable tissue as well as hemorrhage (*asterisk*)

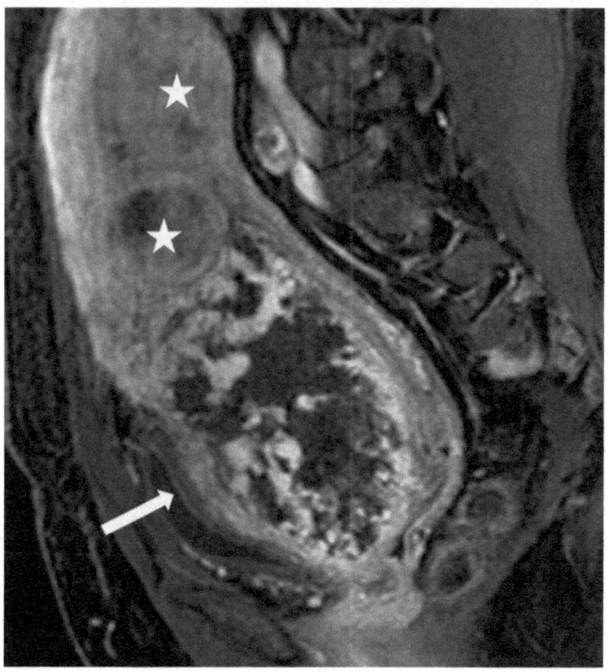

Fig. 6.69 A large mass is seen in the uterus (*arrow*). The mass is highly vascular with areas of irregular enhancement and a central nonenhancing region (*arrow*). Additionally, there are two fibroids (*asterisks*) in the anterior and posterior fundus

abortion or ectopic pregnancy. The incidence is about 2–7 per 100,000 pregnancies and occurs in women between 15 and 49 years of age. Most choriocarcinoma have aneuploid karyotype, and about three-quarters of them contain a Y chromosome.

Patients present with symptoms due to persistent increased hCG or due to metastatic lesions. Choriocarcinoma is suspected if increase in hCG after GTN or any pregnancy is present.

Choriocarcinoma is a rapidly growing, aggressive tumor with extensive necrosis and hemorrhage with tendency for early and extensive vascular invasion. At histologic evaluation, predominant biphasic population of cytotrophoblasts and syncytiotrophoblasts with anaplastic features and few interspersed intermediate trophoblasts can be seen, with absent chorionic villi.

The investigation starts with a pelvic ultrasound and with subsequent CT or MRI for staging. The uterine mass is often very small, measuring about 2–8 mm focus and may not be detectable with imaging. However, size of the lesion does not correlate to the presence of metastases.

Ultrasound findings are quite variable. Choriocarcinoma manifests as a discrete, central infiltrative mass often invading the myometrium with cystic areas and heterogeneity. Doppler study shows high velocity, low-impedance flow. Enlarged cystic ovaries (theca lutein cysts) secondary to increased levels of hCG is also seen.

MRI shows intermediate heterogenous signal depending on the stage of hemorrhage and necrosis, loss of zonal anatomy and increased flow voids. Post contrast T1 study shows nodular and well defined enhancing margins, because tumor usually invades the myometrium through the venous sinuses. The enhancing solid component is usually located in the periphery of the tumor and indicates active foci of tumor. Intratumoral vascularity is minimal in most patients when compared to invasive mole.

CT and MRI imaging helps in studying the extension of tumor beyond the uterus to the pelvic structures and metastases to other organs. Metastases are common to lung, brain and liver and uncommon in bones. The metastatic lesions are often large and heterogenous with hemorrhagic components.

FIGO anatomical staging of uterine choriocarcinoma is as follows: Stage 1: Disease confined to uterus, Stage 2: Extends outside uterus, but limited to pelvis, Stage 3: Extends to lungs, and Stage 4: Extension to all other sites.

Modified WHO prognostic scoring system as adapted by FIGO includes age, antecedent pregnancy, interval months from index pregnancy, pretreatment serum hCG, tumor size, site of metastases, number of metastases and previous failed chemotherapy.

Treatment options include chemotherapy with agents like Methotrexate and actinomycin D. Patients show very good response to chemotherapy, with about 75 % remission even with extensive metastatic disease. Hysterectomy becomes necessary in about one-third of cases, in cases of extensive parametrial invasion, non responsive tumor and uncontrolled bleeding even after embolisation.

Pitfalls Invasive mole and placental site trophoblastic tumor could mimic choriocarcinoma with increased vascularity and myometrial invasion and often needs pathological evaluation to confirm. Histopathologically, invasive mole can be differentiated by the presence of invasive villi and placental site trophoblastic tumor by the presence of predominantly intermediate trophoblasts. Retained products of conception may not show vascularity or myometrial invasion and can be easily differentiated.

Teaching Points

1. Choriocarcinoma is suspected if increased hCG is seen after GTN or pregnancy.
2. Metastases with uterine GTN are more likely choriocarcinoma.
3. Negative pelvic ultrasound does not rule out choriocarcinoma. Size of the uterine lesion is not related to metastases.
4. Invasive mole and placental site trophoblastic tumor may mimic choriocarcinoma and histopathology is confirmatory.

Suggested Readings by Case

Case 6.1

Garel L, Dubois J, Grignon A, Filiatrault D, Van Vliet G. US of the pediatric female pelvis: a clinical perspective. Radiographics. 2001;21(6):1393–407.
Hamm B, Forstner R. MRI and CT of the female pelvis. Springer; Berlin Heidelberg; 2007. p. 388.
Lee TT, Rausch ME. Polycystic ovarian syndrome: role of imaging in diagnosis. Radiographics. 2012;32(6):1643–57.
Merz E. Ultrasound in obstetrics and gynecology. Thieme; Stuttgart, Germany; 2007. p. 326.
Merz E, Miric-Tesanic D, Bahlmann F, Weber G, Wellek S. Sonographic size of uterus and ovaries in pre- and postmenopausal women. Ultrasound Obstet Gynecol. 1996;7(1):38–42.

Case 6.2

Dill-Macky MJ, et al. Ovarian sonography. In: Ultrasonography in obstetrics and gynecology. 4th ed. W.B. Saunders Company; 2000. p. 863–4.
Jain KA. Sonographic spectrum of hemorrhagic ovarian cysts. J Ultrasound Med. 2002;21:879–86.
Jeong YY, Outwater EK, Kang HG. Imaging evaluation of ovarian masses. Radiographics. 2000;20:1445–70.
Reed Dunnick N, et al. Textbook of uroradiology. 5th ed. Lippincott Williams & Wilkins; Philadelphia, USA; 2013. p. 363–6.
Tamai K, Koyama T, Saga T, et al. MR features of physiologic and benign conditions of the ovary. Eur Radiol. 2006;16(12):2700–11.

Case 6.3

Dill-Macky MJ, et al. Ovarian sonography. In: Ultrasonography in obstetrics and gynecology. 4th ed. W.B. Saunders Company; 2000. p. 863–4.
Jeong YY, Outwater EK, Kang HG. Imaging evaluation of ovarian masses. Radiographics. 2000;20:1445–70.
Reed Dunnick N, et al. Textbook of uroradiology. 5th ed. Lippincott Williams & Wilkins; 2013. p. 363–6.
Swire MN, Castro-Aragon I, Levine D. Various sonographic appearance of the hemorrhagic corpus luteum cyst. Ultrasound Q. 2004;20(2):45–58.
Tamai K, Koyama T, Saga T, et al. MR features of physiologic and benign conditions of the ovary. Eur Radiol. 2006;16(12):2700–11.

Case 6.4

Chiang G, Levine D. Imaging of adnexal masses in pregnancy. J Ultrasound Med. 2004;23(6):805–19.
Kier R, McCarthy SM, Scoutt LM, et al. Pelvic masses in pregnancy: MR imaging. Radiology. 1990;176:709–13.
Rahatzad MT, Adamson D. A pictorial essay of pelvic and abdominal masses seen during pregnancy. J Clin Ultrasound. 1986;14:255–67.

Case 6.5

Lee TT, Rausch ME. Polycystic ovarian syndrome: role of imaging in diagnosis. Radiographics. 2012;32(6):1643–57.
Vargas HA, Barrett T, Sala E. MRI of ovarian masses. J Magn Reson Imaging. 2013; 37(2):265–81.

Case 6.6

Darwish A, Amin AF, Mohammad SA. Laparoscopic management of paratubal and paraovarian cysts. JSLS. 2003;7(2):101–6.
Jeong YY, Outwater EK, Kang HG. Imaging evaluation of ovarian masses. Radiographics. 2000; 20:1445–70.
Kim JS, Woo SK, Suh SJ, et al. Sonographic diagnosis of paraovarian cysts: value of detecting a separate ipsilateral ovary. AJR Am J Roentgenol. 1995;164:1441–4.

Case 6.7

Corwin MT, Gerscovich EO, Lamba R, et al. Differentiation of ovarian endometriomas from hemorrhagic cysts at MR imaging: utility of the T2 dark spot sign. Radiology. 2014;271(1):126–32.
Glastonbury CM. The shading sign. Radiology. 2002;224(1):199–201.
Siegelman ES, Oliver ER. MR imaging of endometriosis: ten imaging pearls. Radiographics. 2012;32:1675–91.
Umaria N, Olliff JF. Imaging features of pelvic endometriosis. Br J Radiol. 2001;74(882):556–62.

Case 6.8

Chiou SY, Lev-Toaff AS, Masuda E, et al. Adnexal torsion: new clinical and imaging observations by sonography, computed tomography, and magnetic resonance imaging. J Ultrasound Med. 2007;26(10):1289–301.
Duigenan S, Oliva E, Lee SI. Ovarian torsion: diagnostic features on CT and MRI with pathologic correlation. AJR Am J Roentgenol. 2012;198(2):W122–31.
Huchon C, Fauconnier A. Adnexal torsion: a literature review. Eur J Obstet Gynecol Reprod Biol. 2010;150(1):8–12.
Lourenco AP, Swenson D, Tubbs RJ, et al. Ovarian and tubal torsion: imaging findings on US, CT, and MRI. Emerg Radiol. 2014;21(2):179–87.
Wilkinson C, Sanderson A. Adnexal torsion – a multimodality imaging review. Clin Radiol. 2012;67(5):476–83.

Case 6.9

Jung S, Lee J, Rha S. CT and MR imaging of ovarian tumors with emphasis on differential diagnosis. Radiographics. 2002;22:1305–25.
Outwater EK, Siegelman ES, Hunt JL. Ovarian teratomas: tumor types and imaging characteristics. Radiographics. 2001;5067:475–90.
Pokharel SS, Macura KJ, Ihab R, et al. Current MR imaging lipid detection techniques for diagnosis of lesions in the abdomen and pelvis. Radiographics. 2013;33:681–702.
Saba L, Guerriero S, Sulcis R, et al. Mature and immature ovarian teratomas: CT, US and MR imaging characteristics. Eur J Radiol. 2009;72:454–63.

Case 6.10

Oh SN, Rha SE, Byun JY, et al. MRI features of ovarian fibromas: emphasis on their relationship to the ovary. Clin Radiol. 2008;63(5):529–35.
Paladini D, Testa A, Van Holsbeke C, et al. Imaging in gynecological disease (5): clinical and ultrasound characteristics in fibroma and fibrothecoma of the ovary. Ultrasound Obstet Gynecol. 2009;34(2):188–95.
Shinagare AB, Meylaerts LJ, Laury AR, et al. MRI features of ovarian fibroma and fibrothecoma with histopathologic correlation. AJR Am J Roentgenol. 2012;198(3):W296–303.
Troiano RN, Lazzarini KM, Scoutt LM, et al. Fibroma and fibrothecoma of the ovary: MR imaging findings. Radiology. 1997;204(3):795–8.

Case 6.11

Hart WR. Mucinous tumors of the ovary: a review. Int J Gynecol Pathol. 2005;24(1):4–25.
Imaoka I, Wada A, Kaji Y, et al. Developing an MR imaging strategy for diagnosis of ovarian masses. Radiographics. 2006;26(5):1431–48.
Tamai K, Koyama T, Saga T, et al. MR features of physiologic and benign conditions of the ovary. Eur Radiol. 2006;16(12):2700–11.

Case 6.12

Imaoka I, Wada A, Kaji Y, et al. Developing an MR imaging strategy for diagnosis of ovarian masses. Radiographics. 2006;26(5):1431–48.
Jeong YY, Outwater EK, Kang HK. Imaging evaluation of ovarian masses. Radiographics. 2000;20(5):1445–70.
Jung SE, Lee JM, Rha SE, et al. CT and MR imaging of ovarian tumors with emphasis on differential diagnosis. Radiographics. 2002;22(6):1305–25.
Tamai K, Koyama T, Saga T, et al. MR features of physiologic and benign conditions of the ovary. Eur Radiol. 2006;16(12):2700–11.

Case 6.13

Matsuoka Y, Ohtomo K, Araki T, et al. MR imaging of clear cell carcinoma of the ovary. Eur Radiol. 2001;11(6):946–51.

Montag AG, Jenison EL, Griffiths CT, et al. Ovarian clear cell carcinoma. A clinicopathologic analysis of 44 cases. Int J Gynecol Pathol. 1989;8(2):85–96.

Wagner BJ, Buck JL, Seidman JD, et al. Ovarian epithelial neoplasms: radiologic-pathologic correlation. Radiographics. 1994;14(6):1351–74.

Case 6.14

Azuma A, Koyama T, Mikami Y, et al. A case of Sertoli-Leydig cell tumour of the ovary with a multilocular cystic appearance on CT and MR imaging. Pediatr Radiol. 2008;38(8):898–901.

Cai SQ, Zhao SH, Qiang JW, et al. Ovarian Sertoli—Leydig cell tumors: MRI findings and pathological correlation. J Ovarian Res. 2013;6(1):73.

Jung SE, Rha SE, Lee JM, et al. CT and MRI findings of sex cord-stromal tumor of the ovary. AJR Am J Roentgenol. 2005;185(1):207–15.

Young RH, Scully RE. Ovarian Sertoli-Leydig cell tumors. A clinicopathological analysis of 207 cases. Am J Surg Pathol. 1985;9(8):543–69.

Case 6.15

Kim SH, Kim SH. Granulosa cell tumor of the ovary: common findings and unusual appearances on CT and MR. J Comput Assist Tomogr. 2002;26(5):756–61.

Ko SF, Wan YL, Ng SH, et al. Adult ovarian granulose cell tumors: spectrum of sonographic and CT findings with pathologic correlation. AJR Am J Roentgenol. 1999;172(5):1227–33.

Stein M, Koenigsberg M, Han M. US case of the day. Adult-type granulosa cell tumor. Radiographics. 1996;16(1):200–3.

Van Holsbeke C, Domali E, Holland TK, et al. Imaging of gynecological disease (3): clinical ultrasound characteristics of granulose cell tumors of the ovary. Ultrasound Obstet Gynecol. 2008;31(4):450–6.

Case 6.16

Ha H, Baek S, Kim S, Kim H, Kwon H. Krukenberg's tumor of the ovary: MR imaging features. AJR Am J Roentgenol. 1995;164(6):1435–9.

Imaoka I, Wada A, Kaji Y, et al. Developing an MR imaging strategy for diagnosis of ovarian masses. Radiographics. 2006;26:1431–49.

Kim S, Kim W, Park K, et al. CT and MR findings of Krukenberg tumors: comparison with primary ovarian tumors. J Comput Assist Tomogr. 1996;20:393–8.

Koyama T, Mikami Y, Saga T, et al. Secondary ovarian tumors: spectrum of CT and MR features with pathologic correlation. Abdom Imaging. 2007;32:784–95.

Testa A, Ferrandina G, Timmerman D, et al. Imaging in gynecological disease: ultrasound features of metastases in the ovaries differ depending on the origin of the primary tumor. Ultrasound Obstet Gynecol. 2007;29(5):505–11.

Case 6.17

Pompili G, Munari A, Franceschelli G. Magnetic resonance imaging in the preoperative assessment of Mayer-Rokitansky-Kuster-Hauser syndrome. Radiol Med. 2009;114(5):811–26.

Strübbe EH, Willemsen WN, Lemmens JA, et al. Mayer-Rokitansky-Küster-Hauser syndrome: distinction between two forms based on excretory urographic, sonographic, and laparoscopic findings. AJR Am J Roentgenol. 1993;160(2):331–4.

Case 6.18

Muller GC, Hussain HK, Smith YR, et al. Mullerian duct anomalies: comparison of MRI diagnosis and clinical diagnosis. AJR Am J Roentgenol. 2007;189(6):1294–302.
Olpin JD, Heilbrun M. Imaging of Müllerian duct anomalies. Clin Obstet Gynecol. 2009;52(1):40–56.
Shulman LP. Müllerian anomalies. Clin Obstet Gynecol. 2008;51(2):214–22.

Case 6.19

Mueller GC, Hussain HK, Smith YR, et al. Müllerian duct anomalies: comparison of MRI diagnosis and clinical diagnosis. AJR Am J Roentgenol. 2007;189(6):1294–302.
Troiano RN, Mccarthy SM. Mullerian duct anomalies: imaging and clinical issues. Radiology. 2004;233(1):19–34.

Case 6.20

Behr SC, Courtier JL, Qayyum A. Imaging of müllerian duct anomalies. Radiographics. 2012; 32(6):E233–50.
Brody JM, Koelliker SL, Frishman GN. Unicornuate uterus: imaging appearance, associated anomalies, and clinical implications. AJR Am J Roentgenol. 1998;171(5):1341–7.
Mueller GC, Hussain HK, Smith YR, et al. Müllerian duct anomalies: comparison of MRI diagnosis and clinical diagnosis. AJR Am J Roentgenol. 2007;189(6):1294–302.
Woodward PJ, Sohaey R, Wagner BJ. Congenital uterine malformations. Curr Probl Diagn Radiol. 1995;24(5):178–97.

Case 6.21

Behr SC, Courtier JL, Qayyum A. Imaging of müllerian duct anomalies. Radiographics. 2012;32(6):E233–50.
Deutch TD, Abuhamad AZ. The role of 3-dimensional ultrasonography and magnetic resonance imaging in the diagnosis of müllerian ductanomalies: a review of the literature. J Ultrasound Med. 2008;27(3):413–23.
Mueller GC, Hussain HK, Smith YR, et al. Müllerian duct anomalies: comparison of MRI diagnosis and clinical diagnosis. AJR Am J Roentgenol. 2007;189(6):1294–302.
Woodward PJ, Sohaey R, Wagner BJ. Congenital uterine malformations. Curr Probl Diagn Radiol. 1995;24(5):178–97.

Case 6.22

Charles L. Renell; T-shaped uterus in Diethylstibestrol (DES) exposure. AJR Am J Roentgenol. 1979;132:979–80.
Troiano RN, Mccarthy SM. Mullerian duct anomalies: imaging and clinical issues. Radiology. 2004;233(1):19–34.
Ubeda B, Paraira M, Alert E, et al. Hysterosalpingography: spectrum of normal variants and nonpathologic findings. AJR Am J Roentgenol. 2001;177(1):131–5.

Case 6.23

Aydogdu O, Pulat H. Asymptomatic far-migration of an intrauterine device into the abdominal cavity: a rare entity. Can Urol Assoc J. 2012;6:134–6.
Boortz HE, Margolis D, Ragavendra N. Migration of intrauterine devices: radiologic findings and implications for patient care. Radiographics. 2012;32(2):335–52.
Levsky JM, Herskovits M. Incidental detection of a transmigrated intrauterine device. Emerg Radiol. 2005;11(5):312–4.

Case 6.24

Jha RC, Zanello PA, Ascher SM, et al. Diffusion-weighted imaging (DWI) of adenomyosis and fibroids of the uterus. Abdom Imaging. 2014;39(3):562–9.
Novellas S, Chassang M, Delotte J, et al. MRI characteristics of the uterine junctional zone: from normal to the diagnosis of adenomyosis. AJR Am J Roentgenol. 2011;196:1206–13.
Shwayder J, Sakhel K. Imaging for uterine myomas and adenomyosis. J Minim Invasive Gynecol. 2014;21:362–76.
Takeuchi M, Matsuzaki K. Adenomyosis: usual and unusual imaging manifestations, pitfalls, and problem-solving MR imaging techniques. Radiographics. 2011;31:99–115.

Case 6.25

Armstrong AJ, Hurd WW, Elguero S, et al. Diagnosis and management of endometrial hyperplasia. J Minim Invasive Gynecol. 2012;19(5):562–71.
Jorizzo JR, Chen MY, Martin D, et al. Spectrum of endometrial hyperplasia and its mimics on saline hysterosonography. AJR Am J Roentgenol. 2002;179(2):385–9.
Nalaboff KM, Pellerito JS, Ben-levi E. Imaging the endometrium: disease and normal variants. Radiographics. 2001;21(6):1409–24.

Case 6.26

ACOG Committee Opinion No. 336. Tamoxifen and uterine cancer. Obstet Gynecol. 2006; 107:1475–8.
Ascher SM, Imaoka I, Lage JM. Tamoxifen-induced uterine abnormalities: the role of imaging. Radiology. 2000;214(1):29–38.

Case 6.27

Ciavattini A, Di Giuseppe J, Stortoni P, et al. Uterine fibroids: pathogenesis and interactions with endometrium and endomyometrial junction. Obstet Gynecol Int. 2013;2013:173–84.
Fonseca-Moutinho JA, Barbosa LS, Torres DG, et al. Abnormal uterine bleeding as a presenting symptom is related to multiple uterine leiomyoma: an ultrasound-based study. Int J Womens Health. 2013;5:689–94.
Wilde S, Scott-Barrett S. Radiological appearances of uterine fibroids. Indian J Radiol Imaging. 2009;19(3):222–31.

Case 6.28

Kraljević Z, Visković K, Ledinsky M, et al. Primary uterine cervical cancer: correlation of preoperative magnetic resonance imaging and clinical staging (FIGO) with histopathology findings. Coll Antropol. 2013;37(2):561–8.

Pannu HK, Corl FM, Fishman EK. CT evaluation of cervical cancer: spectrum of disease. Radiographics. 2001;21(5):1155–68.

Sala E, Rockall AG, Freeman SJ, et al. The added role of MR imaging in treatment stratification of patients with gynecologic malignancies: what the radiologist needs to know. Radiology. 2013;266(3):717–40.

Tirumani SH, Shanbhogue AKP, Prasad SR. Current concepts in the diagnosis and management of endometrial and cervical carcinomas. Radiol Clin North Am. 2013 ;51(6):1087–110.

Case 6.29

Barwick TD, Rockall AG, Barton DP, et al. Imaging of endometrial adenocarcinoma. Clin Radiol. 2006;61(7):545–55.

Ortoft G, Dueholm M, Mathiesen O, et al. Preoperative staging of endometrial cancer using TVS, MRI, and hysteroscopy. Acta Obstet Gynecol Scand. 2013;92(5):536–45.

Sala E, Rockall AG, Freeman SJ, et al. The added role of MR imaging in treatment stratification of patients with gynecologic malignancies: what the radiologist needs to know. Radiology. 2013;266(3):717–40.

Tirumani SH, Shanbhogue AKP, Prasad SR. Current concepts in the diagnosis and management of endometrial and cervical carcinomas. Radiol Clin North Am. 2013;51(6):1087–110.

Chapter 7
Male Pelvis

Prostate

Case 7.1

Brief Case Summary 60 year old man with elevated PSA and prior history of intravesical BCG for bladder carcinoma.

Imaging Findings Transrectal ultrasound shows an isoechoic lesion in left lobe of the prostate gland with a contour deformity along the left posterolateral margin of prostate (Fig. 7.1). Contrast enhanced CT shows the same area to be hypo enhancing with loss of the left recto-prostatic angle (Fig. 7.2).

Differential Diagnosis Prostate carcinoma.

Diagnosis and Discussion Granulomatous prostatitis secondary to BCG therapy.

Intravesical BCG is an accepted method of therapy for bladder cancer. About 40 % of these patient will subsequently show elevation of PSA and approximately 10 % will have clinically symptomatic prostatitis which occur due to reflux of BCG into the prostate.

Granulomatous prostatitis may be secondary to BCG or idiopathic (termed non-specific granulomatous prostatitis, NSGP). NSGP usually demonstrates non necrotic lesions with low T2 signal and ADC values mimicking cancer. Prostatitis secondary to BCG usually demonstrates necrosis. Inflammation may spread to peri-prostatic tissues with loss of normal anatomical landmarks such as the recto-prostatic angle.

A prior history of BCG therapy with accompanying imaging findings usually allow for a confident diagnosis. The PSA in most cases returns to normal within 4–6 months of starting anti-tubercular therapy.

Imaging Pitfalls The low T2 signal lesion in the peripheral zone and diffusion restriction may mislead the radiologist into considering malignancy as the diagnosis,

M.G. Harisinghani, A. Rajesh, *Genitourinary Imaging: A Case Based Approach*, DOI 10.1007/978-1-4471-4772-5_7

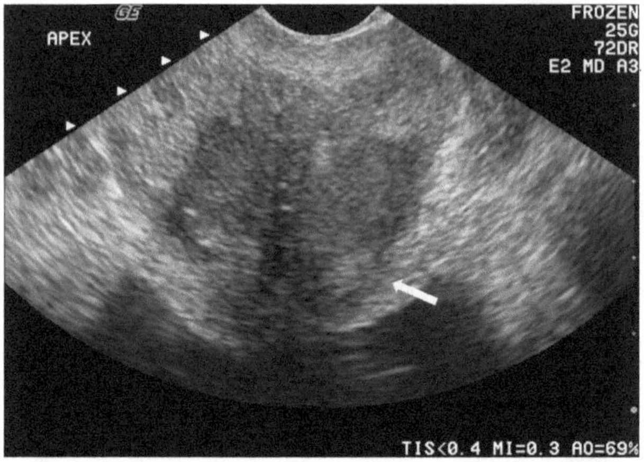

Fig. 7.1 Transrectal ultrasound shows an isoechoic lesion in left lobe of the prostate gland with a contour deformity along the left posterolateral margin of prostate

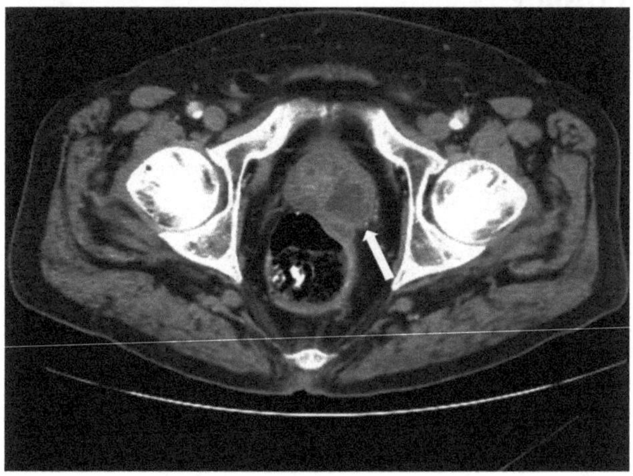

Fig. 7.2 Contrast enhanced CT shows the same area to be hypo enhancing with loss of the left recto-prostatic angle

however the presence of necrosis, lack of rapid wash-out, and high choline peak on MR spectroscopy assist in differentiation.

Teaching Points

- Granulomatous prostatitis can occur secondary to intravesical BCG therapy for bladder carcinoma.
- Prior history of BCG exposure coupled with imaging findings usually point to the correct diagnosis and biopsy is usually unnecessary.

Case 7.2

Brief Case Summary 55 year old male with rising PSA levels and abnormal digital rectal examination (DRE), past h/o tuberculosis.

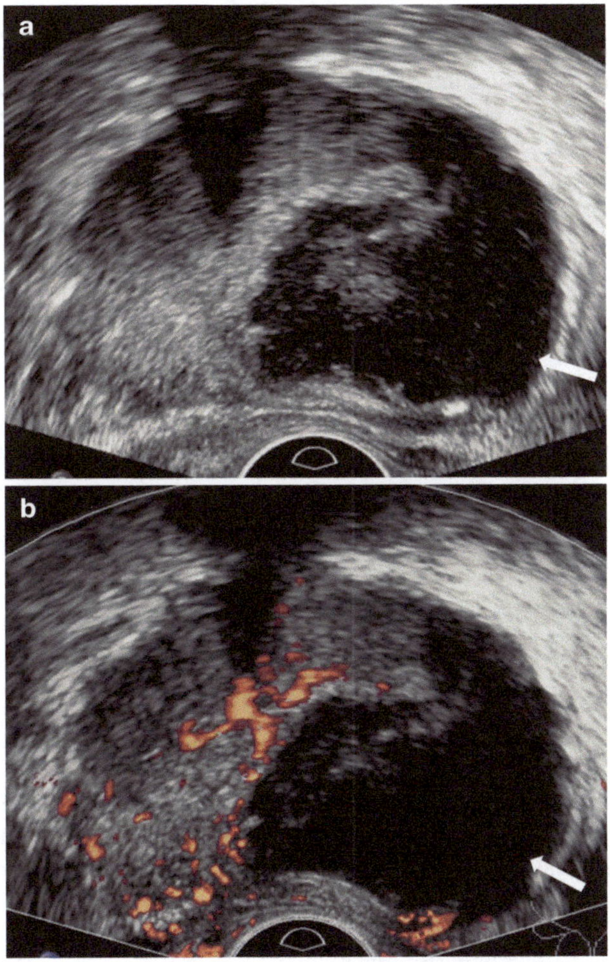

Fig. 7.3 (**a**, **b**) Transrectal ultrasound image demonstrates a well demarcated hypoechoic collection in the left lobe of prostate peripherally placed. It does not show vascularity like the surrounding normal gland

Imaging Findings Transrectal ultrasound image demonstrates a well demarcated hypoechoic collection in the left lobe of prostate peripherally placed. It does not show vascularity like the surrounding normal gland (Fig. 7.3a, b).

Differential Diagnosis Carcinoma prostate.

Diagnosis and Discussion Prostatic tubercular abscess

Genito urinary tuberculosis constitutes 10–14 % of extrapulmonary tuberculosis cases. Prostatic involvement is rare. The usual mode of infection is hematogenous spread or descending infection from the upper urinary tract. Risk factors include prior history of TB, immunocompromised status or intravesical BCG therapy.

Imaging is sought once DRE is abnormal or PSA levels rise. USG is the initial modality of choice. It displays a well marginated hypoechoic collection with no internal vascularity, few internal echoes may be visible. MRI reveals T2 heterogeneity within a well marginated lesion. Diffusion restriction may be present confounding the diagnosis. However post contrast images reveal some amount of necrosis, unusual for a malignancy. Biopsy if often necessary to reach a definite conclusion. Urine PCR has shown good sensitivity and specificity in diagnosis of Genito-urinary TB in general.

Pitfalls Tubercular abscess of the prostate may mimic a malignancy with low T2 signal and ADC values. However presence of necrosis and lack of rapid washout and choline elevation on MRS are clues that help to rule out a malignant lesion.

Teaching Point

- Tubercular abscess in the prostate is rare
- It may closely mimic malignancy on clinical and laboratory examination-multiparametric MRI often allows confident differentiation of these entities.

Case 7.3

Brief Case Summary A 62 year old male with hard prostate on digital rectal examination and elevated PSA levels.

Imaging Findings Axial T2 weighted images (Fig. 7.4a, b) reveal an ill defined hypointense nodule involving the central gland in the mid prostate on left side. There is extension into the peripheral zone as well. The corresponding ADC maps reveal a low ADC, dynamic contrast enhancement color maps show rapid washout kinetics (red) in the region of T2 signal abnormality (Fig. 7.5).

Differential Diagnosis

- benign hypertrophic nodule
- post radiation changes
- chronic prostatitis

Diagnosis and Discussion Carcinoma prostate.

Prostatic cancer is the second most common cause of cancer death among American men, after lung cancer. Imaging and MRI in particular play a key role in identification of the malignancy and its management.

Central gland (transitional zone and central zone combined) tumors pose a unique challenge as the normal T2 hyperintense background of the peripheral zone is absent, moreover there is significant overlap in T2 signals of normal central gland tissue and tumor nodules. Hence imaging multi-parametric MRI (MP-MRI) is paramount. Tumors in this location often present with ill-defined margins and a uniform low T2 signal. Since these tumors are highly cellular they display low ADC values and restricted diffusion. Neovascularity within their substance manifests as rapid wash-in and subsequent wash-out of gadolinium on dynamic contrast enhanced

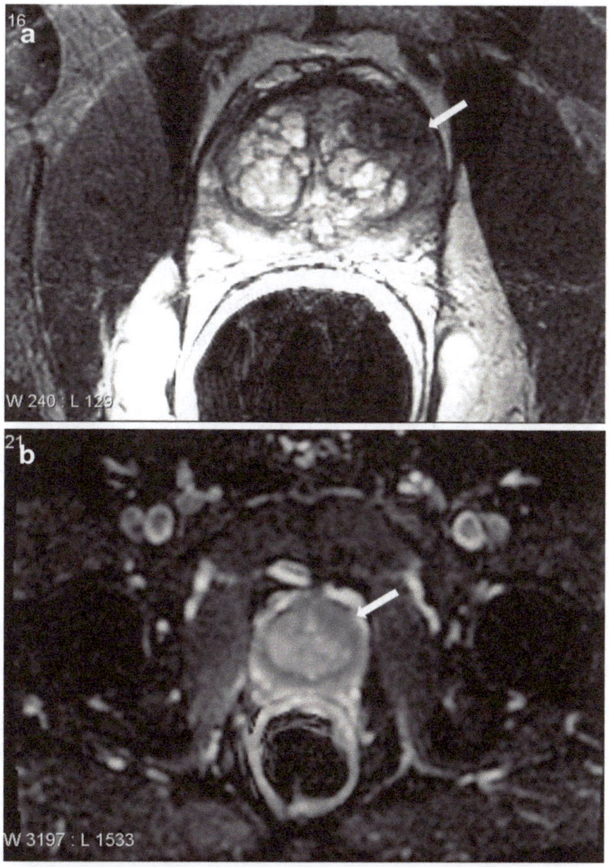

Fig. 7.4 (**a**, **b**). Axial T2 weighted images reveal an ill-defined hypointense nodule involving the central gland in the mid prostate on left side. There is extension into the peripheral zone as well

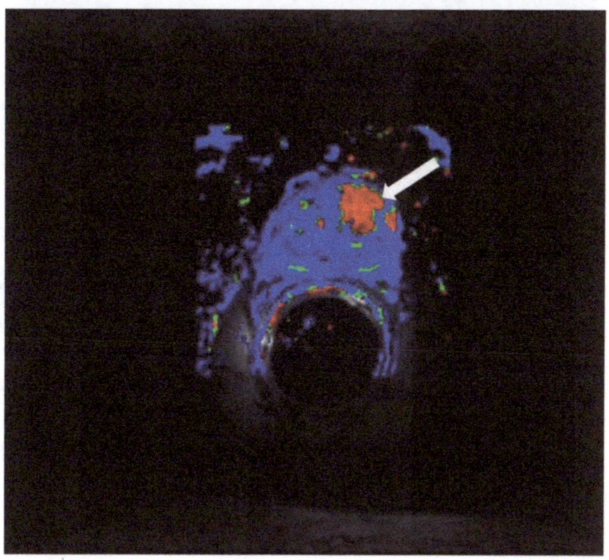

Fig. 7.5 Corresponding ADC maps reveal a low ADC, dynamic contrast enhancement color maps show rapid washout kinetics (*red*) in the region of t2 signal abnormality

(DCE) scans. These generally appear as red areas on post processed color maps (provided there is at least >20 % washout).

Other features of a central gland tumor are lenticular shape, absence of a discernable capsule and invasion of the anterior fibromuscular stroma, asymmetric rapid wash-in/wash-out kinetics and elevated choline on MRS also suggest the diagnosis although no single feature is pathognomonic.

Pitfalls

- Chronic prostatitis may mimic cancer with a low T2 signal and mild diffusion restriction. However it usually doesn't produce mass effect or a contour deformity of the gland. Furthermore the degree of diffusion restriction on DWI and wash-out on DCE are less than that of prostate cancer.
- Hypertrophic nodule – usually arise in central gland, they can be differentiated from cancer by their well defined capsulated margins, they rarely reach the capsule and normal tissue is seen interposed between them and the capsular margin. The MRS generally reveals a normal spectrum. Symmetric contrast enhancement kinetics are usually seen.
- Post radiation changes may also demonstrate a low t2 signal secondary to fibrosis – these foci do not show diffusion restriction, rapid washout or choline peaks on MP-MRI.

Teaching Point

- Interpretation of MP-MRI relies on sound knowledge of normal prostatic zonal anatomy, typical findings of cancer and that its mimics.
- No single imaging finding is pathognomonic for prostatic cancer.

Case 7.4

Brief Case Summary A 70 year old male with rising PSA levels and normal clinical examination.

Imaging Findings Axial T2 weighted image demonstrates a well marginated uniformly hypointense lesion in the mid gland located within the normal T2 hyperintense stroma of the peripheral zone (PZ) (Fig. 7.6).

It is seen to extend up to and beyond the capsular margin into the periprostatic fat. The recto-prostatic angle is obliterated and ipsilateral neurovascular bundle is invaded. Restricted diffusion with is seen with high signal on DWI and corresponding low signal on ADC maps (Figs. 7.7 and 7.8). Color perfusion maps obtained from DCE MRI shows rapid wash-out in the lesion (red) (Fig. 7.9).

Differential Diagnosis

- Benign hypertrophic nodule in PZ.
- Displaced central zone

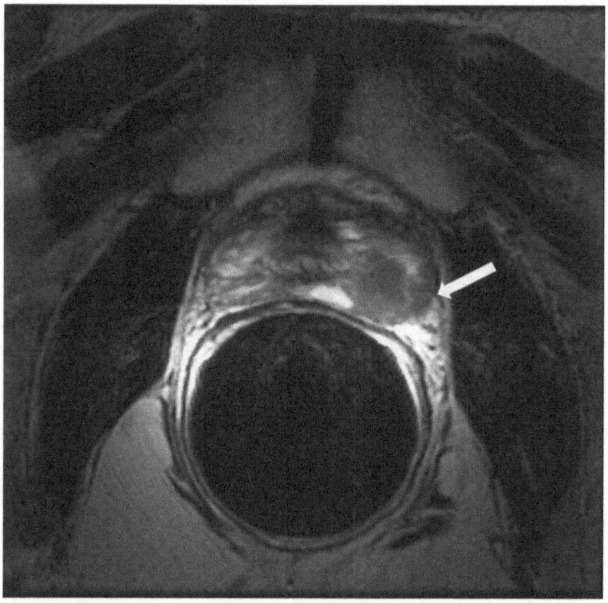

Fig. 7.6 Axial T2 weighted image demonstrates a well marginated uniformly hypointense lesion in the mid gland located within the normal T2 hyperintense stroma of the peripheral zone (PZ)

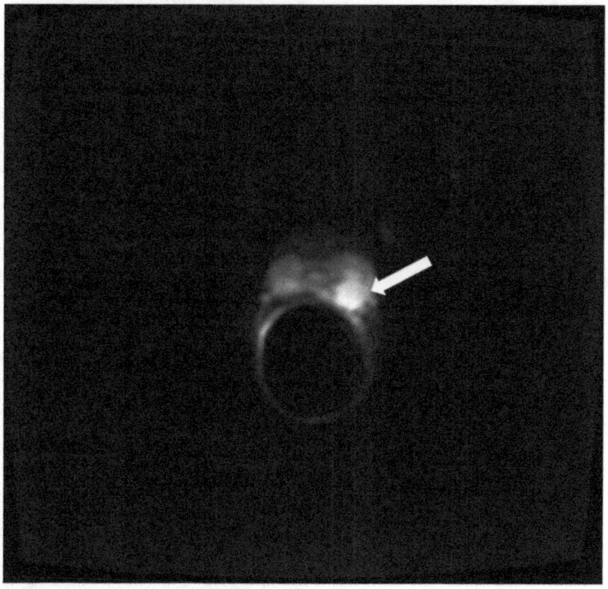

Fig. 7.7 Lesion is seen to extend up to and beyond the capsular margin into the periprostatic fat. The recto-prostatic angle is obliterated and ipsilateral neurovascular bundle is invaded

- Post radiation changes
- Pseudolesion in the midline of PZ

Diagnosis and Discussion Carcinoma prostate in peripheral zone of left lobe mid gland with Extracapsular extension (ECE).

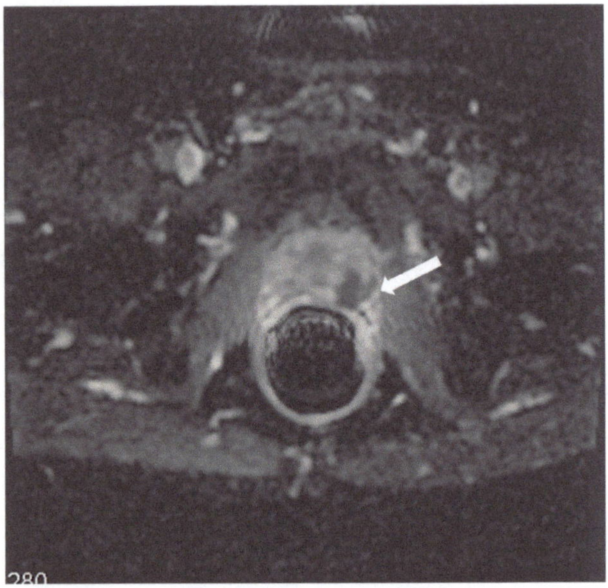

Fig. 7.8 Restricted diffusion which is seen with high signal on DWI and corresponding low signal on ADC maps

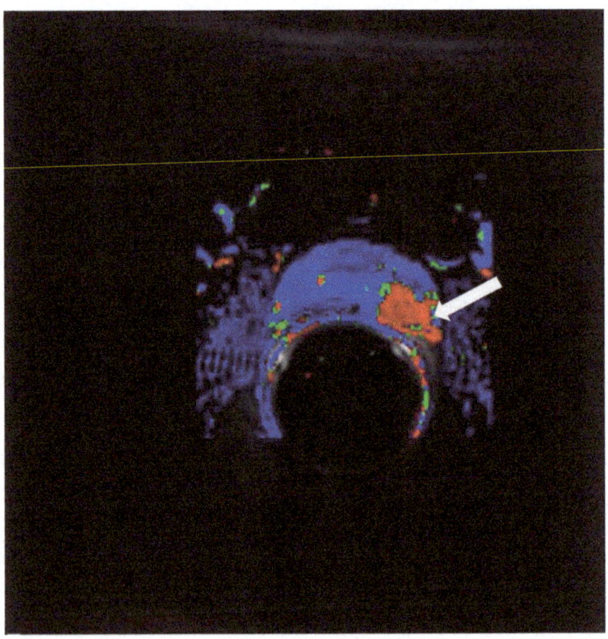

Fig. 7.9 Color perfusion maps obtained from DCE MRI shows rapid wash-out in the lesion (*red*)

The normal peripheral zone displays a relatively high signal on T2 images owing to fluid filled ducal and acinar components. This has the advantage of providing excellent contrast resolution for detection of the T2 hypointense tumours.

Carcinoma appears uniformly low in T2 signal compared to bright surrounding PZ. Hence T2 images are useful for initial localization of the abnormality. But given the myriad mimics of carcinoma, multiparametric imaging is used for further characterization.

Carcinoma usually (in addition to a low T2 signal) demonstrates ill defined margins, low ADC values and rapid wash-out of contrast on DCE scans. They also show raised choline peaks on MRS. Once each of these features are present, the diagnosis can be made with reasonable certainty.

The normal gland capsule is a low signal intensity rim (of about 1 mm thickness) surrounding the gland. Breach of this margin constitutes ECE, this upstages the tumor from one that is localized to the prostate (T2) to one that is locally advanced (T3), in addition to conferring a poorer prognosis. Extracapsular extension is common and exquisitely demonstrated by high resolution t2 images. The primary imaging signs of ECE are:

(a) Asymmetric capsular bulge with irregular margins
(b) Obliteration of normal recto-prostatic angle
(c) Asymmetry or non visualization of the neurovascular bundle
(d) Encasement of the neurovascular bundle
(e) Seminal vesicle invasion.

The implications of detecting ECE on MRI are myriad. Patients with ECE have a higher rate of local recurrence, invasion of neurovascular bundles may alter surgical approach. Some patients may refuse surgery given that it may not be possible to salvage the neurovascular bundles.

Pitfalls

- Post biopsy haemorrhage may appear as a low T2 signal focus, a prior history of biopsy coupled with a hyperintense focus on T1 images avoids an erroneous diagnosis.
- Benign nodule in PZ – usually shows a well defined border, rarely reaches capsule and shows bilateral symmetric wash-out kinetics. The T2 signal of these nodules matches that of the central gland.
- Displaced central zone – may mimic a PZ cancer when it gets displaced by a hypertrophied TZ, it is also of low T2 signal. Typical location at base of prostate and bilateral symmetry help differentiate this entity from malignancy.
- Post radiation changes – result in fibrosis and uniformly low t2 signal in the gland, hence t2 imaging cannot be relied upon. Radiation changes however do not display restricted diffusion, rapid wash-out or elevated choline as malignancies do.
- Pseudolesion in midline of PZ – a focus of low T2 signal and low ADC can often be found in the midline, it is thought to be the point of fusion of the prostatic capsule with the adjacent fascia. Lack of rapid enhancement, concave contour and midline location should aid in differentiation from its sinister counterpart.

Teaching Point

- Carcinoma appears as an ill defined lesion of low T2 signal in a normally hyperintense PZ.
- Detection of ECE, neurovascular invasion and seminal vehicle invasion are essential as they significantly alter patient management and confer a poor prognosis.

Seminal Vesicle and Vas deferens

Case 7.5

Brief Case Summary: 24 year old male with abdominal pain

Imaging Findings CT scan of the abdomen and pelvis without intravenous contrast demonstrates an absent left seminal vesicle. A normal right seminal vesicle is noted (Fig. 7.10, arrow).

Differential Diagnosis Seminal vesicle agenesis, seminal vesicle hypoplasia

Diagnosis and Discussion Seminal vesicle agenesis (in patient with cystic fibrosis).

Seminal vesicle agenesis can occur in two distinct settings. The first setting involves an embryological insult to the mesonephric duct while the second is seen in the setting of mutations involving the cystic fibrosis transmembrane conductance regulator gene (CFTR). Both settings may have corresponding abnormalities of the vas deferens (typically agenesis), with associated renal abnormalities only seen with the former, particularly if the insult takes place before ureteral budding (which occurs at approximately 7 weeks gestation). Seminal vesicle agenesis associated with mutations of the CFTR is thought to occur secondary to intraluminal obstruction by thick and tenacious secretions.

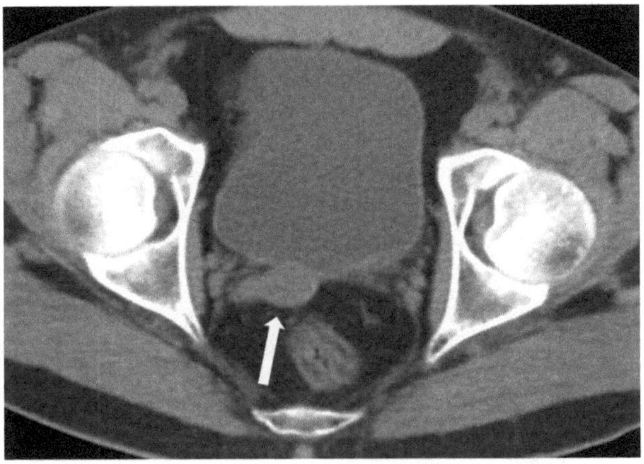

Fig. 7.10 CT scan of the abdomen and pelvis without intravenous contrast demonstrates an absent left seminal vesicle. A normal right seminal vesicle is noted (arrow)

Asymptomatic patients require no treatment. Symptomatic patients typically complain of infertility. On occasion, an ectopic vas deferens may insert into a Mullerian duct remnant resulting in cystic dilatation leading to pain, hematospermia and/or epididymitis. A variety of surgical options may be considered for symptomatic patients including vasoepididymostomy and transuretheral resection of the ejaculatory duct.

Pitfalls Absence of the seminal vesicle is diagnostic for seminal vesicle agenesis. A small seminal vesicle with fewer septa suggests the presence of seminal vesicle hypoplasia, though no diagnostic criteria have been established.

Teaching Points

1. Absence of the seminal vesicle should prompt an evaluation for associated upper urinary tract abnormalities and/or evidence for cystic fibrosis.
2. Absence of the ipsilateral kidney suggests an embryological insult before 7 weeks gestation.
3. The most common symptom is infertility for which a variety of surgical options may be considered.

Case 7.6

Brief Case Summary 42 year old male with abdominal pain

Imaging Findings CT scan of the abdomen and pelvis with intravenous contrast demonstrates an off-midline oval fluid-attenuation mass posterior to the bladder (asterisk, Fig. 7.11). Note is made of an absent right kidney (Fig. 7.12).

Differential Diagnosis Bladder diverticulum, seminal vesicle cyst, cyst of the vas deferens, prostatic utricle cyst, tortuous hydroureter.

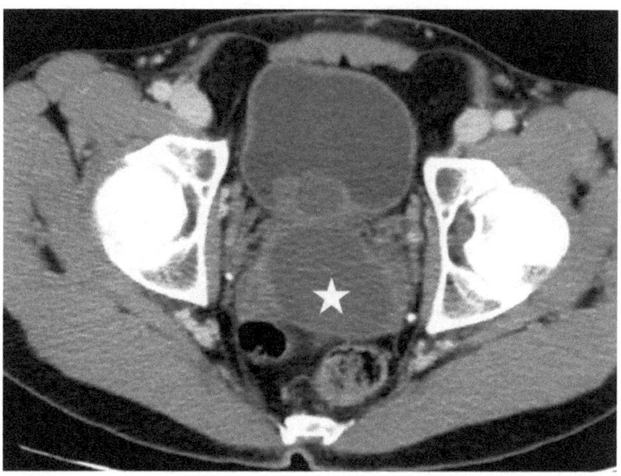

Fig. 7.11 CT scan of the abdomen and pelvis with intravenous contrast demonstrates an off-midline oval fluid-attenuation mass posterior to the bladder (*asterisk*)

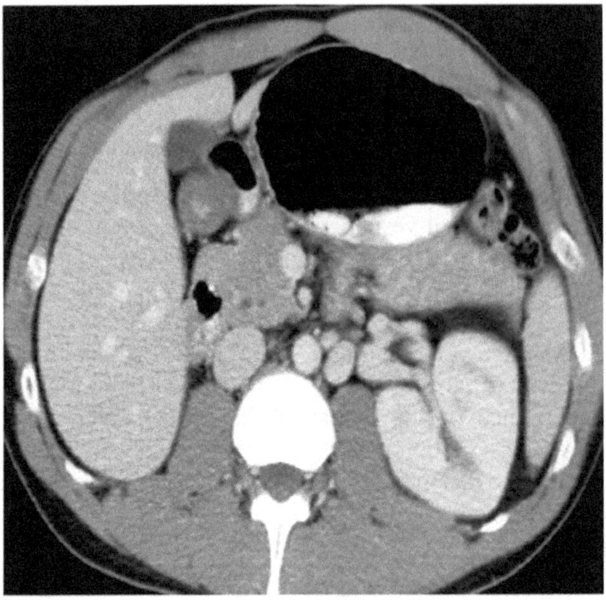

Fig. 7.12 Axial CT demonstrates an absent right kidney

Diagnosis and Discussion Seminal vesicle cyst (with agenesis of the right kidney).

Cysts of the seminal vesicle may congenital or acquired. They are usually discovered between the second and third decades of life and may be related to the onset of sexual activity. Congenital cysts may be isolated findings or may be associated with upper urinary tract abnormalities (such as renal agenesis) or autosomal dominant polycystic kidney disease (particularly with the presence of bilateral cysts). Clinical presentation is variable, ranging from incidental lesions in asymptomatic patients, to pelvic discomfort, recurrent infections (prostatitis, urinary tract infection and/or epididymitis) as well as hematospermia.

CT imaging demonstrates the presence of a well-defined fluid density retrovesicular mass arising in the expected region of the seminal vesicle, above the level of the prostate gland. The majority of the lesion is less than 5 cm in maximal diameter. Seminal vesicle cysts have variable signal intensity on T1 weighted MR images (due to the presence of hemorrhagic and/or proteinacious debris) but typically demonstrate high signal on T2 weighted imaging. No enhancing components are observed after the administration of contrast medium. Sonography demonstrates the presence of a cystic mass, although minimal complexity may be observed due to intraluminal debris.

Asymptomatic lesions require no diagnostic or therapeutic intervention. Excision may be performed for symptomatic lesions, particularly if they present with bowel or bladder obstruction.

Pitfalls There are a number of cystic masses that may arise in a similar location, which can be potentially differentiated by their location and relationship to adjacent structures. Intraprostatic cysts include utricle and Mullerian duct cysts (both of which are midline) as well as ejaculatory duct cysts (off-midline or paramedian) and prostatic retention cysts (lateral location). Extraprostatic cysts include cysts of the vas deferens and Cowper duct cysts, with the latter occurring at the level of the posterior urethra. Bladder diverticulae demonstrate a connection to the bladder lumen while multiplanar imaging can allow differentiation of seminal vesicle cysts from a tortuous hydroureter.

Teaching Points

1. Seminal vesicle cysts are benign findings that are often asymptomatic for which no diagnostic or therapeutic intervention is needed. Excision may be considered if symptoms are present, particularly with the presence of bladder outlet obstruction.
2. Seminal vesicle cysts are commonly associated with upper urinary tract abnormalities such as renal agenesis. The presence of bilateral seminal vesicle cysts should prompt an evaluation for underlying autosomal dominant polycystic kidney disease.
3. There are a number of potential mimickers of this lesion in the pelvis. Categorizing lesions first by their relationship to the prostate gland (intra or extraprostatic) and then their location with respect to the midline (median, paramedian and lateral) allows for an algorithmic approach to the radiologic interpretation.

Case 7.7

Brief Case Summary: 77 year old male with abdominal pain.

Imaging Findings Frontal radiograph of the pelvis demonstrates bilateral, symmetric, and tubular calcifications (Fig. 7.13).

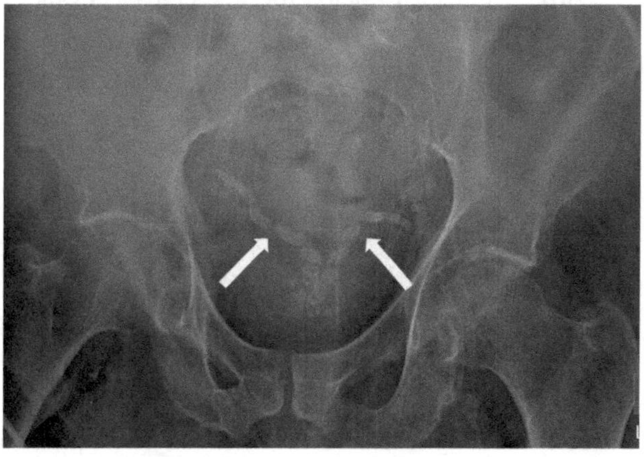

Fig. 7.13 Frontal radiograph of the pelvis demonstrates bilateral, symmetric, and tubular calcifications

Differential Diagnosis Vas deferens calcifications, bladder calculi, calcified pelvic neoplasm, phleboliths.

Diagnosis and Discussion: Vas deferens calcifications

Vas deferens calcifications are benign findings, most often seen in diabetic patients. Other reported associations include secondary hyperparathyroidism as well as chronic infections such as tuberculosis or schistosomiasis. Idiopathic cases are exceedingly rare.

Imaging finding are fairly characteristic with calcifications seen lining the wall of the vas deferens, often bilateral and symmetric. Chronic inflammation from tuberculosis may lead to the deposition of intraluminal or intramural calcifications. As opposed to the more common diabetes related calcifications, findings in tuberculosis tend to be unilateral and segmental in distribution.

Unless there is a strong clinical suspicion for tuberculosis or other inflammatory conditions, no treatment is required. In all other cases, the presence of seminal vesicle calcifications gives insight into concurrent endocrine or metabolic derangements that the patient may have.

Pitfalls Seminal vesicle calcifications have a characteristic pattern allowing for easy differentiation from other causes of pelvic calcifications. A phlebolith is a small calcification found within a vein. On radiographs they often demonstrate a radiolucent center (distinguishing them from ureteral stones) and CT imaging may demonstrate the "comet tail" sign, representing the parent vein.

Teaching Point

1. Seminal vesicle calcifications are benign findings with a characteristic imaging appearance, most often seen in patients with diabetes.
2. Other uncommon causes include secondary hyperparathyroidism as well as tuberculosis. Calcifications associated with chronic inflammation tend to unilateral and segmental.
3. The presence of seminal vesicle calcifications gives insight into concurrent endocrine or metabolic derangements that the patient may have. Unless there is a strong clinical suspicion for tuberculosis or other inflammatory conditions, no treatment is required.

Case 7.8

Brief Case Summary None.

Imaging Findings Axial T2 (Fig. 7.14) and T1 without (Fig. 7.15) and with gadolinium (Fig. 7.16) images show enlargement and thickening of the left seminal vesicles (arrows) with associated enhancement.

Differential Diagnosis Invasion from adjacent prostatic or rectal carcinoma

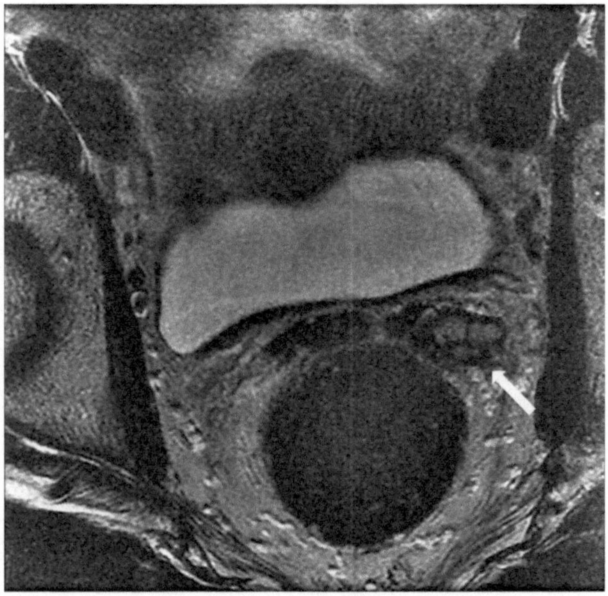

Fig. 7.14 Axial T2 image shows enlargement and thickening of the left seminal vesicles (*arrows*)

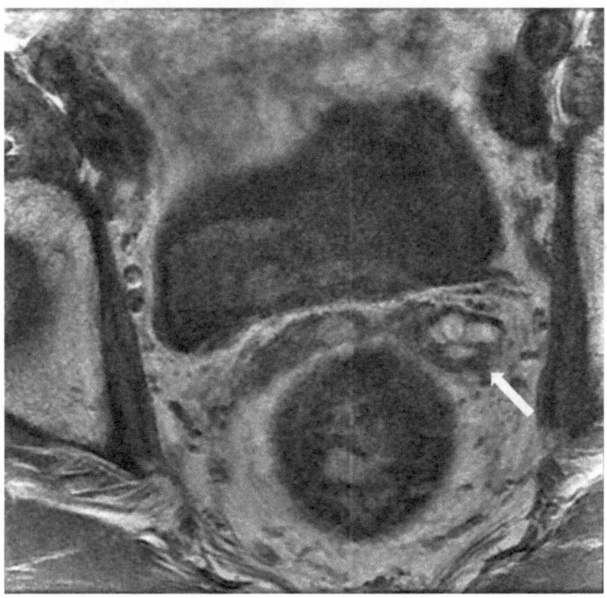

Fig. 7.15 Axial T1, without gadolinium, image shows enlargement and thickening of the left seminal vesicles (*arrows*)

Diagnosis and Discussion Seminal vesicle amyloidosis

Seminal vesicle amyloidosis is a common finding seen on autopsy and is related to aging. The incidence increases with age and is about 21 % in patients above 75 years of age. It may occur as a localized finding or may be associated with systemic amyloidosis, the former being more common. When localized, this condition is

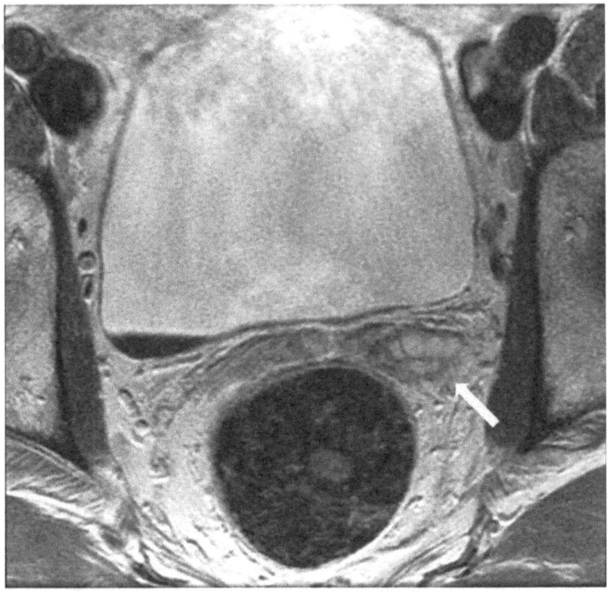

Fig. 7.16 Axial T1, with gadolinium, image shows enlargement and thickening of the left seminal vesicles (*arrows*) with associated enhancement

bilaterally symmetrical with subepithelial amyloid deposits in lamina propria. When related to systemic amyloidosis, the amyloid deposits are seen in blood vessel walls or in muscles.

Patients are generally asymptomatic but rare symptoms include hematospermia and enlargement of seminal vesicles.

Ultrasound may show enlargement of the seminal vesicles. Focal lesions, seen as hypoechoic foci are otherwise indistinguishable from other seminal vesicle masses. CT shows focal or diffuse bilateral enlargement of the gland but is limited in assessing the internal architecture. MRI shows diffuse wall thickening of the seminal vesicle. The amyloid foci are seen as hypointense deposits on T2 and there may be associated areas of hemorrhage which appear hyperintense on T1. The imaging features may simulate tumor deposits, however, contrast enhanced MRI may be able to differentiate the two entities by showing enhancement in latter.

Pitfalls Seminal vesicle amyloidosis is easily confused with primary tumor or tumor invasion from adjacent structures and has been seen to be responsible for upstaging of various adjacent tumors. Normal PSA levels will exclude the possibility of extension of prostatic carcinoma into seminal vesicles. But even in high PSA levels, a diagnosis of amyloidosis cannot be ruled out as it is frequently seen coexisting with prostate and bladder cancer. Though imaging may help ascertain the origin of focal lesion to some extent, the definitive diagnosis is made on histopathological studies.

Teaching Point Due to the considerable overlap between imaging features of seminal vesicle amyloidosis and of primary tumor/tumor invasion into the gland, TRUS guided biopsy should be considered in all masses involving the seminal vesicles wherein there is uncertainty about the origin and nature of mass.

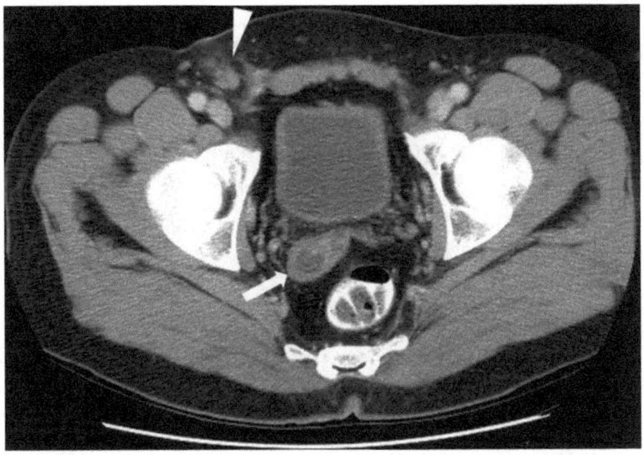

Fig. 7.17 Axial CT scan demonstrates a focal lesion in the right seminal vesicle with central hypodensity (*arrow*) and right inguinal lymph nodes with surrounding fat stranding in the right inguinal area (*arrowhead*). Biopsy of the right inguinal lymph node revealed metastasis from the testicular primary

Case 7.9

Brief Case Summary 34-year-old man with history of seminoma status post right orchiectomy.

Imaging Findings Axial CT scan (Fig. 7.17) demonstrates a focal lesion in the right seminal vesicle with central hypodensity (arrow) and right inguinal lymph nodes with surrounding fat stranding in the right inguinal area (arrowhead). Biopsy of the right inguinal lymph node revealed metastasis from the testicular primary.

Differential Diagnosis Infiltrating carcinoma from adjacent organs like prostate, rectum and urinary bladder; seminal vesicle amyloidosis

Diagnosis and Discussion Seminal Vesicle Neoplasms

Primary tumors of seminal vesicles are an extremely rare entity and metastasis are commoner than primary tumors. Reported benign tumors include cystadenoma, papillary adenoma, leiomyoma, epithelial stromal tumors, neurilemmoma and teratoma. Malignant tumors include adenocarcinoma (most common), leiomyosarcoma, angiosarcoma, mullerian adeosarcoma like tumor, carcinoid, seminoma and cystosarcoma phylloides. There is no specific age limit with cases occurring in patients ranging from 19 to 90 years of age.

Clinical symptoms vary and can include hematuria, hemospermia, dysuria, difficult defecation and general pelvic pain.

Diagnosing seminal vesicle neoplasms is difficult as it may simulate a mass arising from adjacent pelvic structures such as the rectum, bladder and prostate with infiltration into the seminal vesicles. Tumor markers including prostatic specific antigen (PSA), prostatic acid phosphatase (PAP) and carcinogenic embryonic antigen (CEA) should be negative and can help exclude colorectal and prostatic tumors. Recently CA-125 and cytokeratin 7 positivity have been reported to assist in diagnosis with the former being used to assess response to therapy.

Dalgaard and Giertson proposed the following criteria for primary adenocarcinoma of the seminal vesicles:

(a) The tumor should be a microscopically verified carcinoma, localized exclusively or mainly to the seminal vesicle.
(b) The presence of other simultaneous primary carcinoma should be excluded.
(c) The tumor should preferably resemble the architecture of the non-neoplastic seminal vesicle.

Diagnosis is based on clinical, radiological, and histological findings. On imaging, seminal vesicle masses are seen either as retrovesical masses with or without prostatic or urethral obstruction or as infiltrating seminal vesicle lesions with an enhancement pattern similar to advanced prostatic carcinoma.

Rectal ultrasound helps localize the tumor with the added benefit of obtaining biopsy specimens. On US, a cystadenoma may appear as a unilateral multiseptate cystic mass in a characteristic retrovesical location. Solid focal masses may appear mildly echogenic as compared to the rest of the normal parenchyma. Metastasis to seminal vesicles is seen as nonspecific soft tissue masses.

Cross sectional imaging with CT and MRI, in addition to localizing the tumor, also allows for exclusion of carcinoma of adjacent organs in early stages by demonstrating the epicenter of the mass. Also, CT and MR can accurate characterize lesions such as a teratoma which contains cystic and fatty components which can be readily characterized on both CT and MR. Primary adenocarcinoma of the seminal vesicles manifest as solid heterogeneous masses of intermediate signal intensity on T1 and hyperintense on T2. Few helpful imaging features point towards invasion of seminal vesicle rather than a primary tumor including obliteration of the angle between the seminal vesicle and prostate gland and loss of internal architecture of the gland. Rarely the only imaging features visualized may be focal enlargement or wall thickening of seminal vesicles. Metastasis to seminal vesicles are also seen as focal enlargement of the gland or as nonspecific a T2 hypointense soft tissue mass which cannot be differentiated from hemorrhage or radiation changes or senile amyloidosis and thus require a biopsy for definitive diagnosis.

Pitfalls Primary tumors of seminal vesicle are difficult to differentiate from carcinoma originating in adjacent structures with secondary involvement of the seminal vesicles based only on imaging. Tumors of seminal vesicle origin are PSA, PAP and CEA negative whereas these markers are positive in prostatic and colorectal cancers. Primary tumors of seminal vesicle may show cytokeratin 7 and CA-125 positivity which is generally not seen in prostatic, bladder and rectal carcinomas. CK 20 positivity, seen in most rectal tumors, is not a feature of seminal vesicle tumor. A fair degree of overlap and inconsistencies in tumor markers may however still be seen. Poorly differentiated adenocarcinoma of seminal vesicle may be indistinguishable from poorly differentiated prostate carcinoma and certain adenocarcinomas of urinary bladder.

The distinction from amyloidosis cannot be made on imaging alone in cases of localized masses and thus requires biopsy.

Teaching Points Tumors of seminal vesicle are extremely rare with only about 50 cases reported in literature.

Immunohistochemistry may help in an otherwise difficult diagnostic dilemma with certain negative parameters helping in distinguishing carcinomas from adjacent structures.

Testis

Case 7.10

Brief Case Summary 38 year old male with absent left testicle on physical exam.

Imaging Findings Gray scale transverse midline image of the scrotum demonstrates a normal right testicle (arrow, Fig. 7.18) with absence of the left testicle. Gray scale and color Doppler images of the left inguinal canal demonstrate the presence of an ovoid hypoechoic structure with internal vascularity, compatible with an undescended testicle (arrow, Figs. 7.19 and 7.20).

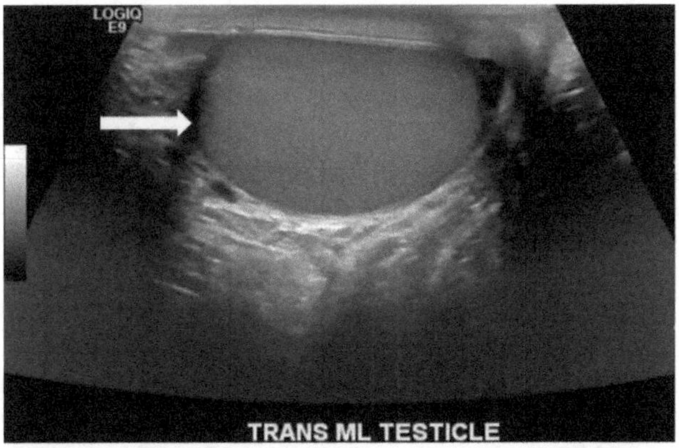

Fig. 7.18 Gray scale transverse midline image of the scrotum demonstrates a normal right testicle (*arrow*) with absence of the left testicle

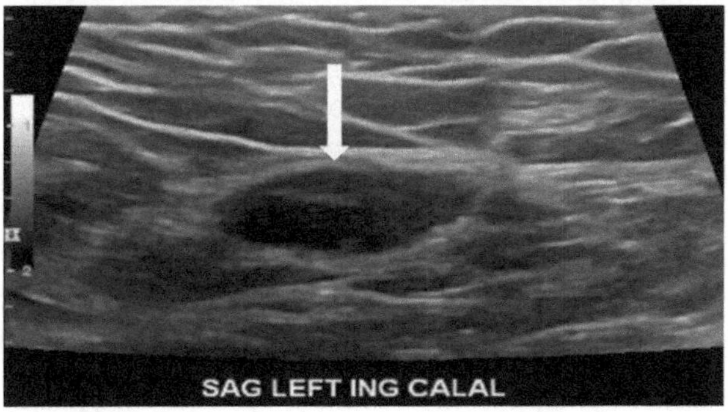

Fig. 7.19 Gray scale image of the left inguinal canal demonstrate the presence of an ovoid hypoechoic structure with internal vascularity, compatible with an undescended testicle (*arrow*)

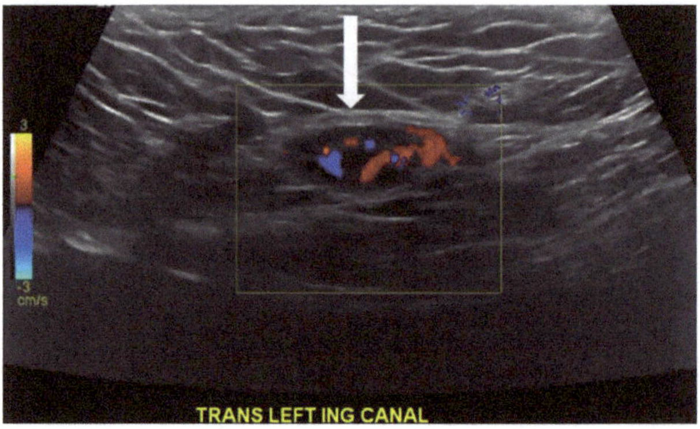

Fig. 7.20 Color Doppler image of the left inguinal canal demonstrate the presence of an ovoid hypoechoic structure with internal vascularity, compatible with an undescended testicle (*arrow*)

Differential Diagnosis Left sided cryptorchidism, left inguinal canal lymph node

Diagnosis and Discussion Left sided cryptorchidism

Cryptorchidism refers to an absence of testes within the scrotum which may be related to an absent testicle from agenesis or atrophy or may be related to failure of embryological descent from an intra-abdominal location. In addition, the terms retractile testes and ascending testes have been coined to refer to entities in which the normal testicle has been either pulled cephalad by the cremesteric reflex but remains reducible (retractile) or has ascended after a normal location in childhood without the ability to reduce into the scrotum (ascending).

Undescended testicles has higher incidence in premature infants and is most often unilateral with a predilection for the right side in approximately 70 % of cases. The etiology is likely multifactorial, although the most common cause is thought to be a defect in prenatal androgen secretion. The final diagnosis should not be made until at least 6 months of age as a small percentage of patients demonstrate gradual testicular descent during the first few months of life.

Imaging may be useful in locating the undescended testicle, though many feel that imaging studies should be bypassed in lieu of laparoscopic or inguinal exploration due to insufficient sensitivity. The most common location is within 2 cm of the internal inguinal ring. On ultrasound, the undescended testicle manifests as a round or oval hypoechoic structure between 7 and 15 mm in diameter. The detection of the mediastinum testis allows specific characterization of the mass as an undescended testicle. CT imaging has limited use in the evaluation of cryptorchidism and may demonstrate the presence of the spermatic cord leading to a mass in the inguinal canal. Despite the improved soft tissue contrast, MR imaging also has a limited role, with non-specific characteristics with the undescended testicle manifesting as an enhancing T1 hypointense mass with variable hyperintense T2 signal depending on the degree of atrophy.

Cryptorchidism is associated with infertility and a 4–7 fold increase in the risk for testicular cancer, with seminoma being the most common tumor. Other complications include an increased risk of torsion, trauma and inguinal hernia. Surgical treatment is the mainstay of therapy with orchiopexy as the treatment of choice for viable testes. If the testicle is non-viable, an orchiectomy is performed. Ascending testes are treated with orchiopexy while retractile testes require close clinical follow up.

Pitfalls Lymph nodes may be impossible to differentiate from an atrophic testicle, though detection of the mediastinum testes confers more specificity. Overall, imaging plays a limited role, particularly in the setting of a non-palpable testicle. Laparoscopic or inguinal exploration is often the diagnostic and subsequent therapeutic treatment of choice.

Teaching Points

1. Cryptorchidism refers to the absence of testes within the scrotum, one cause of which may be an undescended testicle. The most common location is within 2 cm of the internal inguinal ring.
2. The role of imaging is limited in the evaluation of the undescended testicle, with laparoscopic or inguinal exploration usually preferred. US is the imaging modality of choice with the demonstration of the mediastinum testes specific for testicular tissue.
3. Patients with undescended testicles are at an increased risk for infertility and neoplasm. Surgical treatment is the mainstay of therapy with orchiopexy as the treatment of choice for viable testes. If the testicle is non-viable, an orchiectomy is performed.

Case 7.11

Brief Case Summary A 70 year old male with right sided testicular pain.

Imaging Findings Gray scale image of the scrotum demonstrates an abnormal appearance of the right testicular parenchyma which is hypoechic (asterisk, Fig. 7.21a) with respect to the normal appearing left testicle (hollow asterisk, Fig. 7.21a). Color Doppler image demonstrates the presence of increased flow in the right testicle (Fig. 7.21b). Gray scale and color Doppler interrogation of the right epididymis demonstrates the presence of a heterogeneous and hypoechoic epididymis (arrow, Fig. 7.21c) with the presence of increased flow (arrow, Fig. 7.21d).

Differential Diagnosis Testicular torsion, orchitis, seminoma

Diagnosis and Discussion Epididymo-orchitis

Epididymitis is the most common cause of acute scrotal pain in adolescents and men over the age of 35 years. The pathophysiology typically involves inflammation related to an ascending infection from the prostatic urethra and/or seminal vesicles, through hematogenous spread of infection has been reported. Spread to the testicle is commonly seen (referred to as epididymo-orchitis) occurring in 20–40 % of patients with epididymitis. The causative organism is typically bacterial with

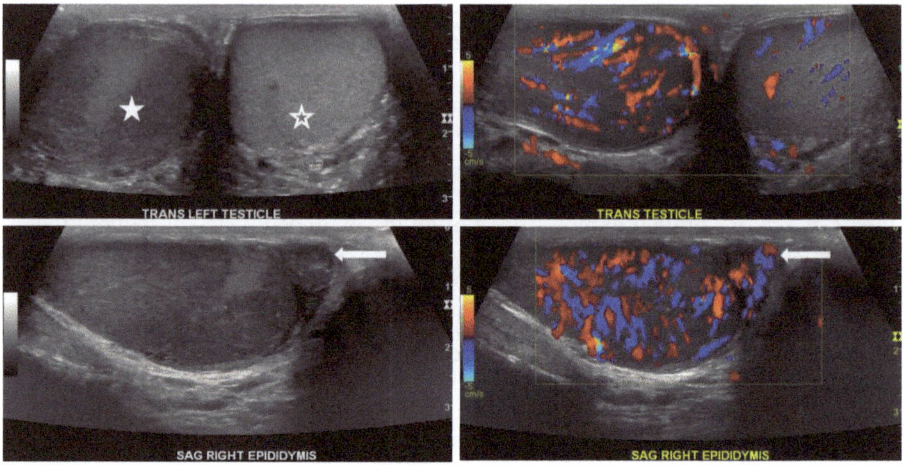

Fig. 7.21 Gray scale image of the scrotum demonstrates an abnormal appearance of the right testicular parenchyma which is hypoechoic (*asterisk*, **a**) with respect to the normal appearing left testicle (*hollow asterisk*, **a**). (**b**) Color Doppler image demonstrates the presence of increased flow in the right testicle. Gray scale and color Doppler interrogation of the right epididymis demonstrates the presence of a heterogeneous and hypoechoic epididymis (*arrow*, **c**) with the presence of increased flow (*arrow*, **d**)

Neisseria gonorrhea and *Chlamydia trachomatis* occurring in sexually active males and *Escherichia coli* affecting young boys and elderly males. Cryptococcosis, tuberculosis and parasitic infections are infrequent etiologies. Non-infectious etiologies include sarcoidosis, Behcets disease and medications (such as amiodarone), though these are exceedingly rare. Patients typically present with fever and scrotal pain.

Ultrasound is the imaging modality of choice, commonly demonstrating the presence of an enlarged, heterogeneous but predominately hypoechoic epididymis. The retrograde transmission of infection from the urinary tract results in initial involvement of the tail prior to the body and head of the epididymis. Spread to the testicle demonstrates similar findings on gray scale imaging. A reactive hydrocele is often present. Color evaluation demonstrates diffuse hyperemia of the inflamed tissue. If left untreated, epididymo-orchitis may be complicated by a pyocele or testicular abscess which manifests as an avascular hypo to anechoic mass with increased peripheral flow on color imaging.

Prognosis for both epididymitis and epididymo-orchitis is generally good, with most cases resolving with antibiotic therapy alone. The presence of an abscess may require surgical drainage.

Pitfalls Epididymo-orchitis needs to be differentiated from testicular torsion as the latter requires prompt surgical treatment. On imaging testicular torsion demonstrates no flow, while hyperemia is present with epididymo-orchitis. Cases of torsion-detorsion may present with increased flow, although patients are typically pain free at the time of detorsion as opposed to epididymo-orchitis where the hyperemic testicle is associated with persistent scrotal pain. Isolated orchitis without involvement of the epididymis is not common, though can be seen in the clinical setting of mumps or HIV infection. On imaging, testicular neoplasms may present as vascular regions of decreased echogenicity, although clinically, they typically present as a painless, palpable mass.

Teaching Points

1. Epididymitis is a common cause of testicular pain. In up to 40 % of patients the testicle may also be involved (epididymo-orchitis). Both conditions are conservatively managed with antibiotics and the presence of an abscess may require drainage.
2. Retrograde transmission of a bacterial urinary tract infection is the most common cause. *Neisseria gonorrhea* and *Chlamydia trachomatis* are common organisms in sexually active males, while *Escherichia coli* is seen in young boys and elderly males.
3. Sonography is the imaging modality of choice with findings demonstrating the presence of a heterogeneous, but predominately hypoechoic epididymis (and testicle in cases of epididymo-orchitis) associated with hyperemia.
4. Torsion-detorsion or a testicular neoplasm may have a similar imaging appearance though patients are pain free at the time of hyperemia in the case of the former, while neoplasms typically present as a painless, palpable mass.

Case 7.12

Brief Case Summary 62 year old male with right testicular pain.

Imaging Findings Ultrasound shows hypoechoic collection (arrow, Fig. 7.22) in the right scrotum inferior to the testis with scrotal thickening and hyperemia (Fig. 7.23) which could represent an abscess.

Differential Diagnosis Epididymo-ochitis, intratesticular/epididymal simple cysts, intratesticular spermatocele, tubular ectasia, epidermoid cyst, tunica albuginea cyst, intratesticular varicocele.

Diagnosis and Discussion Testicular or epididymal abscess is an uncommon manifestation of severe or untreated epididymoorchitis and hence occurs typically in sexually active young adults. Rare causes include secondary bacterial infection of a hematoma or an intratesticular infarct.

The causative organisms are either sexually transmitted from *Neisseria gonorrhea*, *Chlamydia trachomatis* or from other sources like the urinary tract from *Enterococcus spp.*, coliforms. Tuberculous etiology can be considered in endemic countries.

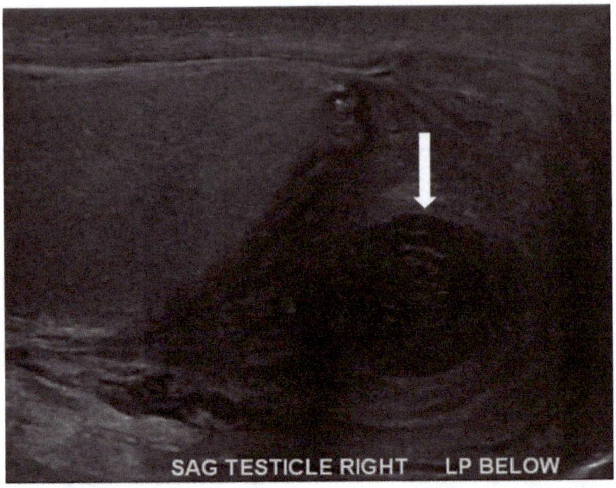

Fig. 7.22 Ultrasound shows hypoechoic collection (*arrow*) in the right scrotum inferior to the testis

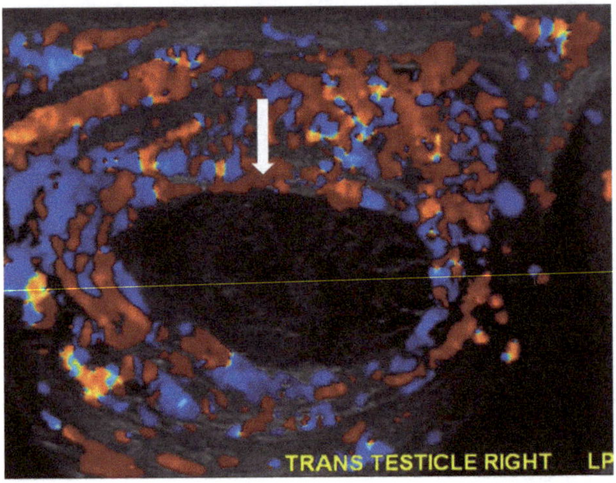

Fig. 7.23 Image shows scrotal thickening and hyperemia, which could represent an abscess

The patient presents with pain and swelling of the involved testis, with fever, often lasting for days. Tuberculous abscesses can be indolent. Examination may reveal a red, enlarged and tender hemiscrotum.

Grayscale and Doppler ultrasound is often the first and last modality to confirm the diagnosis. The abscess itself may be identified as are secondary findings including scrotal thickening and hyperemia. The abscess may be hypoechoic and well defined or an area of heterogeneously altered echotexture in the evolving stage. The abscess is avascular and can be intratesticular or epididymal. The surrounding inflammation or typical imaging signs of epididymo-orchitis including surrounding zone of increased vascularity, diffusely altered echotexture with increased vascularity in the testis and the epididymis, hydrocele/ pyocele and scrotal wall edema help to differentiate this lesion from its differential diagnoses.

CT or MRI do not have a role in the contemporary management of acute scrotum. In a rare instance of a complex abscess with perineal or pelvic extension, MRI may be useful for treatment planning. On MRI, the liquefied portion is hyperintense on T2 and hypointense on T1 with avid enhancement of the surrounding tissues and restricted diffusion.

The presence of long-term scrotal swelling without tenderness and a lower degree of blood flow in the peripheral portion of a large abscess are suggestive of tuberculous abscess.

Treatment of testicular/ epididymal abscess consists of appropriate antibiotics alone or with surgical drainage if necessary. Uncommonly, severe cases may necessitate orchiectomy. If medically managed, the abscess can be followed up on ultrasound for resolution.

Pitfalls An evolving abscess can be difficult to differentiate from isolated epididymo-ochitis. Absence of vascularity in the index area may provide a clue; a follow up ultrasound may be performed in case of a doubt.

Teaching Points

1. Testicular or epididymal abscess is usually a complication of severe or untreated epididymoorchitis.
2. Ultrasound is the diagnostic modality of choice. MRI is used for treatment planning in a complex abscess or as a problem solving tool.
3. A focal avascular zone of hypo or heterogeneous echogenicity with surrounding zone of increased vascularity is the hallmark.

Case 7.13

Brief Case Summary: 24 year old male status post scrotal trauma.

Imaging Findings Color transverse midline images demonstrate the presence of a left sided hydrocele (asterisk, Fig. 7.24). Transverse and sagittal gray scale images of the left demonstrate the presence of a hypoechoic line traversing the left testicular parenchyma (arrow, Fig. 7.25) with extrusion of portions of the left testicle (arrow, Fig. 7.26) through a defect in the tunica albuginea.

Differential Diagnosis Testicular fracture with associated rupture, testicular torsion, seminoma, segmental testicular infarct.

Diagnosis and Discussion: Testicular fracture with associated rupture

Traumatic injuries to the scrotum may result from both blunt and penetrating trauma, with the latter often going to the operating room without an antecedent imaging study. Patients are typically young, ranging from 10 to 30 years of age and the right testicle is more often injured than the left. The spectrum of imaging

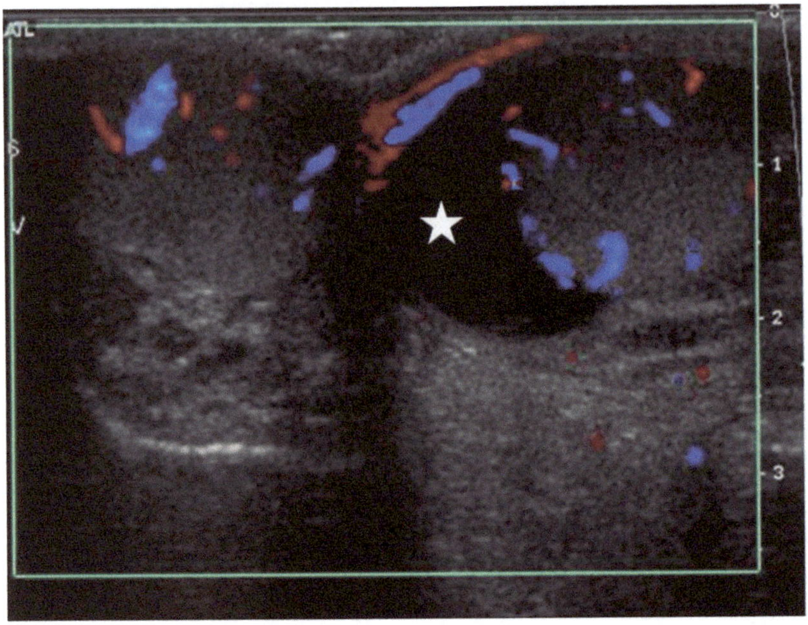

Fig. 7.24 Color transverse midline images demonstrate the presence of a left sided hydrocele (*asterisk*)

Fig. 7.25 Transverse gray scale image of the left demonstrate the presence of a hypoechoic line traversing the left testicular parenchyma (*arrow*)

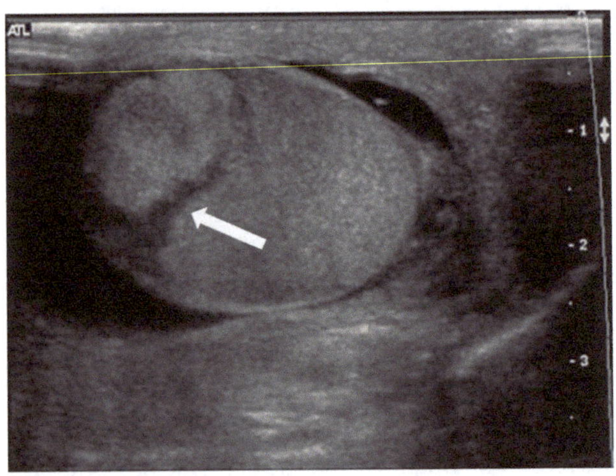

findings includes hydroceles, hematoceles, intratesticular hematomas, testicular fracture or testicular rupture.

Ultrasonography is the imaging study of choice. Hydroceles and hematoceles manifest as avascular, extratesticular hypoechoic collections of variable complexity depending on the presence of underlying fibrin strands or blood products. A fluid-fluid level may be occasionally observed in hematoceles. Intratesticular hematomas

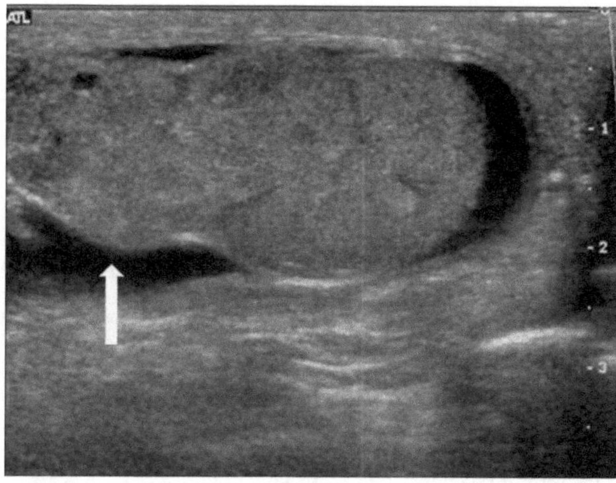

Fig. 7.26 Sagittal gray scale image of the left demonstrate the presence of a hypoechoic line traversing the left testicular parenchyma, with extrusion of portions of the left testicle (*arrow*) through a defect in the tunica albuginea

manifest as an avascular mass of variable echogenicity – hyperechoic to the adjacent parenchyma in acute hematoma and hypo to anechoic in chronic hematoma. Testicular fractures manifest as a linear, avascular, hypoechoic line traversing the testicular parenchyma, though the fracture line may be difficult to visualize. Fractures may or may not be associated with rupture. Testicular rupture is suggested with the presence of a heterogeneous testicular echotexture with associated contour abnormality. Further findings of a disrupted tunica albuginea confer increased specificity. MR imaging may be obtained in equivocal cases of testicular rupture, where imaging findings demonstrate a break in the normal low intensity signal tunica albuginea. Intratesticular hematomas will demonstrate no enhancement and will have characteristic signal findings related to the stage of hemoglobin breakdown.

Testicular rupture, as well as fractures associated with loss of testicular perfusion, requires emergent surgery. Large intratesticular hematomas and hematoceles may also warrant surgical exploration.

Pitfalls In the setting of a conservatively managed intratesticular hematoma, follow-up sonographic imaging is important to ensure resolution to exclude the presence of an underlying neoplasm and to exclude the presence of subsequent infection or necrosis.

Teaching Points

1. Heterogeneous testicular parenchymal echotexture associated with an irregular contour abnormality and a disrupted tunica albuginea are findings indicative of testicular rupture.
2. Testicular rupture and testicular fracture with the loss of perfusion to the testicle require emergent surgical repair. Large intratesticular hematomas and hematoceles may also warrant surgical exploration.
3. A conservatively managed intratesticular hematoma requires sonographic follow-up to resolution to exclude the possibility of an underling neoplasm.

Case 7.14

Brief Case Summary: 20 year old male with 48 h of left testicular pain

Imaging Findings Gray scale image of the scrotum demonstrates an abnormal appearance to the left testicular parenchyma, which is hypoechoic and slightly more heterogeneous when compared to the right testicle (asterisk, Fig. 7.27). No vascular flow is demonstrated on color and power Doppler interrogation (Figs. 7.28 and 7.29).

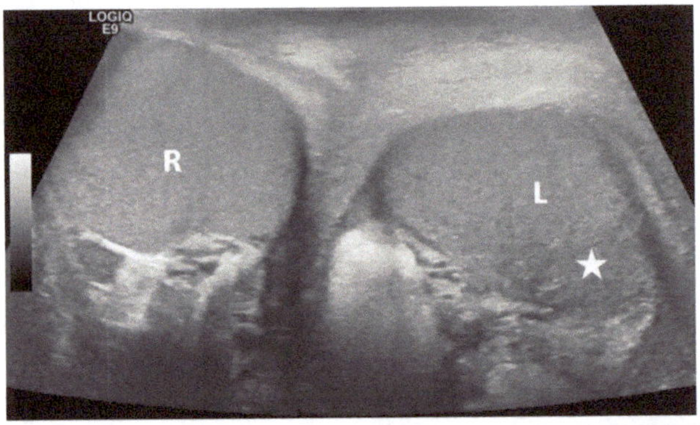

Fig. 7.27 Gray scale image of the scrotum demonstrates an abnormal appearance to the left testicular parenchyma, which is hypoechoic and slightly more heterogeneous when compared to the right testicle (*asterisk*)

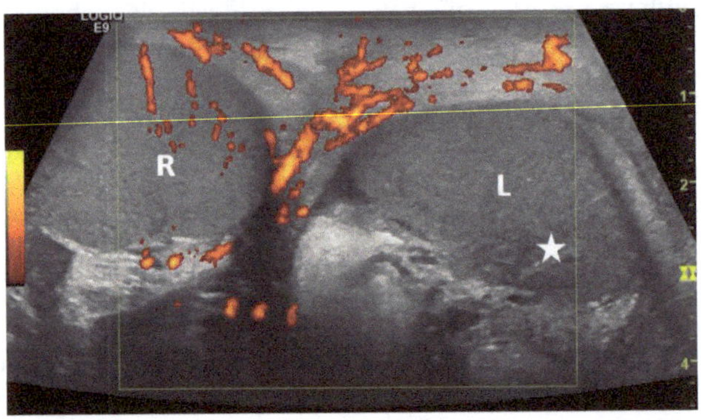

Fig. 7.28 No vascular flow is demonstrated on color interrogation

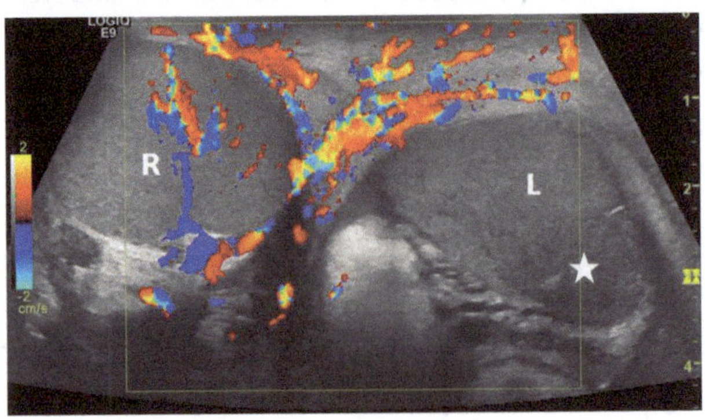

Fig. 7.29 No vascular flow is demonstrated on power Doppler interrogation

Differential Diagnosis Left testicular torsion, orchitis, testicular neoplasm.

Diagnosis and Discussion: Left testicular torsion (intravaginal).

Testicular torsion is a urological emergency and is a relatively common cause of testicular pain, particularly in young males and the pediatric population. Two discrete categories exist: extravaginal and intravaginal. Extravaginal torsion is seen exclusively in prenates and newborns, occurring secondary to lack of fixation of the tunica vaginalis along the scrotal wall. Intravaginal torsion can be seen at any age (but more often in adolescents and young adults) and occurs secondary to a lack of fixation of the testis to the tunica vaginalis Patients with a "bell clapper" deformity where the tunica vaginalis completely surrounds the testicle and the distal spermatic cord (rather than attach along the posterolateral aspect of the testis), are particularly prone to intravaginal torsion. Both intra and extravaginal torsion result in twisting of the spermatic cord causing venous congestion and arterial compromise leading to testicular ischemia. Clinically, patients present with acute onset scrotal pain associated with nausea, vomiting and/or a low grade fever. On physical exam, the hemiscrotum is erythematous, swollen and tender. The cremasteric reflex is absent and the testicle may be high riding and/or have a horizontal lie in the standing position (rather than the normal vertical orientation). Elevation of the hemiscrotum above the level of the pubic symphysis will not relieve the pain (Prehn' s sign).

Ultrasonography is the key diagnostic imaging study, although gray-scale findings may be normal in the early stages (2–4 h after onset of pain). After approximately 4–6 h, the torsed testicle will appear enlarged and hypoechoic (due to edema), eventually becoming increasingly heterogeneous with regions of increased echogenicity due to areas of hemorrhage and infarction (24 h after onset of pain). Evaluation of the twisted spermatic cord may demonstrate an extratesticular mass with concentric layers of variable echogenicity ("whirlpool sign"). A reactive hydrocele and scrotal edema may be present. Evaluation on color Doppler ultrasound demonstrates no detectable flow to the torsed testicle, findings which can be confirmed with power and spectral Doppler tracings. Early cases of torsion may demonstrate a small amount of residual arterial flow, though the presence of high resistance waveforms and an overall decreased amount of flow (evaluated via a side by side comparison to the contralateral testicle) is indicative of underlying torsion. Occasionally, the testicle may undergo spontaneous detorsion and demonstrate paradoxically increased flow on color Doppler interrogation, mimicking orchitis. The clinical history including improvement/lack of pain with the findings of increased flow as well as evaluation of the epididymis is critical in this regard, particularly since isolated orchitis without epididymitis is an uncommon entity, often seen in the setting of mumps. Delayed recognition and treatment of testicular torsion can result in ischemia and infarction with permanent loss of testicular function. Normal gray scale findings are a good indication of testicular viability, while increased heterogeneity increases the chances of testicular infarction.

Initiation of surgical treatment within the first 6 h after onset of pain portends the best prognosis. Surgical detorsion with bilateral orchiopexy is performed for viable testicles, while orchiectomy is performed for a non-viable testicle.

Pitfalls The combination of clinical history with gray-scale and color Doppler findings differentiates testicular torsion from other causes of acute onset scrotal pain. A normal appearing epididymis combined with no history of antecedent mumps and improved/intermittent in scrotal pain aids in differentiating the increased flow seen with torsion-detorsion from orchitis. Testicular neoplasms usually present as painless masses with a discrete, vascular mass seen on sonographic imaging.

Teaching Points

1. Testicular torsion is a urologic emergency. Ultrasonography typically demonstrates a hypoechoic testicle with no detectable flow. Twisting of the spermatic cord ("whirlpool sign") and a reactive hydrocele may be present.
2. Torsion-detorsion may present with paradoxically increased flow. A normal appearing epididymis combined with no history of antecedent mumps and improved/intermittent scrotal pain aids in differentiating the increased flow seen with torsion-detorsion from orchitis.
3. Normal gray scale findings are a good indication of testicular viability, while increased heterogeneity increases the chances of testicular infarction.
4. Treatment within 6 h of onset of pain portends the best chances at preserving testicular viability. Surgical detorsion with bilateral orchiopexy is performed for viable testicles, while orchiectomy is performed for a non-viable testicle.

Case 7.15

Brief Case Summary: 25 year old male with testicular pain.

Imaging Findings Gray scale (Fig. 7.30), power (Fig. 7.31), and color (Fig. 7.32) Doppler sagittal images of the right testicle demonstrate an avascular, hypoechoic, wedge shaped lesion extending to the periphery (arrows). Sagittal T1 weighted post contrast MR of the pelvis demonstrates a wedge shaped region of non-enhancement in the right testicle (arrow, Fig. 7.33) with subtle perilesional enhancement.

Differential Diagnosis Seminoma, focal orchitis, segmental testicular infarct.

Diagnosis and Discussion: Segmental testicular infarct

Segmental testicular infarct is a rare entity which may present with acute or subacute testicular pain. Unlike infarction associated with torsion, segmental infarction affects a slightly older patient population (second through fourth decades of life). The majority of cases are idiopathic, though it has been

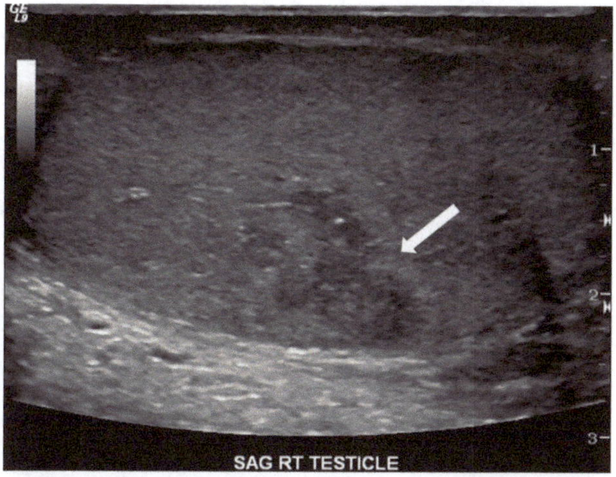

Fig. 7.30 Gray scale Doppler sagittal image of the right testicle demonstrate an avascular, hypoechoic, wedge shaped lesion extending to the periphery (*arrow*)

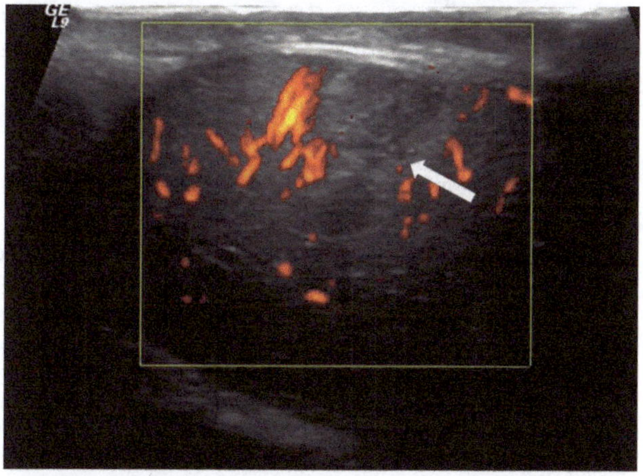

Fig. 7.31 Power Doppler sagittal image of the right testicle demonstrate an avascular, hypoechoic, wedge shaped lesion extending to the periphery (*arrow*)

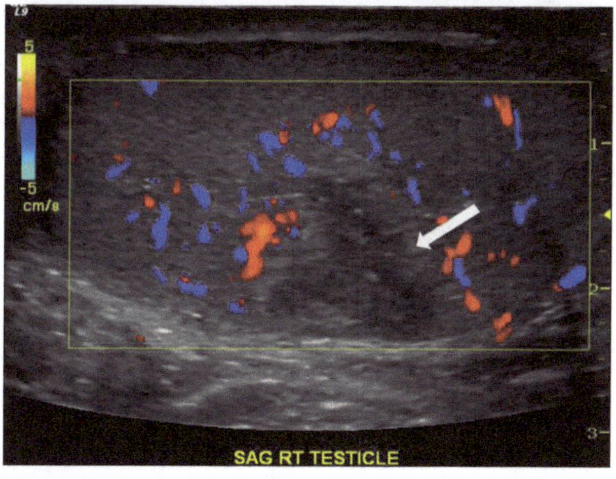

Fig. 7.32 Color Doppler sagittal image of the right testicle demonstrate an avascular, hypoechoic, wedge shaped lesion extending to the periphery (*arrow*)

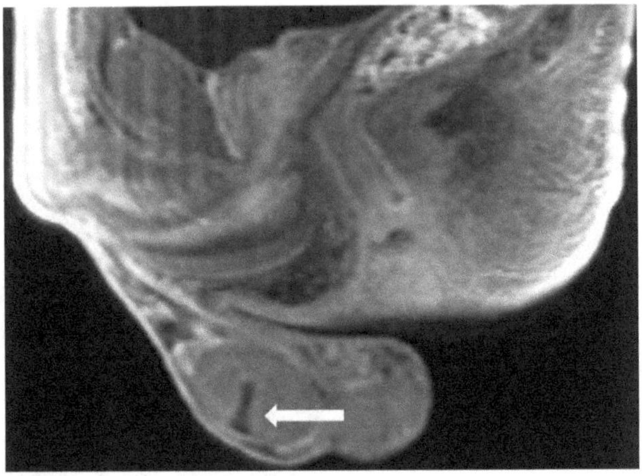

Fig. 7.33 Sagittal T1 weighted post contrast MR of the pelvis demonstrates a wedge shaped region of non-enhancement in the right testicle (*arrow*) with subtle perilesional enhancement

associated with vasculitis, sickle cell disease, hypercoagulable states, incomplete torsion/torsion-detorsion and epididymo-orchitis. Arterial or venous compromise can lead to segmental infarction, though there is a predilection for the upper testicular hemisphere due to a lack of collateral arterial flow involving the anterior branch of the testicular artery.

Ultrasound generally demonstrates a wedge shaped region of decreased echogenicity with the vertex toward the testicular mediastinum. No flow is demonstrated on color or power Doppler imaging. Occasionally, the infarct may appear more rounded and ill-defined with adjacent mass effect, making differentiation from a hypovascular tumor difficult. MR imaging is useful in this regard with the area of infarction appearing as a region of non-enhancement on T1 post contrast imaging often surrounded by a thin rim of perilesional enhancement. The T2 signal is variable and T1 is typically isointense, though high T1 signal may be seen with hemorrhagic infarcts.

Segmental testicular infarcts can be managed conservatively, particularly when the radiologic findings support the clinical suspicion.

Pitfalls Testicular neoplasms or focal orchitis are potential sonographic mimickers, though both typically demonstrate flow on color Doppler and/or power imaging. Orchitis presents with pain, while neoplasms are typically painless.

Teaching Points

1. Segmental testicular infarct is a rare entity which can present with acute or subacute testicular pain.
2. Sonographic findings are characteristic, demonstrating an avascular wedge shaped region of decreased echogenicity. MRI can confirm these findings with the area of infarct appearing as a region of non-enhancement on T1 post contrast imaging often surrounded by a thin rim of perilesional enhancement.
3. Differentiating a segmental testicular infarct from a tumor is critical as the former is treated conservatively, while the latter requires orchiectomy.

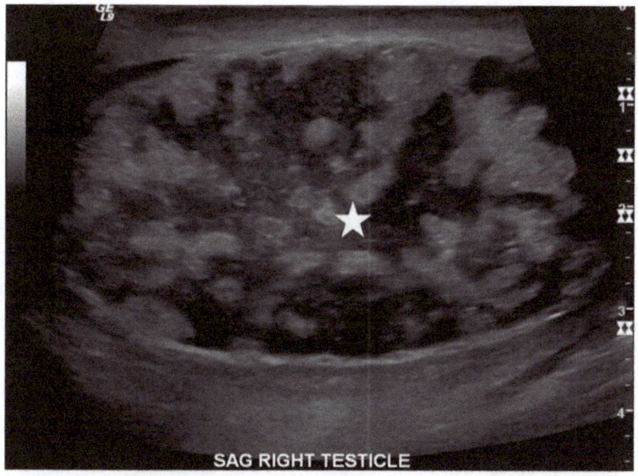

Fig. 7.34 Grayscale ultrasound demonstrates an enlarged, diffusely heterogeneous right testicle measuring 5.4 × 3.1 cm

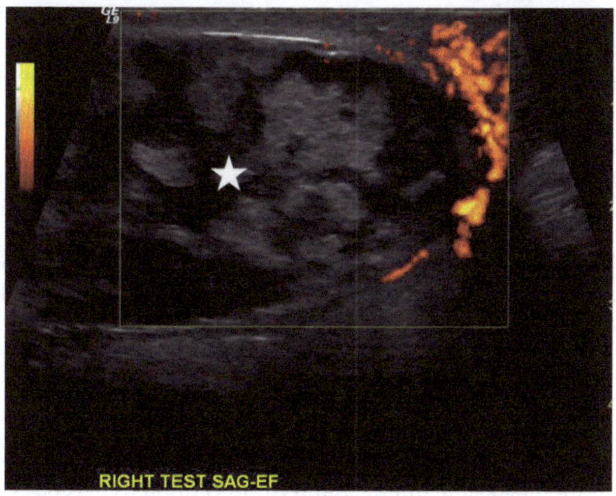

Fig. 7.35 On this image, no vascular flow within the right testicular parenchyma is seen. These findings are consistent with testicular torsion and ischemia/infarction

Case 7.16

Brief Case Summary 47 year old male with right testicular pain.

Imaging Findings Grayscale ultrasound demonstrates an enlarged, diffusely heterogeneous right testicle measuring 5.4 × 3.1 cm (Fig. 7.34). No vascular flow within the right testicular parenchyma is seen (Fig. 7.35). These findings are consistent with testicular torsion and ischemia/infarction.

Differential Diagnosis Orchitis, epididymo-orchitis, testicular abscess.

Diagnosis and Discussion Testicular necrosis or infarction is almost always secondary to torsion of the testis. Less common causes include severe epididymo-orchitis, which causes infarction secondary to increased intratesticular pressures, hypercoagulable states and vasculitis, both of which lead to occlusion of the gonadal vessels.

Testicular torsion presents in adolescents and young adults with an acute scrotum. It is a surgical emergency and prompt recognition and treatment are essential to salvage the testis. The probability of salvage is greatest when treated within 6 h of symptom onset; after 12 h the likelihood of salvage decreases to approximately 20 %. Testicular necrosis is invariably the end result in patients presenting after 24 h.

Ultrasound is the imaging modality of choice for diagnosis of torsion and assessment of vascularity in the testis. In the initial stages, when venous obstruction predominates, there is elevated resistive index (RI > 0.75) in the testicular parenchyma. When the torsion is complete, leading to cessation of arterial inflow, the hallmark is absent vascularity. The demonstration of a "Whirlpool sign", the twisting of the spermatic cord, in both B mode and Doppler ultrasound, is considered highly specific for the diagnosis of torsion.

The infarcted testis is enlarged and avascular with heterogeneous echogenicity, with intermixed hypoechoic (representing infarcted parenchyma) and hyperechoic (representing reperfusion hemorrhage) areas. A peripheral zone of revascularization may be demonstrated after a few days. The scrotal wall is edematous and hyperemic.

The treatment of an infarcted testis involves orchiectomy. Salvage of a torsed testis is dependent on the time of surgical intervention after onset of symptoms and hence timely diagnosis is of utmost importance. Differentiation of the various causes of an infarcted testis is important in protecting the contralateral testicle.

Pitfalls Orchitis or epididymo-orchitis can have a similar imaging appearance and clinical presentation in the setting of a de torsed and hyperemic testicle. A large evolving testicular abscess can mimic an infarcted testis as the affected zone is avascular and the surrounding scrotal structures are hyperemic.

Teaching Points

1. Testicular necrosis is almost always secondary to torsion of the testis. Less common causes include epididymo-orchitis, hypercoagulable states, and vasculitis.
2. Torsion of the testis is a surgical emergency and the salvageability is inversely proportional to the timing of intervention after symptom onset.
3. Ultrasound hallmarks of torsion of the testis include "whirlpool sign", elevated RI in incomplete torsion, absent vascularity in complete torsion.
4. An infarcted testis appears enlarged, and, is avascular, demonstrating shows heterogeneous echogenicity.

Case 7.17

Brief Case Summary: 44 year old male with infertility.

Imaging Findings Grayscale ultrasound demonstrates multiple serpiginous hypoechoic tubular structures (arrows, Fig. 7.36) adjacent to the left testis which show blood flow on the color Doppler (Fig. 7.37) with increased flow after the Valsalva maneuver (Fig. 7.38).

Differential Diagnosis Varicocele

Diagnosis and Discussion: Varicocele

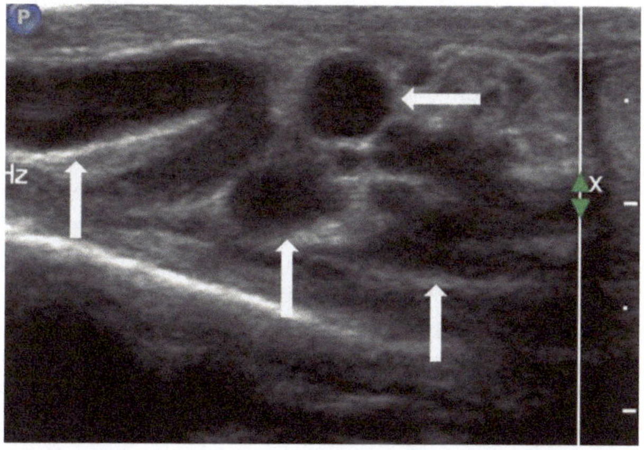

Fig. 7.36 Grayscale ultrasound demonstrates multiple serpiginous hypoechoic tubular structures (*arrows*) adjacent to the left testis

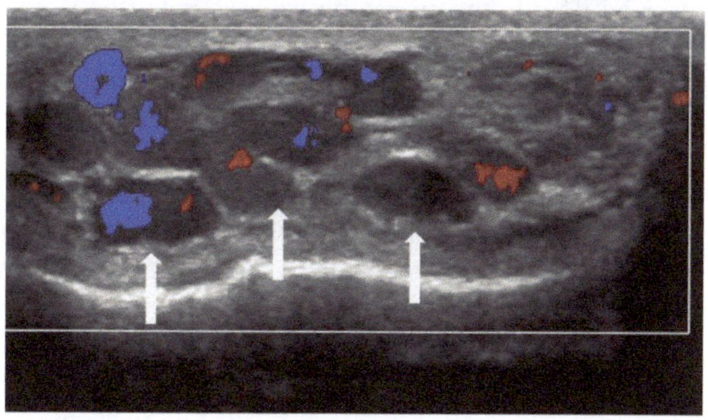

Fig. 7.37 Color Doppler showing blood flow

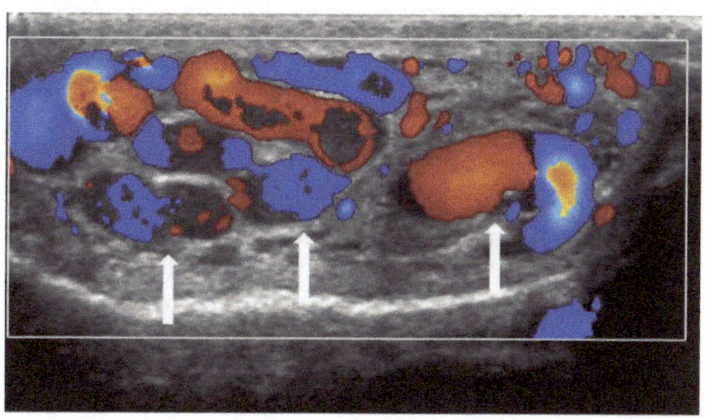

Fig. 7.38 Color Doppler showing increased flow after the Valsalva maneuver

A varicocele refers to abnormal dilatation of the veins of the pampiniform plexus. Varicoceles have a prevalence of 15 % in the general population, though this number escalates as high as 40 % in patients with infertility. Most cases are related to incompetent valves in the spermatic vein. Secondary varicoceles are less common, and result from increased pressure on the spermatic vein from a variety of causes including hydronephrosis and abdominal masses. Presenting symptoms include testicular discomfort with or without the sensation of a mass as well as findings pertaining to infertility. Varicoceles may be suspected and graded on clinical exam but are typically referred to radiology for further evaluation. The left side is more commonly affected for a variety of reasons but is typically attributed to the right angle at which the testicular vein enters the left renal vein and the longer course of the left renal vein.

Ultrasound is the imaging modality of choice. Grayscale imaging demonstrates the presence of multiple hypo to anechoic tubular and serpiginous extratesticular masses measuring greater than 3 mm in size. Low level echoes may be seen due to slow internal flow. Varicoceles increase in size in the upright position or with the patient performing the Valsalva maneuver. Color Doppler imaging demonstrates the presence of flow, with flow reversal/reflux noted during the Valsalva maneuver. Various grading schemes exist which allow classification of findings depending on the length of the lesions, the characteristics of the reflux, and the observed changes on performing the Valsalva maneuver. Varicoceles may be detected as incidental findings on CT and MRI, though these modalities are seldom used in the primary evaluation. Conventional venography may also be used, readily demonstrating the reversed flow in the spermatic veins. While this is considered the best diagnostic test, the advantages are off-set by the associated risks of ionizing radiation, relatively high cost and invasiveness, such that venography is typically used to treat rather than diagnose varicoceles.

Treatment options include a variety of open surgical techniques, laparoscopic varicocelectomy and radiologic embolization (balloon or coil) or sclerotherapy, with the ultimate goal of improving fertility. Common post treatment complications include hydrocele formation and recurrent varicocele which can occur in up to 35 % of patients depending on the technique utilized.

Pitfalls Imaging evaluation is generally straightforward. Careful attention should be made to the presence of an isolated right sided varicocele, a new onset varicocele, or a varicocele which is noncompressible as these findings may be indicative of an underlying mass obstructing gonadal venous return.

Teaching Points

1. Varicoceles are common extratestesticular masses which represent venous dilatation of the pampinoform plexus. Most cases are the result of incompetent valves within the spermatic vein.
2. Secondary varicocele refers to one that forms as a result of increased pressure on the spermatic vein.
3. Sonographic evaluation demonstrates the presence of multiple extratesticular tubular hypo to anechoic masses greater than 3 mm, which increase in size and

demonstrate retrograde flow upon standing and/or performing the Valsalva maneuver.

4. An isolated right sided varicocele, a new onset varicocele or a varicocele which is noncompressible may be indicative of an underlying mass obstructing gonadal venous return for which cross sectional imaging should be considered.

Case 7.18

Brief Case Summary: 30 year old male, with testicular fullness

Imaging Findings Ultrasound of the scrotum demonstrates anechoic fluid (Fig. 7.39, asterisk) surrounding the anterolateral aspect of right testis.

Differential Diagnosis Hydrocele, pyocele, hematocele, epididymal cyst

Diagnosis and Discussion Hydrocele

While a small amount of fluid may be normally seen between the visceral and parietal layers of the tunica vaginalis, a hydrocele refers to a larger accumulation of serous fluid in this space.

Congenital causes are associated with the presence of a patent processus vaginalis, while acquired causes are reactive secondary to infection, trauma, or tumors. Congenital causes may be further classified as communicating (where the processus vaginalis is patent throughout its extent), funicular (processus vaginalis is open to the peritoneal cavity but is closed above the testicle) and encysted (processus vaginalis is closed to the peritoneal cavity and above the testicle).

Imaging demonstrates the presence of simple appearing extratesticular fluid, manifested as avascular and anechoic with increased through-transmission on ultrasound. On MR, the fluid is typically T1 dark and T2 bright without vascularity. Occasionally, a few low level echoes or fibrin strands may be seen on sonographic imaging. Increased heterogeneity of the fluid may suggest the presence of a hematocele, with

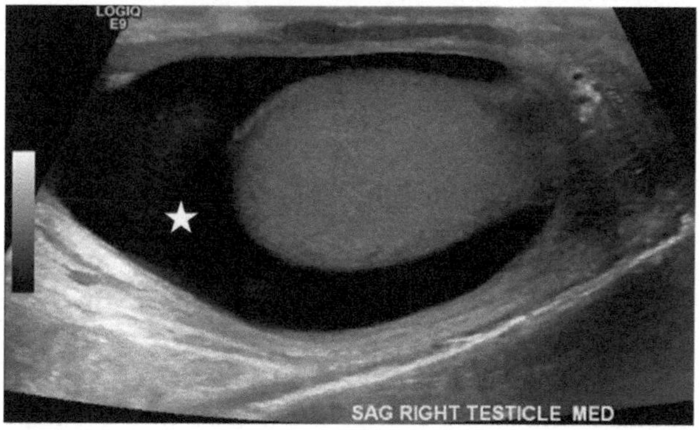

Fig. 7.39 Ultrasound of the scrotum demonstrates anechoic fluid (*asterisk*) surrounding the anterolateral aspect of right testis

potential causes including trauma, post-surgery, tumor and torsion. The presence of gas (as demonstrated by bright echoes with shadowing), particularly in the context of epididymo-orchitis and/or leukocytosis, suggests the presence of a pyocele. The funicular and encysted types of hydrocele demonstrate fluid accumulation cephalad and separate from the testicle in the expected region of the spermatic cord.

Secondary hydroceles are managed by treating the underlying cause. Surgical treatment (hydrocelectomy) or aspiration of fluid with sclerotherapy may be considered for symptomatic congenital hydroceles.

Pitfalls Hydroceles are generally easy to differentiate from epididymal or tunica vaginalis cysts based on location alone. Distinguishing a complex appearing hydrocele from a hematocele or pyocele may be challenging although the clinical picture can help in this regard.

Teaching Points

1. Hydrocele refers to an accumulation of fluid in the tunica vaginalis.
2. Etiologies are classified as congenital or acquired. Congenital causes are related to the presence of a patent processus vaginalis and may be further subdivided into communicating, funicular, and encysted varieties. Acquired causes include trauma, tumor, and infection.
3. Surgical treatment may be considered for symptomatic congenital hydroceles.

Case 7.19

Brief Case Summary: Three different male patients with cystic masses.

Imaging Findings

Patient 1: Gray scale and color Doppler ultrasound images demonstrate a small, well-defined anechoic cyst (arrows, Figs. 7.40 and 7.41) in the right epididymis.
Patient 2: Gray scale and color Doppler ultrasound images show a small anechoic cyst (arrows, Figs. 7.42 and 7.43) on surface of the testis.
Patient 3: Gray scale and color Doppler ultrasound images show a small anechoic cyst (arrows, Figs. 7.44 and 7.45) in right mediastinum testis.

Differential Diagnosis

Patient 1: Epididymal cyst, papillary cystadenoma
Patient 2: Tunica albuginea cyst, adenomatoid tumor
Patient 3: Cystic teratoma, epidermoid, testicular cyst, intratesticular varicocele/aneurysm

Diagnosis and Discussion

Patient 1: Epididymal cyst
Patient 2: Tunica albuginea cyst
Patient 3: Testicular cyst

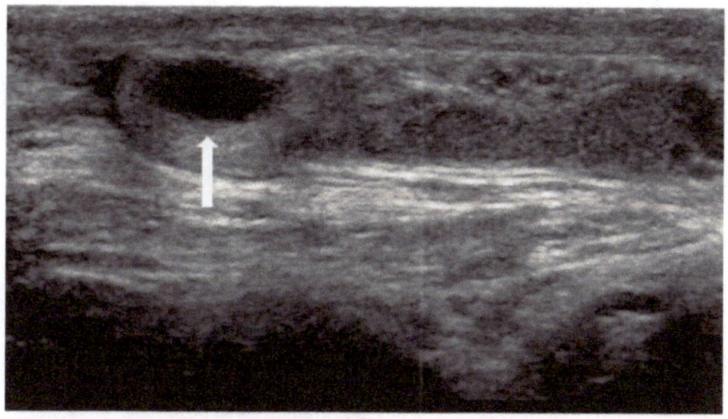

Fig. 7.40 Patient 1: Gray scale ultrasound image demonstrates a small, well-defined anechoic cyst (*arrow*) in the right epididymis

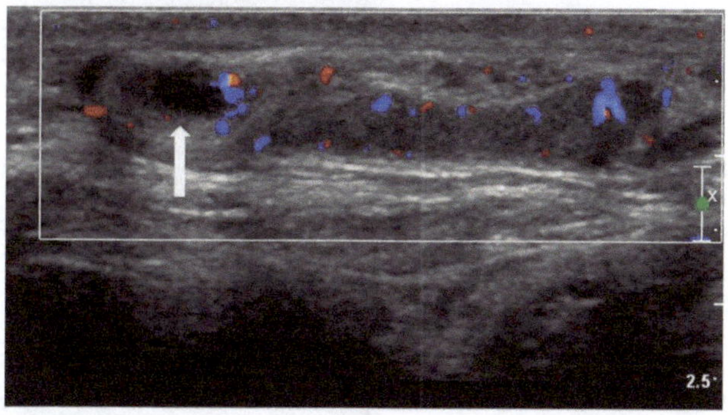

Fig. 7.41 Patient 1: Color Doppler ultrasound image demonstrates a small, well-defined anechoic cyst (*arrow*) in the right epididymis

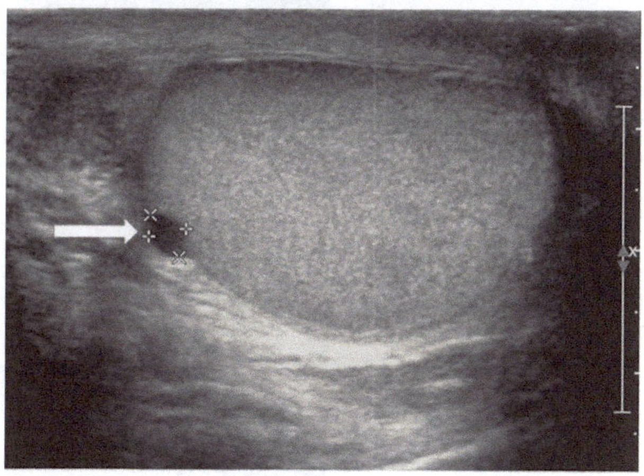

Fig. 7.42 Patient 2: Gray scale ultrasound image shows a small anechoic cyst (*arrow*) on surface of the testis

Epididymal cysts represent the most common epididymal mass, often seen as incidental lesions. These benign masses can either be true epithelial lined cysts, or may represent spermatoceles with the latter typically forming due to outflow obstruction of the efferent ducts. True cysts and spermatoceles are indistinguishable, most often manifesting as avascular, anechoic masses with increased

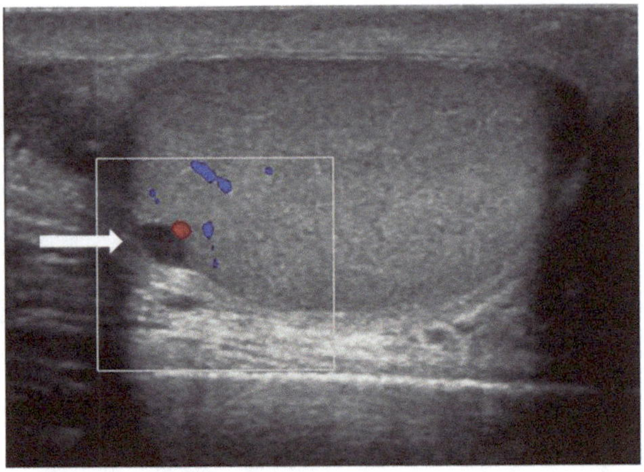

Fig. 7.43 Patient 2: Color Doppler ultrasound image shows a small anechoic cyst (*arrows*) on surface of the testis

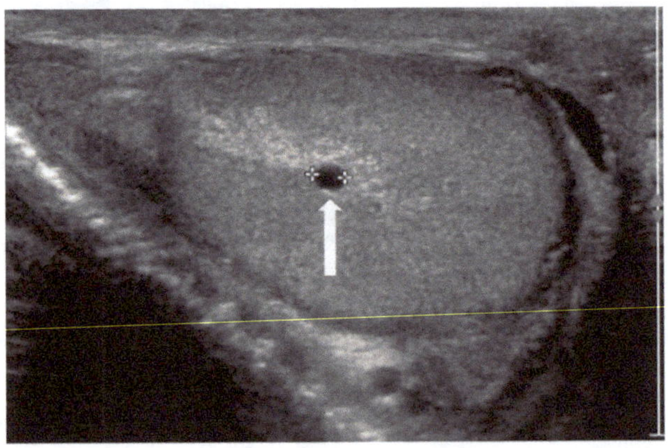

Fig. 7.44 Patient 3: Gray scale ultrasound image shows a small anechoic cyst (*arrow*) in right mediastinum testis

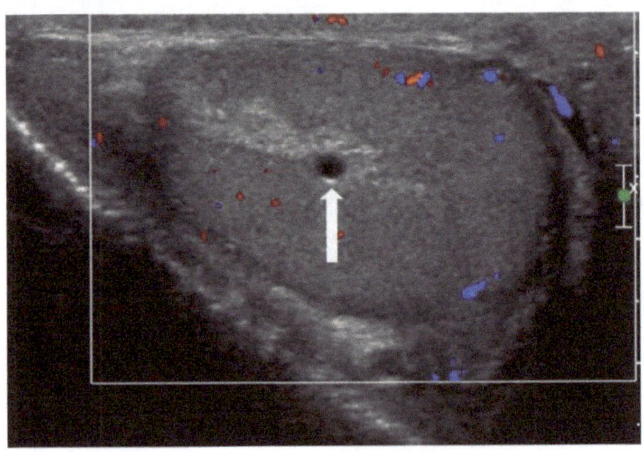

Fig. 7.45 Patient 3: Color Doppler ultrasound image shows a small anechoic cyst (*arrow*) in right mediastinum testis

through-transmission. Larger lesions may appear minimally more complex with the presence of internal septations. Definitive diagnosis may be made by aspiration, though this distinction is seldom needed, given the benign nature of these lesions. Epididymal cysts are more common, though spermatoceles are more often seen in the post-vasectomy patient population.

Tunica albuginea cysts are benign lesions which often manifest as small nodules varying from 2 to 5 mm in size. While their exact etiology remains elusive, they are thought to represent mesothelial embryological remnants. On ultrasound, these lesions are often simple appearing and occur along the upper anterior or lateral aspect of the tunica albuginea. Distinguishing tunica albuginea cysts from testicular or tunica vaginalis cysts may be difficult if the lesions are large. In addition, the lesions may occasionally be complex (due to hemorrhagic or proteinacious debris) in which case the possibility of a neoplasm may be difficult to exclude. MR imaging is useful in both of these circumstances, allowing for accurate localization and to evaluate for the presence of enhancing components.

Testicular cysts are benign lesions which are almost always non-palpable and incidentally detected on sonographic imaging. Once thought to be rare, these lesions are being detected more frequently, likely due to the increased use of ultrasound for scrotal imaging. Their size varies from 2 mm to 2 cm and may be occasionally palpable when located along the periphery of the testicle. Sonographic imaging demonstrates the classic characteristics of a simple cyst (avascular, anechoic with increased through-transmission and imperceptible walls). Any degree of internal complexity should be raise the possibility of a neoplasm for which a contrast enhanced MRI may be useful to exclude the presence of enhancing components. Management of simple appearing testicular cysts is variable. Complex appearing cysts may warrant MR imaging, while a follow-up ultrasound may be considered for symptomatic simple appearing cysts. Asymptomatic simple appearing cysts can likely be dismissed without further follow-up.

Pitfalls Larger epididymal cysts may be confused with hydroceles though the latter envelops the testicle, while epididymal cysts displaces it. Other epididymal masses are typically solid, though papillary cystadenomas (an entity associated with von Hippel-Lindau disease) may have distinct cystic spaces.

Adenomatoid tumors involving the tunica albuginea are rare, solid appearing lesions which allows differentiation from a tunica albuginea cyst. Adenomatoid tumors are the most commonly paratesticular neoplasms and mostly arise from the epididymis but may also be seen in the tunica vaginalis and rete testis.

Both cystic teratomas and epidermoid neoplasms have some degree of internal complexity allowing them to be easily distinguished from a simple parenchymal testicular cyst. An intratesticular aneurysm or varicocele are rare lesions which may mimic a cyst on gray scale imaging. Color imaging, however, will readily demonstrate the presence of flow in the case of aneurysm and varicocele.

Teaching Points

1. Epididymal cysts are the most common mass in the epididymis. They are benign and require no follow-up.
2. Tunica albuginea cysts are benign lesions that often manifests as small nodules and may be palpable.
3. Testicular cysts are uncommon benign lesions that may be dismissed if they are asymptomatic and demonstrate no complex features. Symptomatic simple appearing lesions may require short-term sonographic follow-up, while complex lesions may be evaluated with MRI.

Case 7.20

Brief Case Summary: 45 year old male with painless testicular lump

Imaging Findings Gray scale and color imaging demonstrates the presence of a heterogeneous, predominantly hypoechoic mass (arrows, Figs. 7.46 and 7.47) in the left testicle without internal vascularity. The internal architecture of the lesion suggests the presence of concentric rings of variable echogenicity.

Differential Diagnosis Seminoma, teratoma, dermoid, epidermoid cyst, metastases, testicular infarct.

Diagnosis and Discussion: Epidermoid cyst

Epidermoid cyst is an uncommon, benign testicular tumor, accounting for approximately 1–2 % of all intratesticular lesions. It is most commonly found as a solitary mass in younger males (2nd to 4th decades of life), though bilateral and multifocal lesions have been reported. The tumor may be incidentally discovered or present as a painless mass.

Epidermoid cysts are thought to represent monodermal teratomas containing only ectodermal tissue, with histological analysis demonstrating the presence of a fibrous wall lined by keratinizing squamous epithelium. The sonographic imaging features often mirror these findings with gray scale imaging demonstrating the presence of well-circumscribed masses with hyperechoic walls (which may be calcified) and internal concentric laminations of variable echogenicity giving rise to an "onion-ring" appearance. Alternatively, the lesion may demonstrate a hypoechoic outer ring and a central echogenic center giving rise to a "target" appearance. MR imaging demonstrates similar findings with high T1 and T2 signal seen in lipid and water rich areas and low signal seen corresponding to calcifications and keratin. Despite their solid appearance, these tumors represent cysts and thus do not demonstrate internal vascularity or contrast enhancement.

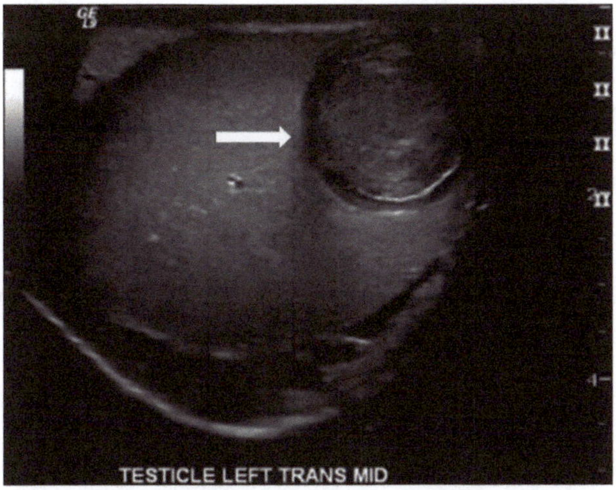

Fig. 7.46 Gray scale imaging demonstrates the presence of a heterogeneous, predominantly hypoechoic mass (*arrow*) in the left testicle without internal vascularity. The internal architecture of the lesion suggests the presence of concentric rings of variable echogenicity

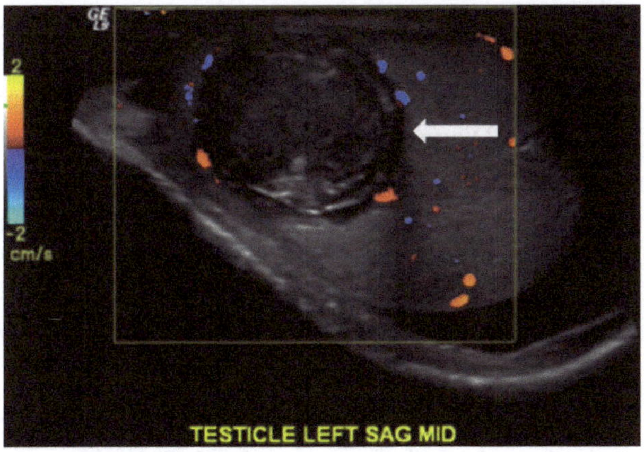

Fig. 7.47 Color imaging demonstrates the presence of a heterogeneous, predominantly hypoechoic mass (*arrow*) in the left testicle without internal vascularity. The internal architecture of the lesion suggests the presence of concentric rings of variable echogenicity

Prospective recognition of an epidermoid cyst can result in conservative surgery with enucleation, avoiding the need for an orchiectomy. Prognosis is excellent with a rare risk of recurrence.

Pitfalls Differentiating a benign epidermoid cyst from other testicular tumors may be challenging. The presence of the classic "target" or "onion ring" appearance, combined with lack of vascularity and negative tumor markers are strongly suggestive of an epidermoid cyst. Metastases are often bilateral and occur in an older age group (above the age of 60). Segmental infarction or hemorrhage typically presents as a non-mass like area of decreased echogenicity without vascularity seen in the context of prior trauma, orchitis or torsion.

Teaching Point

1. Epidermoid cysts are benign lesions with a characteristic appearance of concentric internal rings of variable echogenicity, known as the "target" or "onion ring" sign.
2. The lack of vascularity and negative tumor markers along with the classic gray scale US appearance can help differentiate this benign lesion from malignant testicular neoplasms.
3. Prospective recognition of an epidermoid cyst can result in conservative surgery with enucleation thereby avoiding the need for an orchiectomy.

Case 7.21

Brief Case Summary: 25 year old male with scrotal pain.

Imaging Findings Gray scale ultrasound images of the testicles demonstrate the presence of innumerable punctate non-shadowing echogenic foci bilaterally (Fig. 7.48a, b).

Differential Diagnosis Microlithiasis, burned out germ cell tumor, tuberculosis.

Diagnosis and Discussion: Testicular microlithiasis

Testicular microlithiasis (TM) is a sonographic imaging finding that is most often incidentally discovered in patients undergoing scrotal ultrasound. The exact prevalence is unknown, but is thought to range from 2 to 6 % in asymptomatic patients. Pathologically, TM is thought to represent calcium deposits within the seminiferous tubules, though the entity as such describes radiologic, not pathologic findings.

Sonographically, TM is classically defined as at least 5 intratesticular, non-shadowing echogenic foci measuring 1–3 mm in diameter. The distribution is typically uniform and bilateral, though segmental and unilateral findings can be seen. Limited TM refers to patients with fewer than 5 microliths on sonographic imaging, though the significance of this subclassification is unclear.

The significance of TM lies within the reported increased incidence of associated testicular cancer. In asymptomatic patients who other otherwise healthy, no further imaging follow-up is generally needed. A targeted history and physical by the referring physician to elicit clinical evidence of an underlying testicular dysgenesis syndrome (TDS) or extragonadal germ cell tumor, as well as frequent testicular self-examinations is usually sufficient. Features of TDS include cryptorchidism, subfertility, testicular atrophy and gonadal dysgenesis, all of which are risk factors for testicular germ cell tumors. In patients with features of TDS and TM, regular self-examinations with or without biopsy and/or annual scrotal ultrasound follow-up at the discretion of the referring physician may be considered.

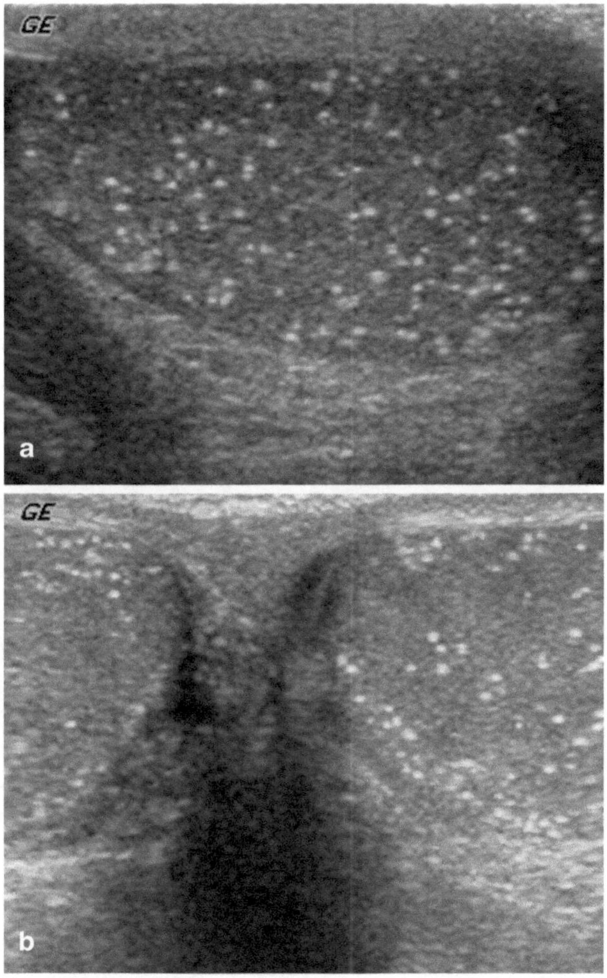

Fig. 7.48 (**a**, **b**) Gray scale ultrasound images of the testicles demonstrate the presence of innumerable punctate non-shadowing echogenic foci bilaterally

Pitfalls Imaging findings are typically pathognomonic. The multiplicity, size and lack of posterior shadowing differentiate this entity from a burned out germ cell tumor. Testicular tuberculosis is rare and is usually presents as hypoechoic masses, with or without calcification in the setting of disease elsewhere.

Teaching Points

1. The presence of multiple, small non-shadowing echogenic foci (typically 1–3 mm) is typically for TM.
2. In asymptomatic patients, no imaging follow-up is needed. Regular testicular self-examinations should be encouraged.
3. In patients with features of TDS, annual sonographic followup may be considered.

Case 7.22

Brief Case Summary: 27 year old male with painless scrotal mass.

Imaging Findings There is a confluence of approximately 5 hypoechoic slightly heterogeneous hypervascular masses (arrows, Fig. 7.49a, b) within the right testicle. The largest measures approximately 2.1 cm in greatest diameter.

Differential Diagnosis Seminomatous germ cell tumor, non-seminomatous germ cell tumor, testicular lymphoma, focal orchitis.

Diagnosis and Discussion Seminomatous germ cell tumor

Primary testicular neoplasms are generally characterized as germ cell or stromal tumors, with germ cell tumors further classified as seminomatous and

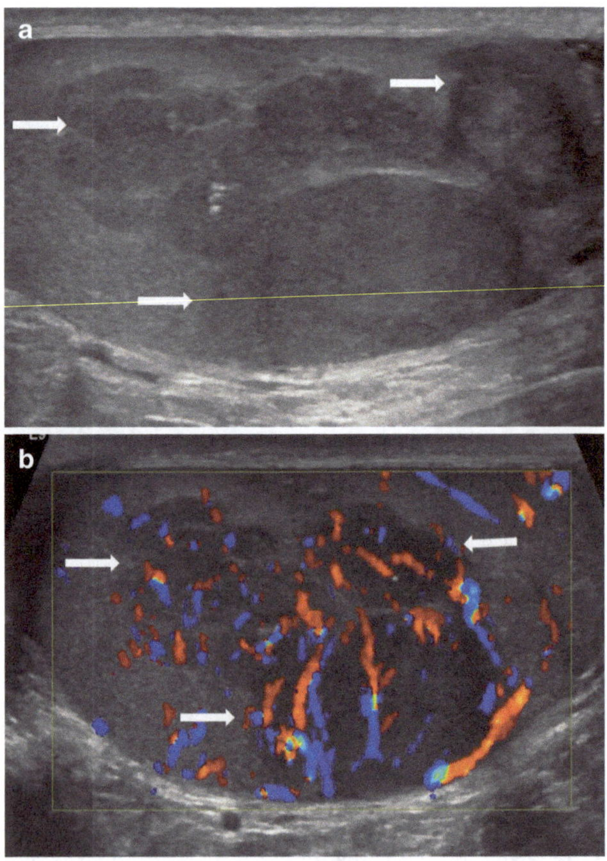

Fig. 7.49 (**a**, **b**). Images show a confluence of approximately 5 hypoechoic slightly heterogeneous hypervascular masses (*arrows*) within the right testicle. The largest measures approximately 2.1 cm in greatest diameter

non-seminomatous neoplasms. Seminoma accounts for the most common germ cell tumor of a single, pure cell lineage, with mixed germ cell tumor (which have elements of both seminomatous and non- seminomatous neoplasms) being the overall most common histology. Non-seminomatous neoplasms include choriocarcinoma, embryonal cell carcinoma, and teratoma and yolk sac tumors. Seminomas are most often seen in young Caucasian males between 25 and 35 years old. Risk factors include a prior history of testicular tumor, a positive family history and cryptorchidism. Clinically, patients present with complaints of a painless, palpable testicular lump, although 10 % of patients may complain of tenderness on physical examination.

Sonography is the initial imaging examination of choice. Seminomatous germ cell neoplasms typically manifest as a uniformly hypoechoic mass with lobulated or multinodular borders. While uncommon, multifocal or bilateral masses may be occasionally seen. Color Doppler imaging demonstrates the presence of increased vascularity. In equivocal cases, MR imaging may be obtained, typically demonstrating a predominantly T2 hypointense mass with inhomogeneous enhancement. CT imaging is reserved for staging purposes with metastases most commonly spreading via the lymphatics to the abdominal retroperitoneal lymph nodes. Contiguous involvement of the skin or epididymis may result in spread of disease to the pelvic lymph nodes. Hematogenous spread to distant organs may occur during the late stages of disease.

Seminomas are radiosensitive tumors, and as such have an excellent prognosis with a combination of orchiectomy followed by radiation. Some centers advocate ongoing surveillance without radiation following radical orchiectomy in patients with stage 1 seminoma.

Pitfalls Non-seminomatous germ cell neoplasms and stromal tumors tend to have a more heterogeneous sonographic appearance although this alone cannot allow confident differentiation from seminoma. Testicular lymphoma is more often seen in patients above the age of 60 and is more likely to manifest as bilateral masses. The clinical picture should allow differentiation of focal orchitis from a testicular neoplasm. In addition, focal orchitis without concomitant epididymitis is uncommon, with exceptions of mumps and HIV. If doubt persists, a MRI or short term follow-up ultrasound may be obtained.

Teaching Points

1. Seminomas are amongst the most common testicular neoplasms, often presenting as a painless scrotal mass in young males 25–35 years old.
2. Imaging findings demonstrate the presence of a uniformly hypoechoic mass with associated vascularity, though imaging along cannot differentiate a seminomatous from a non-seminomatous or stromal tumor.
3. Prognosis is excellent with patients typically undergoing orchiectomy followed by radiation.

Case 7.23

Brief Case Summary: 32 year old male with abdominal pain.

Imaging Findings Gray scale US image of the right lower quadrant lateral to the umbilicus demonstrates the presence of an anechoic mass containing a few low level echoes and internal striations (asterisk, Fig. 7.50). Minimal peripheral vascularity is noted on color imaging (Fig. 7.51). CT scan of the abdomen with intravenous and oral contrast demonstrates the presence of a low density retroperitoneal

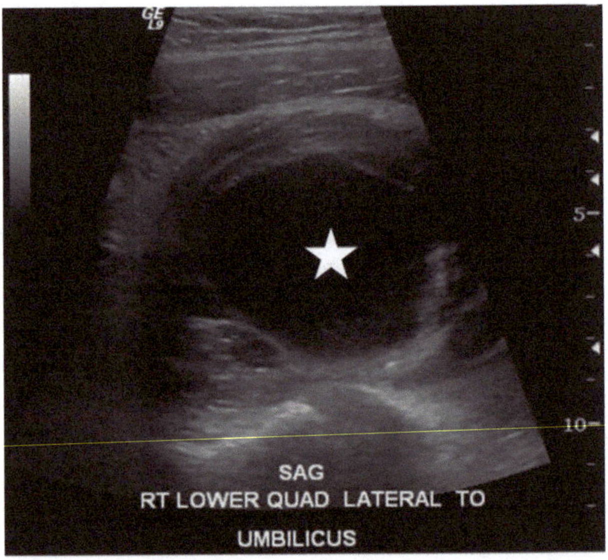

Fig. 7.50 Gray scale US image of the right lower quadrant lateral to the umbilicus demonstrates the presence of an anechoic mass containing a few low level echoes and internal striations (*asterisk*)

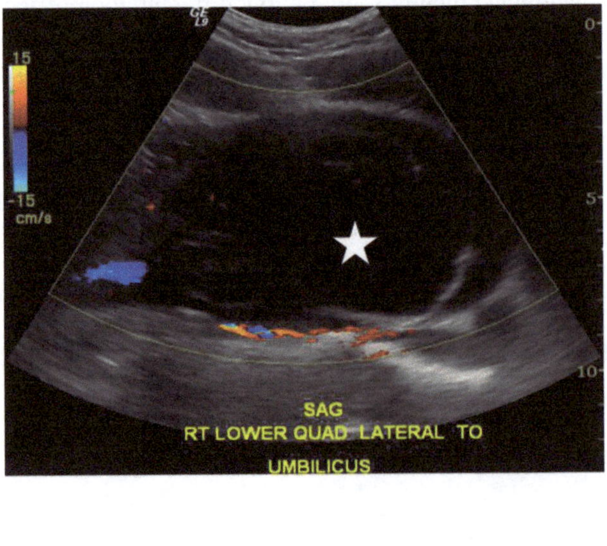

Fig. 7.51 Minimal peripheral vascularity is noted on color imaging

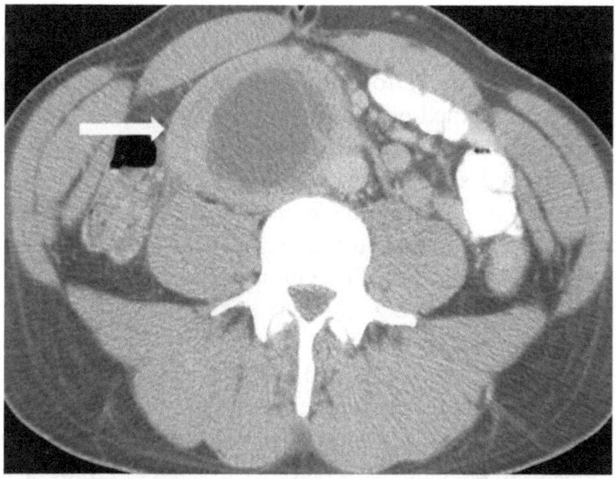

Fig. 7.52 CT scan of the abdomen with intravenous and oral contrast demonstrates the presence of a low density retroperitoneal mass (*arrow*) with a thick peripheral rim

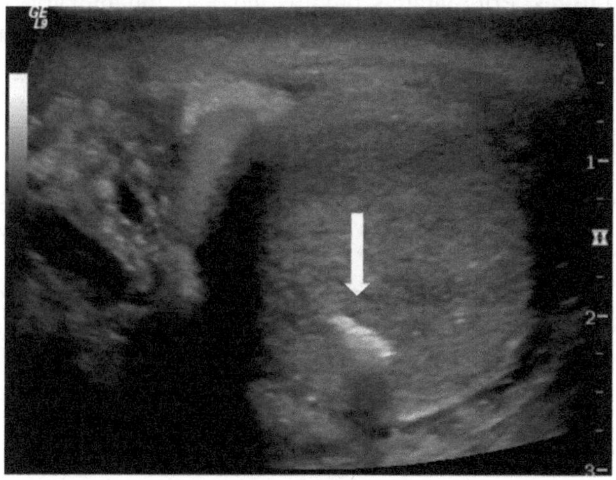

Fig. 7.53 Subsequent gray scale image from a scrotal ultrasound demonstrates the presence of a linear hyperechoic lesion (*arrow*) in the right testicle with posterior shadowing

mass (arrow, Fig. 7.52) with a thick peripheral rim. Subsequent gray scale image from a scrotal ultrasound demonstrates the presence of a linear hyperechoic lesion (arrow, Fig. 7.53) in the right testicle with posterior shadowing.

Differential Diagnosis Burned out germ cell tumor, retroperitoneal sarcoma, testicular microlithiasis

Diagnosis and Discussion: Burned out germ cell tumor

Retroperitoneal extragondal germ cell neoplasms may either arise as primary lesions or represent metastases from a gonadal germ cell tumor (GCT). Primary retroperitoneal GCTs are uncommon and are thought to arise from incompletely migrated germ cell rests. Metastatic retroperitoneal GCTs are more commonly seen, with sonographic imaging typically demonstrating the presence of a discrete testicular mass. Burned out germ cell tumors represent an additional category in which a metastatic retroperitoneal GCT is suspected, without compelling evidence of a discrete testicular mass. Furthermore, patients often present with symptoms pertaining to the retroperitoneal mass without a palpable testicular lump on physical exam. Burned out GCTs have been reported with both seminomatous and non-seminomatous histologies.

Reported sonographic findings include the presence of discrete calcifications, non-mass like hypoechoic regions and scattered echogenic foci. The discrete calcifications are thought to represent areas of scarring in the region of the regressed germ cell neoplasm. While findings are often ipsilateral to the retroperitoneal mass, either testicle may demonstrate the burned out neoplasm. The etiology remains elusive with immune mediated mechanisms thought to be likely involved.

The presence of a burned out GCT requires orchiectomy as chemotherapy alone (with or without radiation) will not cross the blood-testis barrier to treat the underlying primary. The presence of radiological normal appearing testicles may prompt biopsies to exclude the possibility of a small tumor or foci of carcinoma in situ.

Pitfalls Prior infarcts, orchitis and other inflammatory conditions may demonstrate the presence of a focal calcification on sonographic imaging. The possibility of a burned out germ cell tumor should be entertained with the presence of concomitant metastases.

Teaching Points

1. The presence of a retroperitoneal mass and/or lymphadenopathy in a young male should prompt an evaluation of the scrotum to exclude an underlying testicular primary
2. The imaging appearance of a burned out GCT is non-specific with ultrasound demonstrating calcifications, echogenic foci and/or non-mass like area of hypoechogenicity. The presence of concomitant metastases suggests that these non-specific findings may be related to a burned out GCT.
3. Confirmed cases of burned out GCT require both orchiectomy and systemic therapy.

Case 7.24

Brief Case Summary: 76 year old male with history of lymphoma, restaging.

Imaging Findings Axial image from an attenuation corrected F18-FDG PET scan demonstrates the presence of two discrete foci of increased radiotracer uptake in the scrotum (arrow, Fig. 7.54). Gray scale US images of the scrotum demonstrate the presence of multiple bilateral hypoechoic masses (arrows, Fig. 7.55a, b). A representative mass in the left testicle demonstrates the presence of flow on color Doppler imaging (arrow, Fig. 7.56).

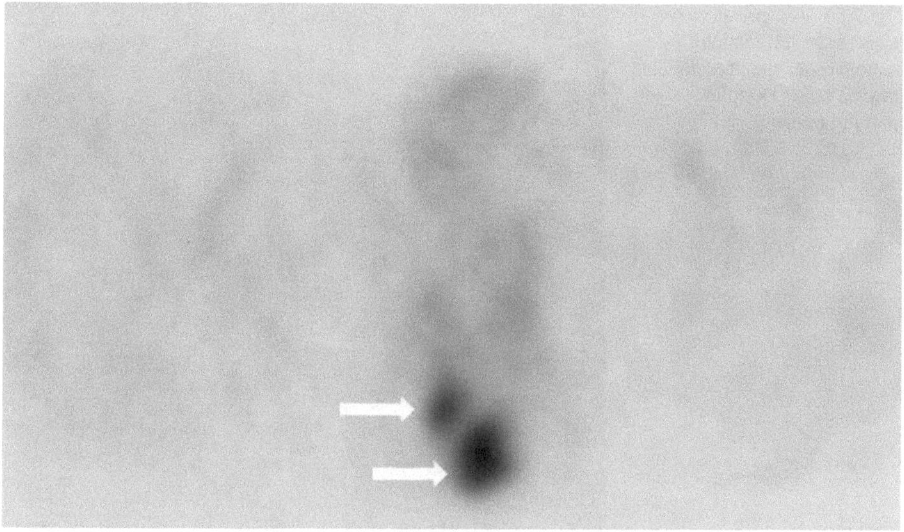

Fig. 7.54 Axial image from an attenuation corrected F18-FDG PET scan demonstrates the presence of two discrete foci of increased radiotracer uptake in the scrotum (*arrow*)

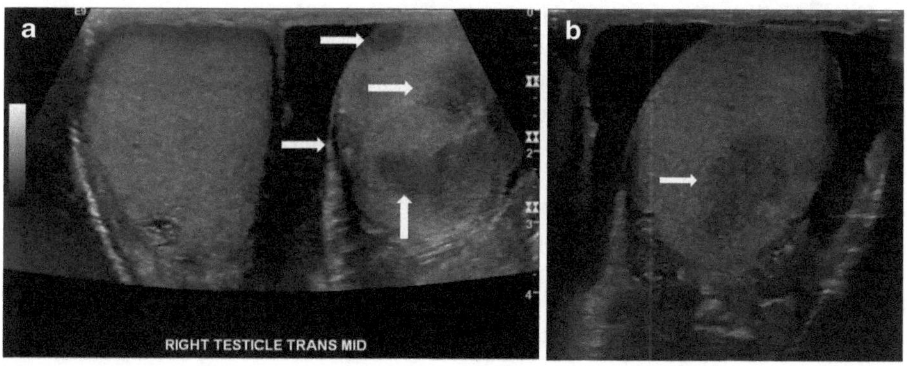

Fig. 7.55 Gray scale US images of the scrotum demonstrate the presence of multiple bilateral hypoechoic masses (*arrows*, **a** and **b**)

Differential Diagnosis Metastatic disease (prostate cancer, testicular lymphoma), testicular germ cell tumor, testicular stromal tumor.

Diagnosis and Discussion: Metastatic disease (testicular lymphoma)

Metastatic disease to the testicles is less common than primary disease, with an incidence ranging from 2.4 to 3.6 %, often seen either in the setting of widely disseminated disease or on autopsy. In approximately 6–7 % of patients, testicular metastases presents as the initial evidence of disease elsewhere, manifesting clinically as palpable masses on scrotal examination. Primary neoplasms which

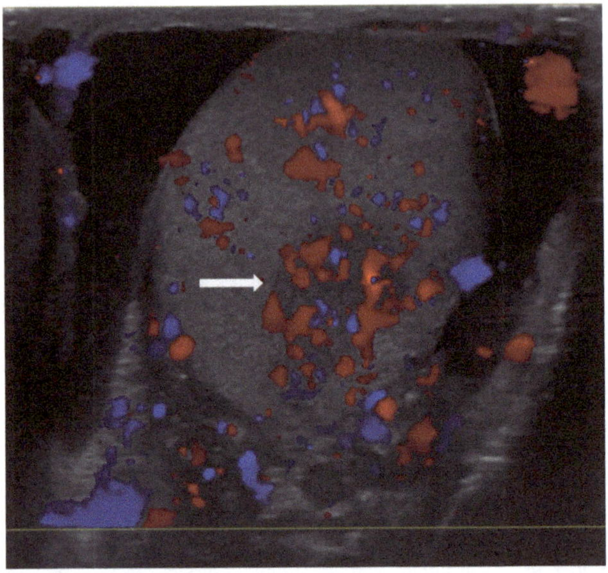

Fig. 7.56 A representative mass in the left testicle demonstrates the presence of flow on color Doppler imaging (*arrow*)

metastasize to the testicle include lymphoma, leukemia, prostate cancer, melanoma and lung. Unlike primary testicular neoplasms, bilateral lesions are more commonly seen with metastatic disease, occurring in 15–20 % of cases.

Testicular lymphoma may occur as a primary tumor, metastatic lesion or site of recurrent disease. Clinically, testicular lymphoma should be suspected in patients above the age of 60 who present with bilateral testicular masses. Unlike germ cell neoplasms, testicular lymphoma does not have a racial predilection. Diffuse large B-cell lymphoma is the most common histologic subtype.

Sonography demonstrates the presence of multiple heterogeneous but predominately hypoechoic masses with vascular flow on color imaging. The prognosis for both metastatic testicular disease and primary testicular lymphoma are poor, with the latter demonstrate a median survival of 13 months.

Pitfalls Sonography alone cannot differentiate primary and secondary testicular neoplasms, though the latter may be suggested if bilateral lesions are seen or if there is a history of a primary neoplasm with a predilection for testicular metastases.

Teaching Points

1. Testicular metastases may be considered if there are bilateral masses in a patient with a history of lymphoma, lung, or prostate cancer. Usually, there is widespread disease at the time of diagnosis.
2. Primary testicular lymphoma is uncommon, but presents as bilateral masses in patients above the age of 60.
3. The prognosis for testicular metastases and primary testicular lymphoma are poor.

Penis

Case 7.25

Brief Case Summary A 24 year old male with neurogenic priapism.

Imaging Findings Pelvis radiograph shows penile erection (arrow, Fig. 7.57). An AP view of the chest showed right lateral dislocation of the T10 vertebral body with associated fracture of the right posterior 11th rib (arrows, Fig. 7.58).

Differential Diagnosis None.

Diagnosis and Discussion Priapism is defined as penile erection that persists for 4 h or longer, is unrelated to sexual activity, and is unrelieved by ejaculation. It is frequently idiopathic but can be secondary to a few pathological states or pharmacological agents. Of these, the most common cause is intracavernosal injection of pharmacostimulants to diagnose or treat erectile dysfunction. Other etiologies include oral pharmaceutical agents used to treat erectile dysfunction (phosphodiesterase inhibitors), sickle cell disease (SCD), genital trauma, cocaine, high spinal cord injury, Peyronie's disease, and malignancy.

The most clinically relevant classification for priapism is classified as ischemic (low flow/veno-occlusive) and non-ischemic (high flow/arterial) categories. "Time is tissue" is an important concept in priapism, especially the ischemic type, where early intervention improves the functional outcome.

Ischemic priapism, which is responsible for 95 % of the cases, is a urological emergency; more than 24 h without intervention results in corporal fibrosis and permanent erectile dysfunction. It is usually due to sinusoidal thrombosis and

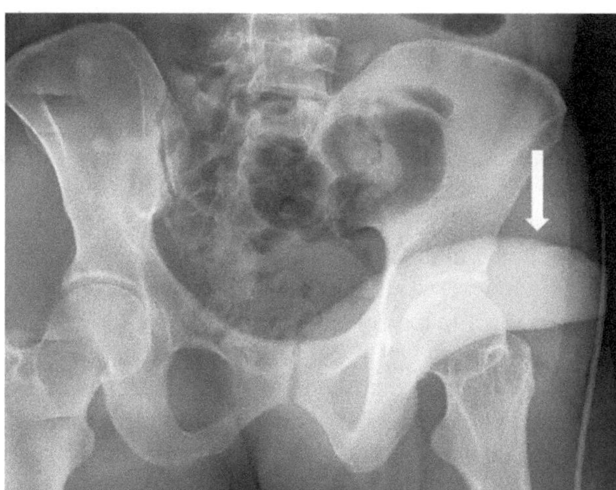

Fig. 7.57 Pelvis radiograph shows penile erection (*arrow*)

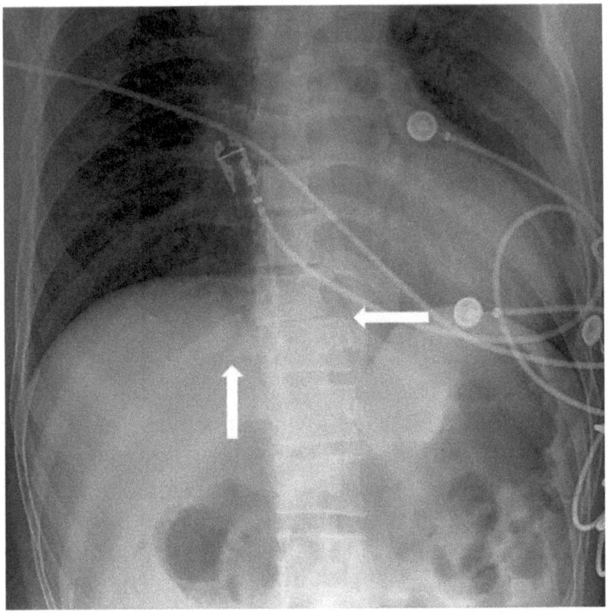

Fig. 7.58 AP view of the chest shows right lateral dislocation of the T10 vertebral body with associated fracture of the right posterior 11th rib (*arrows*)

veno-occlusion with little or no cavernosal blood flow. Non-ischemic priapism is usually a result of trauma, coital or a straddle injury, resulting in arterio-sinusoidal fistulae which lead to an increase in arterial cavernosal flow; the flow is oxygenated and does not need emergent intervention. Stuttering (intermittent) priapism is a variant of ischemic priapism characterized by recurrent episodes of self-limiting painful erections typically lasting less than 4 h duration, historically described in patients with SCD.

Patients with ischemic priapism present acutely with a rigid, painful penis, whereas those with non-ischemic type have a delayed presentation with a painless, non-rigid penis and often have a history of trauma.

The key radiological tool is the penile Doppler study (PDS), which along with clinical assessment and cavernosal blood gas analysis, are used to differentiate the two types of priapism. In the ischemic type, cavernosal flow is either absent or of low velocity – high resistance type, with absent or diminished flow in the dorsal vein. Sinusoids are engorged, thrombosed and non-compressible. A fluid-fluid level may be noted in the corpora cavernosa. In the non-ischemic variant, there is a high velocity, low resistance cavernosal flow pattern with compressible sinusoids and increased flow in the dorsal vein. A penile angiography may be helpful in localizing a fistula.

MRI is useful in the ischemic group for detection and quantification of cavernosal infarction. If there is significant infarcted material, evacuation of the corpora should be considered with insertion of a penile prosthesis. MRI can also determine if metastasis are present as a cause of priapism.

Intervention for ischemic priapism should begin within 4–6 h and include decompression of the corpora cavernosa by aspiration and intracavernous injection of sympathomimetic drugs. When conservative management fails, surgical shunting or evacuation of the necrosed corpora should be considered with insertion of a penile prosthesis. High-flow priapism necessitates transcatheter embolization of either the internal pudendal or cavernosal artery. The main therapeutic goal for stuttering priapism is prevention of future episodes, which may be achieved pharmacologically.

Pitfall A subgroup of ischemic priapism is recognized where there remains high cavernosal arterial flow (often >1–2 m/s) but with high resistance.

Teaching Points

1. Priapism is defined as a penile erection that persists for 4 h or longer, is unrelated to sexual activity, and is unrelieved by ejaculation.
2. Most cases are idiopathic, with most secondary cases occurring due to intracavernosal injection of pharmacostimulants.
3. The role of the radiologist is to help differentiate non-ischemic priapism from the ischemic type, which is a urological emergency.
4. Penile Doppler study is the key radiological investigation. Absent or low velocity – high resistance cavernosal flow is noted in the low-flow type. Conversely, a high velocity – low resistance flow is noted in the high flow type.

Case 7.26

Brief Case Summary A 58 year old male with penile induration

Imaging Findings Gray scale US images (Fig. 7.59a, b) of the penis demonstrate the presence of multiple curvilinear echogenic plaques with posterior shadowing along the dorsal aspect of the tunica albuginea (arrows).

Differential Diagnosis Peyronie's disease, dorsal vein thrombosis, epithelioid sarcoma of the penis, congenital curvature of penis

Diagnosis and Discussion Peyronie's disease

Peyronie's disease (PD) is a rare condition resulting in penile deformity related to the deposition of fibrous plaque within the tunica albuginea. While epidemiologic data are variable, multiple studies suggest a higher incidence in patients above the age of 50 with a statistically significant correlation with the presence of underlying diabetes. The etiology remains elusive, though current thinking suggests that PD results from the deposition of fibrin as a result of acute or chronic penile trauma (due to sexual intercourse or surgical procedures). Clinically, patients complain of abnormal penile curvature, erectile dysfunction, painful erection or a palpable plaque. PD generally demonstrates an acute phase (in which penile pain

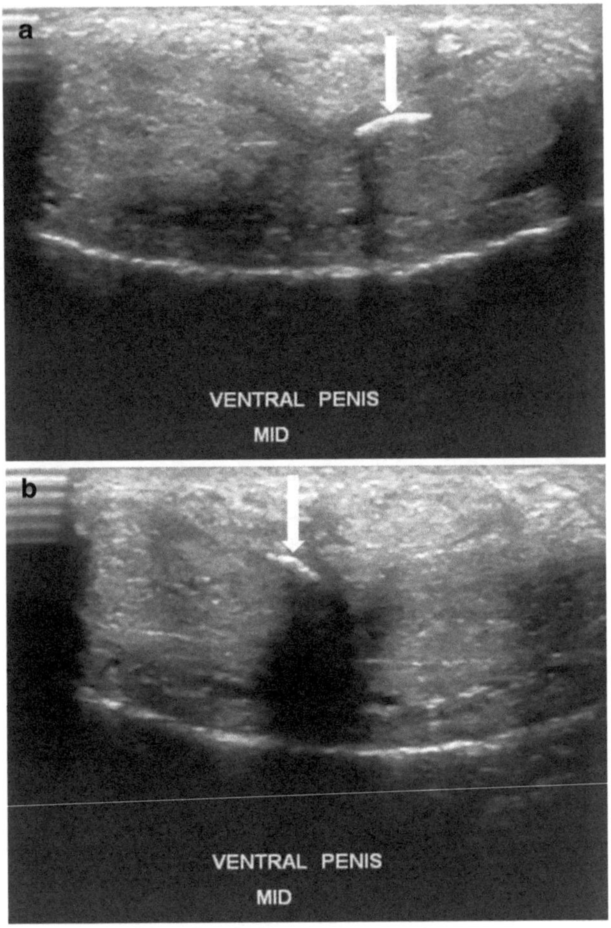

Fig. 7.59 (**a, b**) Gray scale US images of the penis demonstrate the presence of multiple curvilinear echogenic plaques with posterior shadowing along the dorsal aspect of the tunica albuginea (*arrows*)

predominates with active changes of penile malformation) and a chronic phase in which the pain subsides and the malformation becomes stable. Most patients have stable or progressive disease with spontaneous improvement reported in 3–13 % of cases.

Sonographic evaluation of the penis may be obtained to confirm the clinical diagnosis and to evaluate the extent of disease before and after therapy. Non-calcified plaques manifest as focal areas of iso to slightly hyperechoic tunical thickening measuring greater or equal to 1 mm. While hypoechoic plaques may be encountered in the very early stages of disease, care must be taken to confirm that the decreased echogenicity is not related to incorrect insonation of the sonographic beam. Calcified plaques are echogenic and demonstrate posterior shadowing. Plaques are most often located along the dorsal aspect of the penis, but may extend laterally or to the ventral surface and may occasionally involve the penile septum. Circumferential involvement can reduce the girth of the corpora cavernosa at the site of the plaque giving rise to the "hourglass" deformity, which is particularly evident in the erect penis. The relationship of the plaques to the neurovascular bundles should also be delineated, particularly if surgical correction is considered. Concomitant complaints of erectile dysfunction may be evaluated with color Doppler imaging after the intracavernosal injection of vasoactive drugs. Imaging findings may demonstrate the presence of veno-occlusive dysfunction (manifested as high end-diastolic velocity with low resistance waveforms in the cavernosal arteries) or the presence of localized venous leakage at the level of the plaque. MRI may also be used in the evaluation of PD, where plaques manifest as thickened and irregular areas of dark T1 and T2 signal. CT is limited in the setting of non-calcified plaques and are further disadvantaged by the use of ionizing radiation.

Treatment may be triaged according to the phase of disease. Conservative treatment is favored in the acute phase (oral pharmacotherapy, injections or topical treatments) while surgery is offered for the chronic/stabilized phase of the disease.

Pitfalls Dorsal vein thrombosis may give rise to penile pain with focal induration, though distinguishing these findings from tunica albuginea thickening is usually straightforward. Epithelioid sarcoma of the penis is a rare neoplasm which may manifest with findings of focal induration and should be considered in the differential of a growing plaque on sonographic imaging. PD is an acquired condition as opposed to congenital curvature of the penis which is not infrequently associated with hypo or epispadias.

Teaching Points

1. PD is a benign condition thought to be secondary to the presence of penile trauma with subsequent fibrin deposition. Common symptoms include palpable plaque, penile deformity, erectile dysfunction and/or painful erection.
2. Clinically, PD has acute and chronic phases which have management implications.
3. Ultrasound demonstrates the presence of plaque like thickening involving the tunica albuginea ($\geq$1 mm) with or without calcifications. Plaques are most often found along the dorsal aspect of the penis. The relationship of these plaques to the adjacent vessels should be noted.

Case 7.27

Brief Case Summary 76 year old male with penile pain and mass.

Imaging Findings There is a 4.6 × 3.8 cm enhancing mass (Fig. 7.60, arrow) centered within the glans penis that is T2 hypointense (Fig. 7.61) The mass invades the corpora cavernosa, left greater than right, and extends approximately half the length of the penile shaft. There is mass effect on the distal urethra with proximal dilatation (Fig. 7.62, dashed arrow).

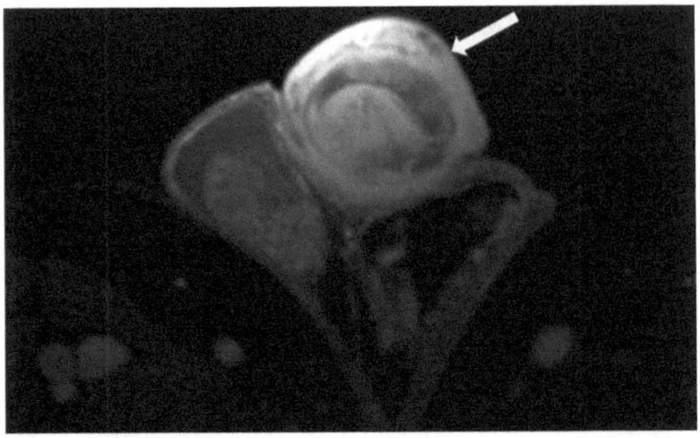

Fig. 7.60 A 4.6×3.8 cm enhancing mass (*arrow*) centered within the glans penis

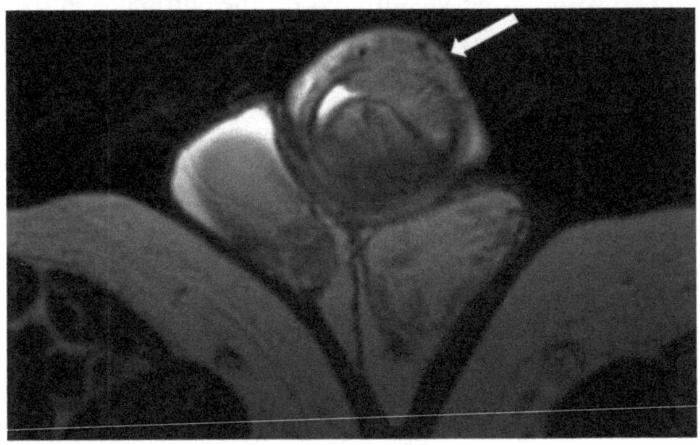

Fig. 7.61 Mass is T2 hypointense and invades the corpora cavernosa, left greater than right, and extends approximately half the length of the penile shaft

Differential Diagnosis Urethral tumor, metastasis, non-epithelial tumors (lymphoma, sarcoma), non-neoplastic lesions (epidermoid cyst, Peyronie's disease, post traumatic fibrosis)

Diagnosis and Discussion Penile cancer is relatively rare in the developed world, accounting for 10–20 % of all malignancies in males in Asia, Africa, and South America but only 1 % in Western countries. The extent of tumor invasion and the status of the locoregional lymph nodes determine the prognosis. Penile cancer can either be primary and metastatic neoplasms. Primary tumors of penis include squamous cell carcinoma, sarcoma, melanoma, basal cell carcinoma, and lymphoma, in which squamous cell carcinoma accounting for more than 95 %. Metastatic penile tumors are most commonly secondary to urogenital tract malignances.

Based on the high soft tissue resolution and multi-planar imaging technique, MRI is the most valuable imaging method to assess the penile tumors. Penile MRI requires special scanning position in the supine with penis dorsiflexed against the lower abdomen in the midline and taped in position. Imaging should be done with a high quality surface coil. Imaging sequences including axial, sagittal, and coronal fat-suppression T2-weighted and enhanced T1-weighted are typically obtained.

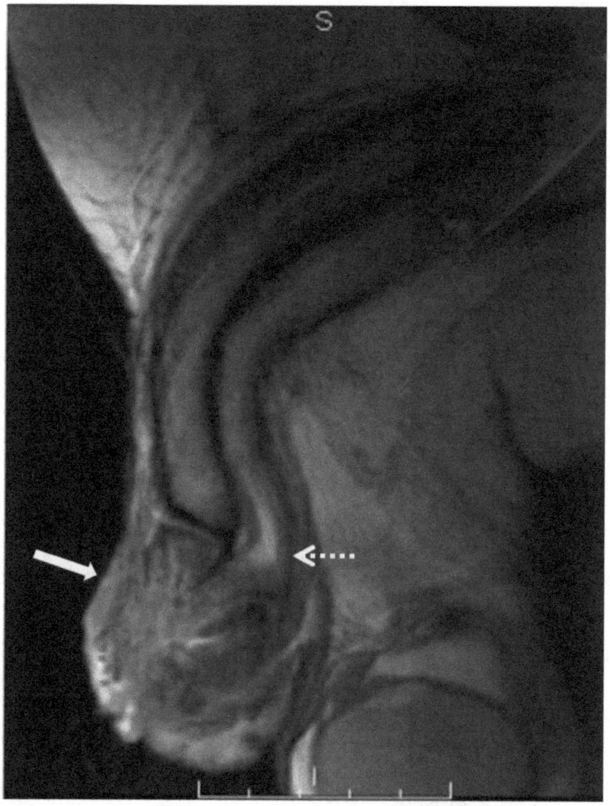

Fig. 7.62 Mass effect on the distal urethra with proximal dilatation (*dashed arrow*)

The most common location of penile squamous cell carcinoma is glans penis (48 %), following by prepuce, coronal sulcus, and shaft. MR is used assess the T staging of the primary tumor, including the involvements of tunica albuginea, corpora, and urethra. Primary tumor manifests as a solitary, ill-defined infiltration lesion that shows hypointense relative to the corpora on both T1- and T2-weighted images with a lesser extent than the corpora cavernosa on T1-weighted enhanced images. The appearances of penile metastatic tumor usually are multiple discrete masses in the corpora cavernosa and corpus spongiosum with relative low signal intensity on both T1- and T2-weighted images. The sensitivities and specificities of MRI for T1-T3 stage of penile cancer range from 75 to 88 % and 83 to 98 %, respectively. Penile cancer spreads via lymphatics with Buck fascia acting as a barrier to corporal invasion and hematogenous spread.

The lymphatic drainage is to the superficial and deep inguinal nodes and the iliac lymph nodes.

Prophylactic inguinal lymphadenectomy is associated with major morbidity in the form of lymphedema and skin flap necrosis with a reported mortality of 1–3 %. The associated morbidity and mortality highlights the need for accurate differentiation of metastatic and reactive lymph nodes to minimize morbidity and mortality.

The lymph node status is assessed with size criteria and morphological features like lobulated contour and necrosis on a CT or MRI. The pelvic lymph nodes can be simultaneously assessed, however, accurate differentiation between malignant and reactive nodes is not found to be accurate. Lymphotrophic nanoparticle–enhanced MR imaging with Ferumoxtran-10 allows accurate characterization of lymph nodes which allows detection of the metastatic nodes, regardless of their size. The modality, although promising, is still under investigation. PET/CT is a sensitive modality although its sensitivity is low in nodes less than 0.5 cm though. Dynamic sentinel lymph node biopsy and intraoperative lymphatic mapping have also been used to detect lymph node metastases to varying degrees of success.

Pitfalls Urethral tumors and non-epithelial penile tumors are histopathological diagnoses and are difficult to differentiate from primary epithelial neoplasm on imaging alone. Metastases, usually from a genitourinary or rectal primary, involve the mid-portion of the corpora, as opposed to peripheral location of the epithelial penile neoplasm, and can present with priapism.

Teaching Point

1. Assessments of local invasion range and lymph node metastasis are essential in treatment planning and predicting prognosis in patients with penile cancer;
2. MRI is the most important imaging modality in penile cancer as it can provide accurate T staging information of primary tumors as well as detecting involved malignant local and distant nodes.
3. CT and MRI can manifest the inguinal, pelvic and retroperitoneal lymphadenopathy caused by penile cancer but the diagnostic accuracy of nodal metastasis is compromised.

Suggested Readings by Case

Case 7.1

Bour L, Schull A, Delongchamps NB, et al. Multiparametric MRI features of granulomatous prostatitis and tubercular prostate abscess. Diagn Interv Imaging. 2013;94(1):84–90.

Gupta N, Mandal AK, Singh SK. Tuberculosis of the prostate and urethra: a review. Indian J Urol. 2008;24(3):388–91.

Suzuki T, Takeuchi M, Naiki T, et al. MRI findings of granulomatous prostatitis developing after intravesical Bacillus Calmette–Guérin therapy. Clin Radiol. 2013;68(6):595–9.

Warrick J, Humphrey PA. Nonspecific granulomatous prostatitis. J Urol. 2012;187:2209–10.

Case 7.2

Bour L, Schull A, Delongchamps N, Beuvon F, Muradyan N, Legmann P, et al. Multiparametric MRI features of granulomatous prostatitis and tubercular prostate abscess. Diagn Interv Imaging. 2013;94:84–90.

Gupta N, Mandal AK, Singh SK. Tuberculosis of the prostate and urethra: a review. Indian J Urol. 2008;24:388–91.

Suzuki T, Takeuchi M, Naiki T, Kawai N, Kohri K, Hara M, et al. MRI findings of granulomatous prostatitis developing after intravesical Bacillus Calmette–Guérin therapy. Clin Radiol. 2013;68:595–9.

Warrick J, Warrick J, Humphrey PA, Humphrey PA. Nonspecific granulomatous prostatitis. J Urol. 2012;187:2209–10.

Case 7.3

Hedgire SS, Eberhardt SC, Borczuk R, McDermott S, Harisinghani MG. Interpretation and reporting multiparametric prostate MRI: a primer for residents and novices. Abdom Imaging. 2014;39(5):1036–51.

Verma S, Rajesh A. A clinically relevant approach to imaging prostate cancer. Am J Roentgenol. 2011;196:S1–10.

Yu J, Fulcher AS, Turner MA, Cockrell CH, Cote EP, Wallace TJ. Prostate cancer and its mimics at multiparametric prostate MRI. Br J Radiol. 2014;87:20130659.

Case 7.4

Hedgire SS, Hedgire ES, Oei TN, McDermott S, Cao K, Patel MZ, et al. Multiparametric magnetic resonance imaging of prostate cancer. Indian J Radiol Imaging. 2012;22:160–9.

Hedgire SS, Eberhardt SC, Borczuk R, McDermott S, Harisinghani MG. Interpretation and reporting multiparametric prostate MRI: a primer for residents and novices. Abdom Imaging. 2014.

Hegde JV, Mulkern RV, Panych LP, Fennessy FM, Fedorov A, Maier SE, et al. Multiparametric MRI of prostate cancer: an update on state-of-the-art techniques and their performance in detecting and localizing prostate cancer. J Magn Reson Imaging. 2013;37:1035–54.

Yu J, Fulcher AS, Turner MA, Cockrell CH, Cote EP, Wallace TJ. Prostate cancer and its mimics at multiparametric prostate MRI. Br J Radiol. 2014;87:20130659.

Case 7.5

Arora SS, Breiman RS, Webb EM, et al. CT and MRI of congenital anomalies of the seminal vesicles. AJR Am J Roentgenol. 2008;189(1):130–5.

Kim B, Kawashima A, Ryu JA, et al. Imaging of the seminal vesicle and vas deferens. Radiographics. 2009;29(4):1105–21.

Saxon P, Badler RL, Desser TS, et al. Segmental testicular infarction: report of seven new cases and literature review. Emerg Radiol. 2012;19(3):217–23.

Case 7.6

Arora SS, Breiman RS, Webb EM, et al. CT and MRI of congenital anomalies of the seminal vesicles. AJR Am J Roentgenol. 2008;189(1):130–5.

Kim B, Kawashima A, Ryu JA, et al. Imaging of the seminal vesicle and vas deferens. Radiographics. 2009;29(4):1105–21.

Saxon P, Badler RL, Desser TS, et al. Segmental testicular infarction: report of seven new cases and literature review. Emerg Radiol. 2012;19(3):217–23.

Case 7.7

Jung YY, Kim JK, Cho KS. Genitourinary tuberculosis: comprehensive cross-sectional imaging. AJR Am J Roentgenol. 2005;184(1):143–50.
Kim B, Kawashima A, Ryu JA, et al. Imaging of the seminal vesicle and vas deferens. Radiographics. 2009;29(4):1105–21.

Case 7.8

Kim B, Kawashima A, Ryu JA, et al. Imaging of the seminal vesicle and vas deferens. Radiographics. 2009;29(4):1105–21.

Case 7.9

Egevad L, Ehrnstrom R, Hakansson U, et al. Primary seminal vesicle carcinoma detected at transurethral resection of prostate. Urology. 2007;69:778311–3.
Kim B, Kawashima A, Ryu JA, et al. Imaging of the seminal vesicle and vas deferens. Radiographics. 2009;29(4):1105–21.
Ohmori T, Okada K, Tabei R, et al. CA 125-producing adenocarcinoma of the seminal vesicle. Pathol Int. 1994;44:333–7.
Tarjan M, Ottlecz I, Tot T. Primary adenocarcinoma of the seminal vesicle. Indian J Urol. 2009;25(1):143–5.

Case 7.10

Krishnaswami S, Fonnesbeck C, Penson D, et al. Magnetic resonance imaging for locating nonpalpable undescended testicle: a meta-analysis. Pediatrics. 2013;131(6):31908–16.
Özden E, Turgut AT, Dogra VS. Imaging the undescended testis. In: Scrotal pathology. Berlin/Heidelberg: Springer; 2012. p. 301–12.
Tasian GE, Copp HL, Baskin LS. Diagnostic imaging in cryptorchidism: utility, indications, and effectiveness. J Pediatr Surg. 2011;46(12):2406–13.

Case 7.11

Avery LL, Scheinfeld MH. Imaging of penile and scrotal emergencies. Radiographics. 2013;33(3):721–40.
Shah A, Kooiman GG, Sidhu PS. Imaging acute scrotal pain in adults-2: inflammation and other disorders. In: Scrotal pathology. Berlin/Heidelberg: Springer; 2012. p. 111–24.

Case 7.12

Berman JM, Beidle TR, Kunberger LE, et al. Sonographic evaluation of acute intrascrotal pathology. AJR Am J Roentgenol. 1996;166(4):857–61.

Dogra VS, Gottlieb RH, Rubens DJ, et al. Benign intratesticular cystic lesions: US features. Radiographics. 2001;21 Spec No suppl 1:S273–81.

Yang DM, Yoon MH, Kim HS, et al. Comparison of tuberculous and pyogenic epididymal abscesses: clinical, gray-scale sonographic, and color Doppler sonographic features. AJR Am J Roentgenol. 2001;177(5):1131–5.

Case 7.13

Avery LL, Scheinfeld MH. Imaging of penile and scrotal emergencies. Radiographics. 2013; 33(3):721–40.

Bertolotto M, et al. Imaging scrotal trauma. In: Scrotal pathology. Berlin/Heidelberg: Springer; 2012. p. 73–84.

Valentino M, et al. Scrotal trauma. In: Abdominal imaging. Berlin/Heidelberg: Springer; 2013. p. 1887–96.

Case 7.14

Aso C, et al. Gray-scale and color Doppler sonography of scrotal disorders in children: an update. Radiographics. 2005;25(5):1197–214.

Turgut AT, Dogra VS. Imaging acute scrotal pain in adults: torsion of the testis and appendages. In: Scrotal pathology. Berlin/Heidelberg: Springer; 2012. p. 99–109.

Case 7.15

Aquino M, Nghiem H, Jafri SZ, et al. Segmental testicular infarction sonographic findings and pathologic correlation. J Ultrasound Med. 2013;32(2):365–72.

Fernández-Pérez GC, Tardaguila FM, Velasco M, et al. Radiologic findings of segmental testicular infarction. AJR Am J Roentgenol. 2005;184(5):1587–93.

Saxon P, Balder RL, Desser TS, et al. Segmental testicular infarction: report of seven new cases and literature review. Emerg Radiol. 2012;19(3):217–23.

Case 7.16

Bird K, Rosenfield AT. Testicular infarction secondary to acute inflammatory disease: demonstration by B-scan ultrasound. Radiology. 1984;152:785–8.

Vijayaraghavan SB. Sonographic differential diagnosis of acute scrotum: real-time whirlpool sign, a key sign of torsion. J Ultrasound Med. 2006;25(5):563–74.

Case 7.17

Cayan S, Shavakhabov S, Kadioglu A. Treatment of palpable varicocele in infertile men: a meta-analysis to define the best technique. J Androl. 2009;30(1):33–40.
Dogra VS, Gottlieb RH, Oka M, et al. Sonography of the scrotum. Radiology. 2003; 227(1):18–36.
Liguori G, et al. Imaging the infertile male-1: varicocele. In: Scrotal pathology. Berlin/Heidelberg: Springer; 2012. p. 261–73.

Case 7.18

Bhosale PR, Patnana M, Viswanathan C, et al. The inguinal canal: anatomy and imaging features of common and uncommon masses. Radiographics. 2008;28(3):819–35.
Singh AK, Kao S, D'Allesandro M, et al. Case 164: funicular type of spermatic cord hydrocele. Radiology. 2010;257(3):890–2.
Woodward PJ, Schwab CM, Sesterhenn IA. From the archives of the AFIP extratesticular scrotal masses: radiologic-pathologic correlation. Radiographics. 2003;23(1):215–40.

Case 7.19

Al-Jabri T, Misra S, Maan ZN, et al. Ultrasonography of simple intratesticular cysts: a 13 year experience in a single centre. Diagn Pathol. 2011;6:24.
Martinez-Berganza MT, Sarria L, Cozcolluela R, et al. Cysts of the tunica albuginea: sonographic appearance. AJR Am J Roentgenol. 1998;170(1):183–5.
Valentino M, et al. Imaging scrotal lumps in adults-2: cysts and fluid collections. In: Scrotal pathology. Berlin/Heidelberg: Springer; 2012. p. 179–89.
Woodward PJ, Schwab CM, Sesterhenn IA. From the archives of the AFIP extratesticular scrotal masses: radiologic-pathologic correlation. Radiographics. 2003;23(1):215–40.

Case 7.20

Arellano CM, Kozakewich HP, Diamond D, et al. Testicular epidermoid cysts in children: sonographic characteristics with pathological correlation. Pediatr Radiol. 2011;41(6):683–9.
Loya AG, Said JW, Grant EG. Epidermoid cyst of the testis: radiologic-pathologic correlation. Radiographics. 2004;24 Suppl 1:S243–6.
Park SB, Lee WC, Kim JK, et al. Imaging features of benign solid testicular and paratesticular lesions. Eur Radiol. 2011;21(10):2226–34.

Case 7.21

Richenberg J, Brejt N. Testicular microlithiasis: is there a need for surveillance in the absence of other risk factors? Eur Radiol. 2012;22(11):2540–6.
Tan M-H, Eng C. Testicular microlithiasis: recent advances in understanding and management. Nat Rev Urol. 2011;8(3):153–63.

Case 7.22

Kreydin EI, Barrisford GW, Feldman AS, et al. Testicular cancer: what the radiologist needs to know. AJR Am J Roentgenol. 2013;200(6):1215–25.
Krohmer SJ, McNulty NJ, Schned AR. Testicular seminoma with lymph node metastases. Radiographics. 2009;29(7):2177–83.
Woodward PJ, Sohaev R, O'Donoghue MJ, et al. From the archives of the AFIP tumors and tumor-like lesions of the testis: radiologic-pathologic correlation. Radiographics. 2002;22(1):189–216.

Case 7.23

Comiter CV, Renshaw AA, Benson CB, et al. Burned-out primary testicular cancer: sonographic and pathological characteristics. J Urol. 1996;156(1):85–8.
Fabre E, Jira H, Izard V, et al. 'Burned-out' primary testicular cancer. BJU Int. 2004;94(1):74–8.
Tasu JP, Faye N, Eschwege P, et al. Imaging of burned-out testis tumor five new cases and review of the literature. J Ultrasound Med. 2003;22(5):515–21.

Case 7.24

Morichetti D, Mazzucchelli R, Lopez-Beltran A, et al. Secondary neoplasms of the urinary system and male genital organs. BJU Int. 2009;104(6):770–6.
Verma N, Lazarchick J, Gudena V, et al. Testicular lymphoma: an update for clinicians. Am J Med Sci. 2008;336(4):336–41.
Woodward PJ, Sohaev R, O'Donoghue MJ, et al. From the archives of the AFIP tumors and tumorlike lesions of the testis: radiologic-pathologic correlation. Radiographics. 2002;22(1):189–216.

Case 7.25

Bassett J, Rajfer J. Diagnostic and therapeutic options for the management of ischemic and nonischemic priapism. Rev Urol. 2010;12(1):56–63.
Halls JE, Patel DV, Patel U. Priapism: pathophysiology and the role of the radiologist. Br J Radiol. 2012;85(Spec No 1):S79–85.
Salonia A, Eardley I, Giuliano F, et al. European Association of Urology guidelines on priapism. Eur Urol. 2014;65(2):480–9.

Case 7.26

Bertolotto M, Pavlica P, Serafini G, et al. Painful penile induration: imaging findings and management. Radiographics. 2009;29(2):477–93.
Kalokairinou K, Konstantinidis C, Domazou M, et al. US imaging in Peyronie's disease. J Clin Imaging Sci. 2012;2:63.
Pavlica P, et al. Peyronie's disease. In: Abdominal imaging. Berlin/Heidelberg: Springer; 2013. p. 1947–60.

Index

M.G. Harisinghani, A. Rajesh, *Genitourinary Imaging: A Case Based Approach*, DOI 10.1007/978-1-4471-4772-5

FSC
www.fsc.org
MIX
Papier | Fördert
gute Waldnutzung
FSC® C083411

Kolibri 360 GmbH
Ferdinand-Jühlke-Straße 7
99095 Erfurt, Deutschland
produktsicherheit@kolibri360.de